Anesthetic Equipment Made Easy®

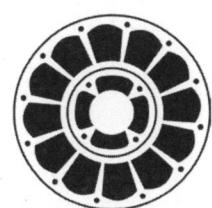

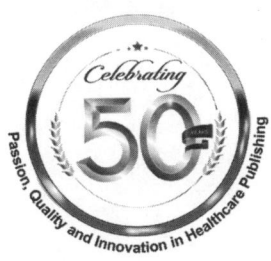

Anesthetic Equipment Made Easy®

S Ahanatha Pillai MD DA
Emeritus Professor
The Tamil Nadu Dr MGR Medical University
Chennai, Tamil Nadu, India
Visiting Consultant
Aravind Eye Hospital and Postgraduate Institute of Ophthalmology
Madurai, Tamil Nadu, India
Formerly, Professor
Department of Anesthesiology
Madurai Medical College and Government Rajaji Hospital
Madurai, Tamil Nadu, India

Foreword
J Renganathan

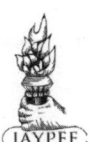

JAYPEE BROTHERS MEDICAL PUBLISHERS
The Health Sciences Publisher
New Delhi | London | Panama

Jaypee Brothers Medical Publishers (P) Ltd

Headquarters
Jaypee Brothers Medical Publishers (P) Ltd
4838/24, Ansari Road, Daryaganj
New Delhi 110 002, India
Phone: +91-11-43574357
Fax: +91-11-43574314
Email: jaypee@jaypeebrothers.com

Overseas Offices

J.P. Medical Ltd
83 Victoria Street, London
SW1H 0HW (UK)
Phone: +44 20 3170 8910
Fax: +44 (0)20 3008 6180
Email: info@jpmedpub.com

Jaypee-Highlights Medical Publishers Inc
City of Knowledge, Bld. 235, 2nd Floor
Clayton, Panama City, Panama
Phone: +1 507-301-0496
Fax: +1 507-301-0499
Email: cservice@jphmedical.com

Jaypee Brothers Medical Publishers (P) Ltd
Bhotahity, Kathmandu, Nepal
Phone: +977-9741283608
Email: kathmandu@jaypeebrothers.com

Website: www.jaypeebrothers.com
Website: www.jaypeedigital.com

© 2019, Jaypee Brothers Medical Publishers

The views and opinions expressed in this book are solely those of the original contributor(s)/author(s) and do not necessarily represent those of editor(s) of the book.

All rights reserved. No part of this publication may be reproduced, stored or transmitted in any form or by any means, electronic, mechanical, photocopying, recording or otherwise, without the prior permission in writing of the publishers.

All brand names and product names used in this book are trade names, service marks, trademarks or registered trademarks of their respective owners. The publisher is not associated with any product or vendor mentioned in this book.

Medical knowledge and practice change constantly. This book is designed to provide accurate, authoritative information about the subject matter in question. However, readers are advised to check the most current information available on procedures included and check information from the manufacturer of each product to be administered, to verify the recommended dose, formula, method and duration of administration, adverse effects and contraindications. It is the responsibility of the practitioner to take all appropriate safety precautions. Neither the publisher nor the author(s)/editor(s) assume any liability for any injury and/or damage to persons or property arising from or related to use of material in this book.

This book is sold on the understanding that the publisher is not engaged in providing professional medical services. If such advice or services are required, the services of a competent medical professional should be sought.

Every effort has been made where necessary to contact holders of copyright to obtain permission to reproduce copyright material. If any have been inadvertently overlooked, the publisher will be pleased to make the necessary arrangements at the first opportunity. The **CD/DVD-ROM** (if any) provided in the sealed envelope with this book is complimentary and free of cost. **Not meant for sale.**

Inquiries for bulk sales may be solicited at: jaypee@jaypeebrothers.com

Anesthetic Equipment Made Easy®

First Edition: **2019**

ISBN 978-93-5270-607-5

Printed at Rajkamal Electric Press, Kundli, Haryana.

Dedicated to

My teacher

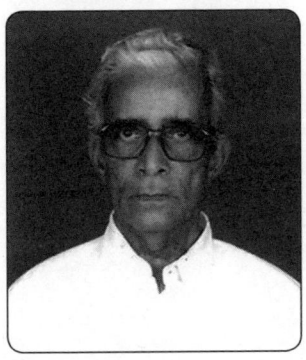

Prof Dr S Viswanathan BSc MD DA
Formerly, Professor and Head
Department of Anesthesiology
Madurai Medical College and Government Rajaji Hospital
Madurai, Tamil Nadu, India
(1974 to 1989)

A renowned, highly talented, excellent, inspiring teacher
Hundreds of his students occupy prestigious positions in India and abroad
I had the fortune to be his student and to work under him for 15 years

Foreword

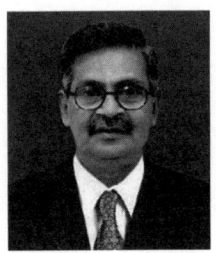

I sincerely congratulate Professor Dr S Ahanatha Pillai for bringing out the book, *Anesthetic Equipment Made Easy*.

This book precisely deals with the basic principles of each component of the anesthesia machine. Starting from the conventional Boyle's machine to the modern anesthesia workstation, the components are discussed. It is interesting to note that the relevant short history of each equipment is discussed in the beginning. The breathing systems and airway management accessories have been dealt with meticulously.

Essential monitors have been discussed separately.

Every chapter has been written in a very simple, easy-to-understand language with adequate illustrations and figures that make easy understanding of the principles.

The author is a good teacher with vast teaching experience of more than 40 years of teaching undergraduate students, postgraduate students, nurses and technicians.

I am sure this book will be useful to the postgraduate students as well as practicing anesthesiologists.

J Renganathan MD DA
Dean, Dhanalakshmi Srinivasan Medical College and
Hospital, Perambalur, Tamil Nadu, India
Formerly, Professor and Head
Department of Anesthesia
Government Mohan Kumaramangalam Medical College
Salem, Tamil Nadu, India
Formerly, Professor, Government Stanley Medical College
Chennai, Tamil Nadu, India
Past President, Indian Society of Anaesthesiologists

Preface

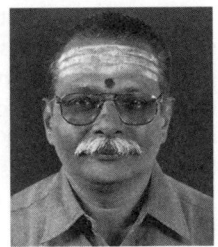

Many excellent books are available on anesthetic equipment that are too good and deal with the subject elaborately in depth which serve as reference books for specialists. But there is no simple book that deals with the fundamentals of anesthetic equipment in an easy way to understand. The purpose of this book is to deliver the fundamentals without any confusion, so that the reader is very clear with the concepts.

The term *Anesthesia Equipment* refers to the anesthesia machine as well as monitoring devices associated with it. The modern trend is to have both the anesthesia machines and the monitors integrated as an *anesthesia delivery system* or *anesthesia workstation*. Regardless of how it is presented, it is useful to consider each component as a separate entity and discuss in order to understand them.

By the term *anesthesia machine*, we mean the assembly of devices that help to prepare a mixture of oxygen, other gases and volatile anesthetic agents, so as to deliver inhalational anesthetics to the patient.

Anesthesia machine or anesthesia workstation is probably the only equipment that an anesthesiologist consistently uses everyday in the operating room. These machines incorporate different devices performing individually different functions. It is not uncommon to see many physicians using their equipment without knowing how they works—the principle of their functioning.

Anesthesiologists may use either an old generation *anesthetic machine* or one of the new generation *anesthetic workstations*. The differences between the two are enormous. In a basic anesthetic machine components that are essential to make the machine fit to deliver the anesthetic gas mixture are incorporated. In anesthetic workstations, modern technological advancements are incorporated lavishly in the essential components, safety devices and monitors that make them highly sophisticated. As expected, inevitably it makes them complicated too. The similarity between the two is the presence of the essential components those are absolutely necessary for administration of anesthesia.

Advancements in medical electronics have grossly modified the structure of a modern anesthetic workstation. *While using any electronic device, we must remember that it is enough to know what the device can do and not how it does that.* The fundamental principles of functioning of the essential components remain the same. It is mandatory that the basic principles are clearly understood for using the equipment effectively and safely. Very few components such as *electronic flow meters* present in some of the latest workstations entirely depend on electronics that is not within the purview of the anesthesiologist.

The anesthesiologist must have a thorough knowledge of the functioning principle of every component of the machine. In the event of any malfunction, he/she must be able to quickly troubleshoot and fix the problem. Wherever possible he/she must be able to rectify the problem immediately or replace the malfunctioning unit so as to continue the anesthesia without causing any harm to the patient.

It is a pleasure to use any equipment after understanding its functions based on the simple principles of physics and mechanics. The book tries to fulfill that pleasure.

Students learn very intricate details by words of mouth from the teachers that could not be found in general texts and hence interacting with the teachers may enhance the degree of understanding the subject.

It is my great fortune that I had the opportunity to teach and train postgraduate students in anesthesiology for nearly 4 decades. I had the passion for training the postgraduate students directly in every step of their work, with the application of the relevant basic sciences. This had given me a lot of insight to deliver the vital details of equipment which should be remembered and never forgotten. Incidentally, in their examinations, the questions are always directed to these aspects only.

In every chapter, relevant history of the equipment is discussed briefly for making the reading interesting and complete.

Checking the anesthetic machine, organizing and keeping ready every piece of the required accessories well before starting the anesthesia is the basic principle of safety, *which is very similar to the pilot checking the cockpit of an aircraft sufficiently before takeoff*. It has been established that failure to do this check has caused disasters. Nonavailability of a piece of equipment, even an *endotracheal connector* and an empty oxygen cylinder are the simple examples.

The subject is presented and explained in simple language with very clear illustrations and figures which help the reader to understand and remember the subject without difficulty.

The applied physics related to the practice of anesthesia are dealt within a very simple, easy-to-understand way in the beginning.

I sincerely hope that this book will prove a useful primer supplement to the excellent textbooks on this subject already available.

S Ahanatha Pillai

Acknowledgments

I am extremely grateful to all my teachers, who always made me realize and feel that teaching is a wonderful, pleasurable experience and inspired me to learn that art from them. It is often quoted 'Teaching is the best way of learning'.

My loving students, both undergraduates and postgraduates consistently inspired me to teach. That strong inspiration is the reason for me to continue teaching for more than four decades. I am grateful to them for their love to me.

With a lot of gratitude, I make special mention about the contribution from my loving wife, Mrs Neelam Ahanathan, being a constant source of inspiration and encouragement in all my endeavors particularly those related to academic ventures. My children gave me the loving care and support so that I could continue teaching. My love and gratitude are due to them.

My thanks are due to my younger colleagues Professor Dr UG Thirumaaran, *Formerly*, Professor of Anesthesiology, Madras Medical College, Chennai, Tamil Nadu, India, and Professor Dr A Paramasivan, Professor of Anesthesiology, Madurai Medical College, Madurai, Tamil Nadu, who have rendered their help in this work. My dear friend Dr K Boominathan, MBBS, DA, *Formerly*, Senior Anesthesiologist, Railway Hospital, Madurai, has done the proof correction of the entire script. I am extremely grateful to him.

My dear colleagues in various surgical specialties have contributed to my development in very many ways for the past four decades and more. Most of them loved me and encouraged me in every endeavor.

Professor Dr J Renganathan, MD, DA, Dean, Dhanalakshmi Srinivasan Medical College, Perambalur, Tamil Nadu, India, had taken pain to go through the whole script and give a Foreword for this book. I am extremely grateful to him for his fine gesture.

I am grateful to Mr VS Vijayasarathy, R&D Engineer and Mr Stanley of Staan Biomed, Engineering Private Limited, Coimbatore, Tamil Nadu, India, for providing the pictures of workstation and other details.

Anaesthetics India Pvt Ltd, Mumbai and Meditech India Ltd, New Delhi have permitted me to use the figures published by them. I am very grateful to them.

I am very grateful to all those patients, the faces of whom I could not remember who submitted themselves for anesthesia and permitted me to learn anesthesiology for the past four decades and for all that they taught me.

I am very grateful to the whole team of M/s Jaypee Brothers Medical Publishers (P) Ltd, New Delhi, India, who helped and guided me, Shri Jitendar P Vij (Group Chairman), Mr Ankit Vij (Managing Director), Mr MS Mani (Group President), Ms Pooja Bhandari (Production Head), Ms Sunita Katla (Executive Assistant to Group Chairman and Publishing Manager), Ms Seema Dogra (Cover Visualizer), and Mr Rajesh Sharma (Production Coordinator), for all their support to work in this project and make it a success. Without their cooperation, I could not have completed this project.

Contents

1. Applied Physics — 1
- Introduction 1
- Matter 1
- Avogadro's Hypothesis 3
- Heat 4
- Vapor and Gases 7
- Pressure 12
- Gas Laws 16
- Poynting Effect 21

2. Anesthesia Machine — 27
- Introduction 27
- History 28
- Modern Workstations 31
- Oxygen Failure Alarm 48
- Scavenging System 57
- Safety Features in Workstations 61
- Checking the Anesthesia Machine 63
- Self-inflating Resuscitator Bag 64

3. Medical Gas Cylinders — 70
- Introduction 70
- History 70
- Parts of a Cylinder 74

4. Medical Gas Pipeline System — 93
- Pipeline of Medical Gases 93
- Manifold Room 94
- Indicators and Alarms 100
- Pipelines and Isolation Valves 102
- Central Vacuum 107
- Compressed Medical Air 108
- Liquid Oxygen 109

5. Pressure Reducing Valves (Pressure Regulators) — 113
- Purpose 113
- Pressure Reducing Valve 113
- Modern Valves 118
- Types of Pressure Reducing Valves 120

6. Flow Meters — 123
- Principles and Types 123
- Rotor 131
- Flow Meter Bank 131
- Variable Orifice Type 135

7. Vaporizers — 142
- Introduction *142*
- History *142*
- Vaporizers *158*
- Boyle's Bottle Vaporizer *159*
- Copper Kettle Vaporizer *160*
- Goldman Vaporizer *161*
- Temperature Compensated Vaporizers *161*
- TEC 4 *164*
- TEC 5 *164*
- TEC 6 *165*
- TEC 7 *166*
- Select-a-tec System *168*

8. Anesthetic Breathing Systems — 173
- History *173*
- Definition *174*
- Classification *175*
- Facemasks *209*

9. Laryngoscopes Endotracheal Tubes and Airways — 217
- Laryngoscopes *217*
- Fiber-optic Intubating Bronchoscope *224*
- Endotracheal Tubes *227*
- Other Less Commonly Used Tubes *238*

10. Laryngeal Mask Airway — 257
- Standard Laryngeal Mask Airway *257*
- Modified Versions of LMA *262*

11. Monitors — 273
- Pulse Oximeter *273*
- Capnography *280*
- Electrocardiogram Monitor *285*
- Monitoring Neuromuscular Block *293*

12. Equipment for Spinal and Epidural Anesthesia — 301
- Techniques of Regional Anesthesia *301*
- Spinal Anesthesia *301*
- Lumbar Puncture *303*
- Positioning for Giving Spinal Anesthesia *304*
- Spinal Needles *304*
- Epidural Anesthesia *307*
- Epidural Needles *307*

Index *317*

Applied Physics

chapter 1

INTRODUCTION
The applied physics discussed in this chapter is related to the fundamental principles of functioning of various components of an anesthesia machine. The relevant applications in the working of the equipment and their practical significance are discussed in appropriate places.

MATTER

Element
It is a substance that has the smallest particle known as atom. Atom is the smallest part to which an element can be subdivided that retains the properties of the substance. Atom cannot be further divided by ordinary means. *Examples:* hydrogen, helium, oxygen, carbon, chlorine.

Compound
It is composed of two or more elements, united chemically. This forms a substance with different properties from that of those individual elements composing it. *Example:* ether is a compound of carbon, hydrogen and oxygen. Nitrous oxide is a compound of nitrogen and oxygen. So, a compound can be divided into *molecules without losing its identity.*

Molecule
A *molecule* is the smallest particle of a substance which still possesses the distinctive properties of the substance. For example, oxygen does not exist as a single atom. It combines with another oxygen atom to form oxygen molecule (O_2). The oxygen gas that we know consists of molecules of oxygen. If oxygen atom combines with atoms of other elements a new compound will be formed. For example, $(C_2H_5)_2O$ is ether—two ethyl groups with one atom of oxygen—(C_2H_5) O (C_2H_5). It is a compound of one atom of oxygen with 4 atoms of carbon and 10 atoms of hydrogen. If a molecule is subdivided, it loses its properties.

Molecular Movement
- All substances, *solids, liquids,* or *gases* are composed of molecules. These molecules are in a state of incessant motion. The ability of the molecules to alter their position varies according to its state, solids, liquids or gases.
- In a solid state, as the density is very high the molecules cannot alter their relative positions, and merely oscillate about a fixed point. The relative volume of the solid is small **(Fig. 1.1)**.

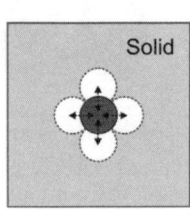 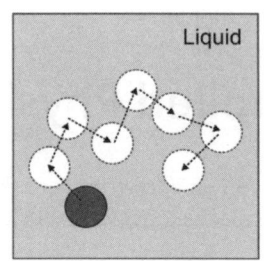 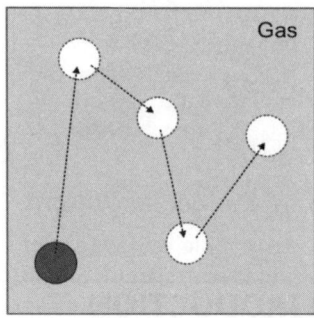

Fig. 1.1: The molecule in a solid, liquid and gas. • *Solid*: The molecule does not change the position, but oscillates about a fixed point in all directions; • *Liquid:* The molecule constantly changes position and moves slowly a short distance within the container; • *Gas:* The molecules are in violent movement, change their position faster and to a greater distance within the container

- The molecules in a liquid are mobile and gradually shift their position throughout the whole liquid as the density is relatively less. The free path of a molecule in the liquid, however, is very short before it collides with its neighbours **(Fig. 1.1)**.
- In the gaseous state the molecules have a much greater degree of mobility, and travel longer distances before colliding with others **(Fig. 1.1)**.
- The relative status of molecules in solid, liquid and gases is shown in **Figure 1.2**.
- Owing to the mobility of its molecules, a liquid or gas has no fixed shape like solid and so assume the shape of the container.
- All gases and many liquids mix readily with their fellows.

Atomic Weight

- Atomic weight of oxygen is used as the basis on which atomic weight of other elements are determined.
- Atomic weight of oxygen is 16.
- Hydrogen is 16 times lighter than oxygen, so the atomic weight is 1.
- Carbon atom has 3/4th of the weight of oxygen, so the atomic weight is 12.

Molecular Weight

- The molecular weight of a substance is the sum of the atomic weights of the elements of which it is composed.

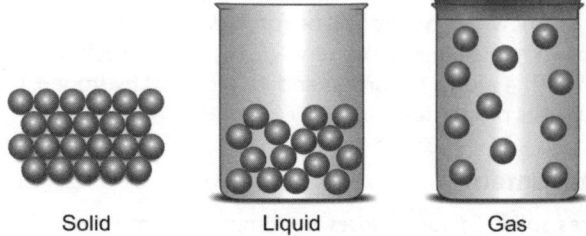

Fig. 1.2: The molecule of a solid, liquid and gas and their relative movements. In solid, the molecules are compact, the volume is small. Do not change position but oscillate in its place; • In liquids the molecules are loose and the volume is relatively bigger. Molecules move very slowly throughout the liquid; • In gases the molecules are very loose, volume is very large. They move very fast and travel long distance within the container

- Oxygen with formula O_2 has a molecular weight of 32.
- Ether $(C_2H_5)_2O$ has molecular weight of 74 ($12 \times 4 + 1 \times 10 + 16$).
- Nitrous oxide N_2O has molecular weight of 44.

This explains that 74 g of ether contains the same number of molecules as in 44 g of nitrous oxide.

Gram Molecular Weight

The term 'mole' is used to refer to what was known earlier as 'gram molecular weight'. One 'mole' of a substance is the molecular weight of the substance expressed in grams. So, one 'mole' of all substances contain the same number of molecules. The number of molecules per 'mole' is known as 'Avogadro's constant'.

It is defined that the mass of one mole of a substance, expressed in grams, is equal to the mean relative molecular mass of the substance. For example, the mean relative molecular mass of natural water is about 18.015, therefore, one mole of water has a mass of about 18.015 grams.

AVOGADRO'S HYPOTHESIS

Equal volumes of all gases under the same condition of temperature and pressure contain the same number of molecules.
- It is shown that a *'mole'* (gram molecular weight) of any gas at the same temperature and pressure occupies the same volume.
- At 0°C temperature and 760 mm Hg pressure (normal temperature and pressure or NTP) this volume is 22.4 L.

Figure 1.3 explains Avogadro's hypothesis and shows how equal volumes of two different gases O_2 and H_2 under the same temperature and pressure have same number of molecules.

Density

The *density* of a gas is usually expressed as the *weight of 1 L of gas in gram*.
- The weight of 22.4 L of the gas is the gram molecule of the gas.
- So the weight of 1 L of a gas = molecular weight/22.4 g.
- Molecular weight of ether is 74.

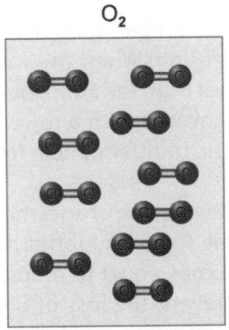
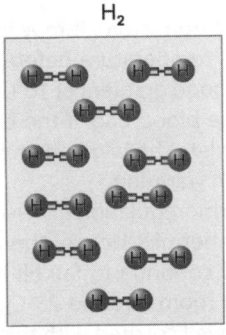
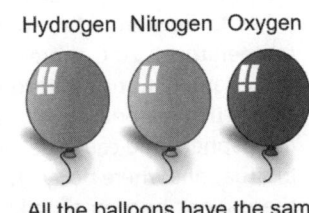

All the balloons have the same volume. This means they all contain the same number of molecules

Equal volumes and the same temperature and pressure

Fig. 1.3: Avogadro's hypothesis. • Equal volumes of oxygen and hydrogen under same temperature and pressure have same number of molecules

- So, the weight of 1 L of ether vapor = 74/22.4 = 3.31 g/L.
- Similarly, the density of nitrous oxide = 44/22.4 = 1.96 g/L.

For practical purposes, air contains 1 volume of oxygen and 4 volumes of nitrogen. (20% + 80%)

At normal temperature and pressure (NTP),

- The weight of 1/5 L of oxygen   = 32/22.4 × 1/5 g   = 0.29 g
- The weight of 4/5 L of nitrogen   = 28/22.4 × 4/5 g   = 1.0 g
- So, the weight of 1 L of air   = 0.29 g + 1.0 g   = 1.29 g
- Therefore, the density of air is   =   1.29 g/L

The *density of a gas* is expressed in relation to the *density of air* which is given the value of 1.

- Thus, the relative density (specific gravity) of nitrous oxide is 1½, ether vapor is 2½. (Ether vapor settles on the floor because it is 2½ times heavier than air).
- Though the term *'density'* is used popularly to denote the weight of a given volume of gas, the proper scientific term is *'specific weight'*.

Specific Weight

Weight per unit volume.

Liquids: The ratio of the specific weight of the liquid at any given temperature to that of water at 4°C.

Gases: The ratio of specific weight of the gas to that of air; both given at NTP (0°C and 760 mm Hg).

HEAT

Heat is an energy that can be given to a substance or abstracted from it.

Heat and *temperature* are different.

Temperature is the thermal status of a substance which determines whether it will give heat or receive heat from another substance when brought in contact with it.

Always heat is transferred from a substance of higher temperature to a substance of lower temperature. This difference in temperature between the two is known as *temperature gradient*. Heat may be transferred by three means *conduction, convection and radiation*.

Practical application:
- When a blood bag is removed from store, it may have the temperature of 10°C. It has to be warmed to room temperature before transfusion. When the room temperature is 20°C, there is a good gradient of 10°C for heat from the atmosphere to be rapidly transferred to the blood bag. If the bag is covered with a towel or some such material, it will insulate the bag and prevent the transfer of heat from atmosphere and cause delay in warming.
- In situations where body's thermoregulation fails—as in deep plane of anesthesia the patient becomes 'poikilothermic'. Hence, the patient suffers hypothermia. The body temperature would continue to fall till it becomes equal to ambient temperature of the operating room (around 23°C). To prevent the loss of body heat to the atmosphere, he is well covered with thick insulating covers. A radiant heater will be placed at a suitable distance to transfer heat and raise the body temperature.

Unit of Heat

Calorie
- It is defined as the quantity of heat required to raise the temperature of 1 g of water by 1°C.
- This is the unit of measuring heat (cal).

Example: The heat required to raise the temperature of 1 L (1000 g or mL) of water from 18°C to 37°C.

1 g of water	raised 1°C	1 cal	
1000 g of water	raised 1°C	1000 cal	
1000 g of water	raised 19°C	19000 cal	= 19 kcal

The larger heat unit kilocalorie (kcal) is usually used to express the caloric value of food.

Specific Heat

The *specific heat* of a substance is the number of calories required to raise the temperature of 1 g of the substance (ideally it is 1 cm^3 of the substance) by 1°C.
- Since the temperature of 1 g of water is raised by 1°C by 1 calorie, *the specific heat of water is 1*.
- The specific heat of ether is 0.5 cal/g (Considering 1 cm^3 of the liquid).
- But the specific heat of ether vapor is 0.0016 (Considering 1 cm^3 of the vapor).

Critical Temperature

Critical temperature of a gas:

Gases become more difficult to liquefy as the *temperature* increases because the kinetic energies of the particles that make up the gas also increase. The *critical temperature* of a substance is the *temperature* at and above which vapor of the substance cannot be liquefied, no matter how much pressure is applied.

For example water can exist only as water vapor above 374°C. Hence, the critical temperature of water is 374°C.

The critical temperature of a gas is the temperature to which it must be cooled before it can be liquefied by the pressure:

It is defined as the temperature above which a liquid cannot continue to be in that state.

In other words, above this temperature gases cannot be liquefied (Compressed into liquid).

Still more simple explanation is; the temperature to which the gas to be brought before it can be liquefied by pressure.

- The lower the temperature, the more the *latent heat* is needed to vaporize the liquid.
- The higher the temperature, the less the *latent heat* is required until a critical temperature is reached.
- At the critical temperature of the liquid the *latent heat* of vaporization is zero.
- Above this temperature the *liquid changes spontaneously into vapor without heat being required* for the change.
- Above this temperature the substance cannot exist in the liquid state.

Critical Temperature of Various Gases

- Air — 141°C
- N$_2$ — 147°C
- O$_2$ — 119°C
- N$_2$O — 36.5°C

The critical temperature should not be confused with the boiling points of the liquid gases.

It may be recalled that *boiling point* is the temperature in which the vapor pressure of the gas equals the atmospheric pressure.

Boiling Points of Various Gases

- Air — 194°C
- N$_2$ — 196°C
- O$_2$ — 183°C
- N$_2$O — 88°C

Practical application:
If a gas is to be liquefied for storing in cylinders, it must be brought below the critical temperature. Otherwise liquefaction is not possible. Critical temperature of N$_2$O is 36.5°C. So above this temperature, the N$_2$O in the cylinder may be in gaseous form—not liquid. In hot climates, it is unsafe to expose the cylinders to direct sun as the whole liquid nitrous oxide is converted into gas and dangerous pressure inside the cylinder may be caused.

At this point of discussion, it is necessary to know about critical pressure of gases.

Critical Pressure

The critical pressure of a gas is the minimum pressure required to liquefy the gas at its critical temperature.

Example: Critical pressure of N$_2$O is 71.6 atm.

Cyclopropane has a critical temperature of 125°C. But at room temperature of 20°C the pressure required to liquefy cyclopropane is only 5 atm pressure (75 psi). Hence, the gas was supplied in light aluminum alloy cylinders.

(1 atm pressure is = 760 mm Hg = 14.7 psi = 33.9 ft of H$_2$O—1.3 kg/cm^2)

Critical temperatures and critical pressures of various gases have been tabulated below.

Gas	Critical temperature	Critical pressure	Boiling point
O$_2$	118°C	50 atm	182°C
N$_2$	140°C	75 atm	195°C
N$_2$O	36.5°C	71.6 atm	89°C
CO$_2$	31°C	72.9 atm	78°C
Ethylene	13°C	51.5 atm	104°C
Cyclopropane	125°C	54 atm	33°C

The *critical temperature* should not be confused with the *boiling point* of the liquid.

	Critical temperature	Boiling point
Water	374°C	100°C
Ether	194°C	34.6°C
N$_2$O	36.5°C	88°C
Halothane	296°C	50°C

Example:
Water boils at 100°C and becomes water vapor and when the temperature falls the vapor condenses into water. But above 374°C water vapor cannot become water again even if pressure is applied to liquefy the vapor.

This means that these substances cannot exist in liquid state above their *critical temperature*.

The liquid that is being converted into gaseous form (vapor) also has the same phenomenon. Ideally the liquid must be at a temperature near its boiling point.

Boiling Point

Boiling point of a liquid is the temperature at which the vapor pressure is equal to the atmospheric pressure.

Example:
Commercially, O_2 is prepared by fractional distillation of liquid air using the difference in the boiling points of O_2 (–183°C) and N_2 (–196°C).

Standard Conditions of Temperature and Pressure

The volume of a gas is often corrected to that it could occupy at 'standard temperature and pressure' (STP)—the volume it occupies at 760 mm Hg and 0°C.

VAPOR AND GASES

Vapor is the gaseous state of a substance which at room temperature and pressure is a liquid.

Example: Ether vapor, Water vapor, etc.

Gas is a substance, which is in gaseous state at room temperature and liquefaction at this temperature is not possible as the room temperature is very much above the critical temperature of the gas.

Example: Oxygen and nitrogen.

Vaporization

- The molecules of a liquid are in constant motion, but there is a strong mutual attraction of the closely packed molecules (cohesion). Some of the molecules on the surface of the liquid move vertically with sufficient speed to overcome the force of cohesion with which their neighbors tend to pull them back into the liquid.
- The molecules escape into the surrounding atmosphere, where it is called *the vapor* of the liquid. This process is named as *'vaporization'* or *evaporation* **(Fig. 1.4)**.
- In the process of evaporation, there is an expenditure of energy by the molecule to overcome the force of cohesion or mutual attraction of the molecules. This expenditure of energy causes drop in the temperature of the liquid.
- This loss of energy is termed as *the latent heat of vaporization* and is derived from the liquid itself and also from the surrounding structures—the container and the air around it.
- Hence, the temperature of the liquid falls initially followed by that of the container.

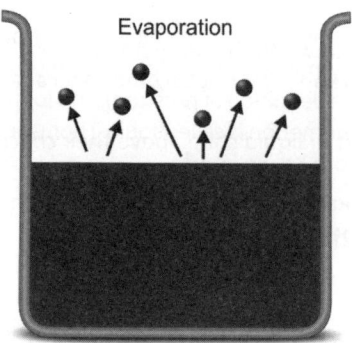 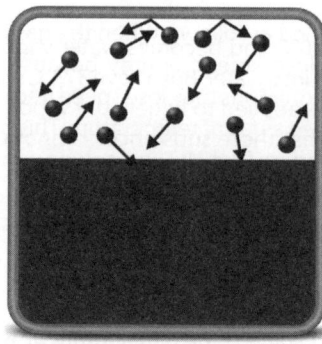

Fig. 1.4: Vaporization and saturated vapor. • Molecules from the liquid surface escape into the atmosphere to form vapor; • The escaped molecules in a closed container reach a point where no further molecules can escape (Saturated vapor); • If some molecules escape at this point equal number of molecules re-enter the liquid; These molecules exerting pressure on the wall of container is *saturated vapor pressure*

- If the liquid is heated and the temperature is raised the movement of molecules becomes more violent and more number of molecules escape out into the atmosphere above the liquid and the rate of vaporization increases.
- Conversely when the temperature of the liquid falls, there will be corresponding decrease of the vapor above the liquid.

Evaporation of Liquid in a Closed Container

- When the liquid is in a closed container the molecules escape out of the liquid in the same way.
- But after certain period of time, when the concentration of vapor above the liquid (the number of molecules in the space) becomes constant—a certain value for the given temperature-evaporation stops. This is the point of equilibrium when there will be a fixed number of molecules above the liquid.
- Even at state of equilibrium, the molecules do escape into the space above the liquid but equal number of molecules will re-enter into the liquid to maintain equilibrium. This point where the number of molecules in the space becomes constant is called *saturated vapor* for that temperature. At this time, the pressure exerted on the walls of the container is known as *the saturated vapor pressure* for the temperature **(Fig. 1.4)**.

Latent Heat of Vaporization

The latent heat of vaporization of a liquid is the amount of heat in calories required to convert 1 g of the liquid at its boiling point into its vapor without altering the temperature of the liquid (heat is to be supplied).

The Joule–Kelvin Principle or Joule–Thomson's Effect

If a compressed gas expands against atmospheric pressure or a lower pressure, it will become cooler (because the gas has done some amount of work) equivalent to the product of reduction in pressure and change of volume.

This is explained as follows: When the gas is released, the molecules recede from each other and lose kinetic energy because they move against forces of mutual attraction (cohesion). Thus they lose speed (recall the definition of pressure). This loss of speed is manifested as fall of temperature. This phenomenon is called Joule-Thomson's effect. (Nomenclature: Prof. W Thomson became Lord Kelvin later).

Explanation of Latent Heat of Vaporization
Ether and N_2O

When ether evaporates from the Boyle bottle vaporizer (glass bottle), initially the latent heat of vaporization is derived from the liquid ether itself. As the liquid becomes cooler, then the latent heat is derived from the bottle and the bottle becomes cooler. Later on, the heat is derived from the surrounding atmosphere so that the water vapor in the atmosphere condenses on the surface of the bottle as dues.

Similarly, when a cylinder of N_2O in the anesthetic machine is opened for use, gaseous nitrous oxide escapes out of the cylinder. This causes a reduction in *the pressure of the gas* (vapor) above the liquid in the cylinder. To compensate this and to raise the pressure, the liquid N_2O starts evaporating. As molecules leave the liquid, *the latent heat of vaporization* is derived from the liquid and the temperature of the liquid drops rapidly. After sometime the latent heat of vaporization is derived from the cylinder and it gets cooled. In course of time the surrounding atmospheric air gets cooled and consequently the water vapor in the atmospheric air gets condensed on the cylinder as due. If carefully watched this condensation of water vapor is confined more to the level of liquid N_2O inside the cylinder. In cold countries the level of condensation is seen on the surface as white snow **(Fig. 1.5)**.

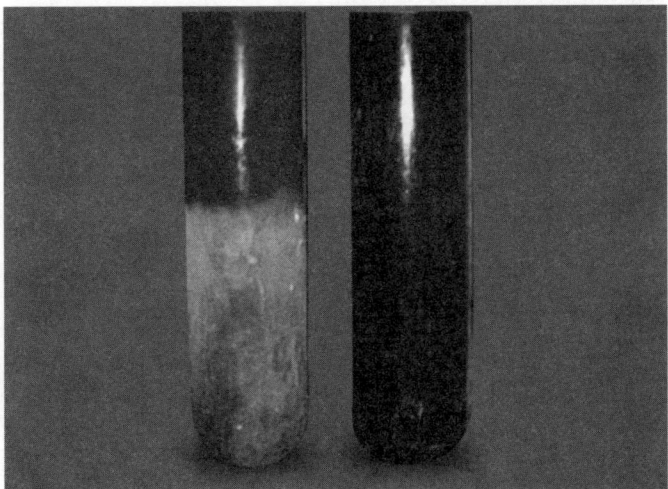

Fig. 1.5: Condensation of water vapor on N_2O cylinder in use. • The latent heat of vaporization is derived from the cylinder and it is cooled rapidly; • Surrounding atmospheric air also gets cooled; • Water vapor from the air gets condensed on the surface of cylinder; • When the ambient temperature is very low it forms snow on the surface; • The snow settles up to the level of liquid N_2O in the cylinder

As vapor is defined as the gaseous form of a substance it is essential to remember the following points.
- Liquids can be converted into gaseous form (vapor). That process is known as *Vaporization*.
- Usually, the solids *melt* into liquids and then *vaporize* into gas form. Example: ice, water, water vapor. Both the processes need heat energy—'latent heat'.
- When the reverse process happens, the vapor condenses into liquid and then the liquid is changed to solid, heat energy (latent heat) is released. Example: water vapor, water, ice.
- Some substances can be converted from solid state into gaseous state without passing through liquid state. That process is known as *sublimation*. Example: camphor, naphthalene.
- Therefore, as it is known that heat can either be given to a substance or abstracted from it, taking water as example, there can be; *latent heat of melting, latent heat of vaporization* which need heat to be supplied and *latent heat of condensation, latent heat of crystallization, latent heat of fusion (solid)* which release heat.
- When a solid sublime into a vapor, *latent heat of sublimation* to be supplied to it.
- The latent heat of vaporization, latent heat of condensation and latent heat of sublimation are schematically represented in **Figure 1.6**.

Sublimation

- Sublimation is the direct change from solid to vapor without going through the liquid stage.
- Solids can also lose molecules (particles) from their surface to form a vapor. In this case we call the effect as *sublimation* rather than evaporation. The reverse phenomenon is also possible.
- In most cases, at ordinary temperatures, the saturated vapor pressures of solids range from low to very, very, very low.
- This is because the forces of attraction among molecules in many solids are too high to allow much loss of particles from the surface.
- However, there are some which do easily form vapors. For example, naphthalene ('mothballs') and camphor have quite a strong smell. Molecules must be

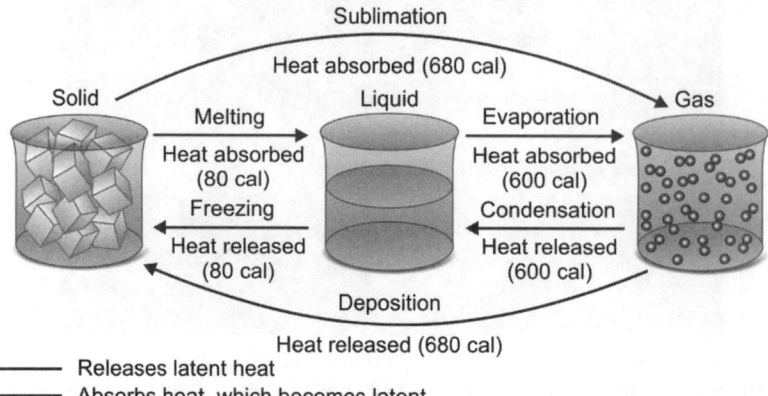

Fig. 1.6: Latent heat of vaporization, condensation, sublimation. • The latent heat of vaporization being used in vaporization and being released in condensation; • Similarly latent heat of sublimation used in formation of vapor is released in the reverse process

breaking away from the surface as a vapor, otherwise the smell would not emanate from it.
- Another fairly common example is solid carbon dioxide—*dry ice*. This never forms a liquid at atmospheric pressure and always converts directly from solid to vapor. That is why it is known as *dry* ice.

Latent Heat of Condensation

The latent heat of condensation is defined as the heat released when one mole of the substance condenses.
- The condensation is the opposite process of evaporation.
- If the vapor *condenses* to a liquid on a surface, then the vapor's *latent energy absorbed* during evaporation is *released*.
- Hence, *latent heat of condensation* is energy released when water vapor condenses to form liquid droplets.

Latent Heat of Crystallization

It is the amount of heat given out or liberated when 1 g of the substance is changed from the liquid to the solid state without alteration of the temperature.
For water it is about 585 calories at room temperature.

Latent Heat of Melting (Latent Heat of Liquefaction)

For converting solid into its liquid state, latent heat of liquefaction is *supplied*.
It is the amount of heat energy required in calories to convert 1 g of solid into its liquid form without altering its temperature.
It is amount of heat that must be supplied to the substance to change into its liquid form without change of temperature. For water it is the same; about 585 calories.

Examples:
- About 580 calories are *required* to convert 1 g of water into vapor without changing the temperature.
- So also, 580 calories are *liberated* when 1 g of water gets condensed (Latent heat of condensation)
- Water has the highest latent heat of vaporization than any other liquid.
- Latent heat of vaporization of ether is 63 calories.

Fall of Temperature of Evaporating Liquid

In vaporizing volatile anesthetic agents:
- When a gas flows over the surface of a liquid, the vapor of the liquid is carried away and is replaced by fresh vapor. This continuous process of vaporization is accompanied by corresponding loss of heat; as the *'latent heat of vaporization'* is being derived from the liquid. So when a volatile anesthetic is used in a vaporizer, as time passes, the temperature of the liquid falls and there will be progressive reduction in vaporization unless heat is supplied.
- When the liquid becomes very cold, the heat may be derived from the surrounding structures or air. The water vapor in the air around the container gets condensed on the surface of the container.
- To prevent this phenomenon and to make the vaporization constant, various temperature compensation devices are used (Discussed in Chapter 7 on vaporizers).

Adiabatic Compression

The process of sudden release of gases and instant recompression without allowing the time for dissipation of *the heat of compression* is known as *Adiabatic compression*. Adiabatic means—without the loss of heat to the outside.

Practical Significance

When a cylinder of oxygen in the yoke of the anesthetic machine is opened, the gas under pressure (2000 lb/sq inch) is released quickly; it gets cooled as latent heat of vaporization is used. But the released gas is instantly recompressed into the pressure reducing valve where enormous amount of latent heat of compression is released and there is no time for dissipating it. This heat is sufficient enough to ignite a combustible material like oil if present resulting in a disaster of fires or explosion. That is why 'Danger—Use No Oil' sign is used wherever compressed gases are used, especially oxygen cylinder.

PRESSURE

Pressure is defined as force per unit area.
By definition, pressure is = *force × area*. It may be expressed as lbs/sq. inch or kg/cm^2, kPa.

- Pressure of a gas is a measure of the molecular bombardment on each unit area of the wall of its container. The closer the molecules the greater the number which strikes each unit area, and therefore the greater pressure exerted.
- *Except at – 273°C (absolute zero) all gases exert pressure.* Such pressure is due to the force exerted by molecules as they bombard the walls of the space of container in which they are confined. This happens because the molecules are in rapid constant motion, at the temperatures usually existing **(Fig. 1.7)**.

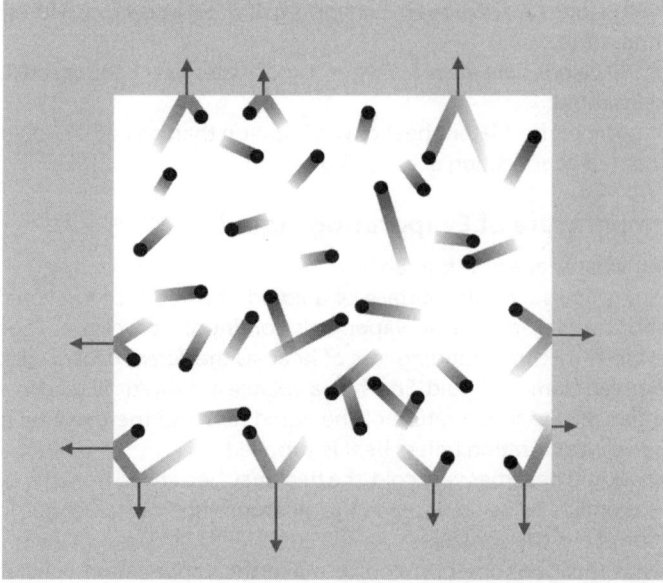

Fig. 1.7: Pressure exerted by the bombardment of molecules on the walls of a closed container

- The standard unit for pressure is the Pascal (Pa), which is a Newton per square meter.
- The SI unit of pressure (the Newton per square meter) is called after the seventeenth-century philosopher and scientist Blaise Pascal as Pascal (Pa)
- A pressure of 1 Pa is too small, hence everyday pressures are often stated in kilopascals (1 kPa = 1000 Pa).

Partial Pressure

- When gases associate as mixture, the pressure of each gas is entirely independent.
- The total pressure exerted by a mixture of gases equals the arithmetic sum of individual pressures exerted by each of the constituent of the mixture.
- It was discussed earlier that under the same conditions of temperature and pressure, equal volumes of all gases contain same number of molecules (Avogadro's hypothesis).
- Air contains 80% nitrogen and 20% oxygen. So in a container of air 20% (1/5) volume is occupied by oxygen and 80% (4/5) volume is occupied by nitrogen.
- Therefore, oxygen exerts 1/5th of the total pressure and nitrogen exerts 4/5th of the total pressure. This is known as 'partial pressure' of the gas in a mixture **(Figs 1.8A to C)**.
- In a mixture of gases, each gas will exert the same pressure which it exerts if it occupies the container alone.

Dalton's law of partial pressures states that in a mixture of non-reacting gases, the total pressure exerted is equal to the sum of *the partial pressures* of the individual gases. (John Dalton in 1801).

This is explained as follows:
- In a mixture of gases, the pressure exerted by each gas is called its *partial pressure* the total pressure exerted equals the arithmetic sum of individual pressures exerted by each of the constituent of the mixture.

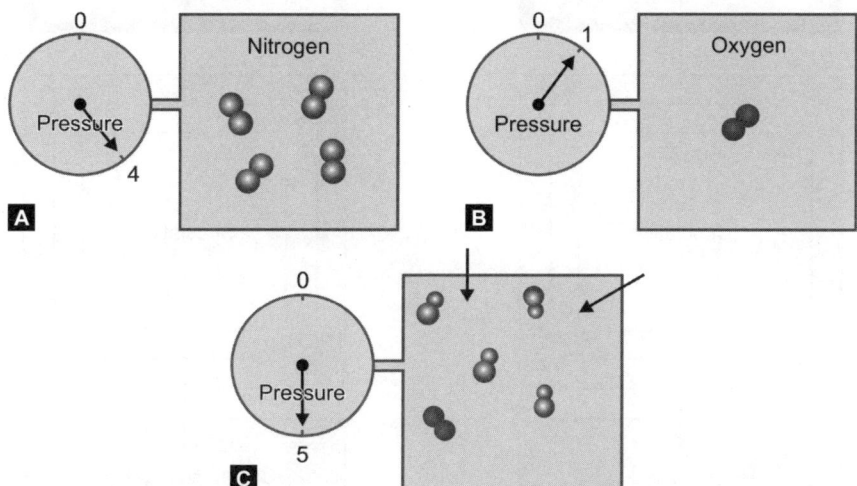

Figs 1.8A to C: Partial pressure of gases in Air. • Chamber A contains 4 molecule of nitrogen and exerts a pressure of 4 units; • Chamber B contains 1 molecule of oxygen and exerts a pressure of 1 unit; • The contents A and B are transferred to chamber C; • Chamber C has total of 5 molecules and exerts pressure of 5 units

- In such a mixture, each gas exerts the same proportion of the total pressure as its volume of total volume.
- Thus, in a mixture of 25% cyclopropane, 25% O_2 and 50% helium, having a total pressure of 800 mm Hg. Partial pressures of O_2 = 200 mm Hg; cyclopropane = 200 mm Hg and helium = 400 mm Hg.

Fick's Law

This law states that the rate of diffusion of gas is proportional to the *gradient of concentration*. When the concentration gradient is high the rate of diffusion is fast.

Application of Dalton's Law and Fick's Law partial pressure in the diffusion of gases

- If a gas exists on either side of a diffusible membrane, the direction of its diffusion is determined by the differences in its partial pressure it exerts on either side of the membrane—(not by the difference in its amount).
- The gas diffuses from the side of higher partial pressure to the side of lower partial pressure till the equilibrium of partial pressure is reached.
- The difference in the partial pressure is the *pressure gradient* that drives the gas across the membrane (diffusion).
- This is the mechanism by which the diffusion of O_2 and CO_2 occurs across alveolar capillary membrane in the lung as well as in the tissue level **(Fig. 1.9)**.
- In the alveoli the percentage of oxygen is 14. Therefore, the partial pressure of this gas is 14% of 760 mm = 100 mm Hg.

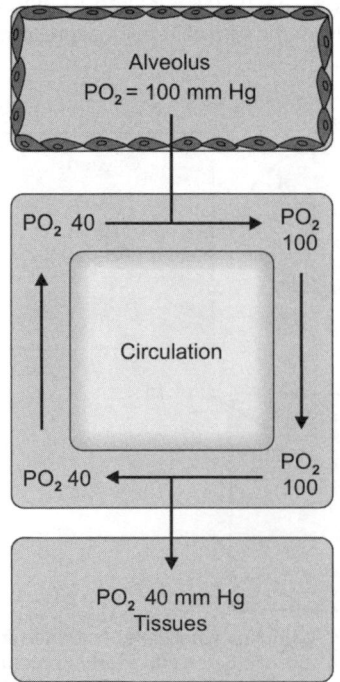
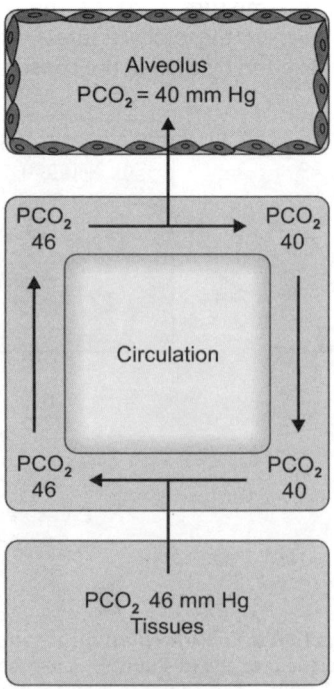

Fig. 1.9: Diffusion of gases aided by gradient in partial pressure

- The tension of oxygen (partial pressure) in the capillaries of the lungs is approximately 40 mm Hg. There is a pressure gradient of 60 mm Hg.
- The oxygen from alveoli diffuses rapidly to the venous blood and this raises the tension of arterial blood leaving the alveoli to 95 mm Hg.

Atmospheric Pressure

It is the pressure exerted by the column of air in the atmosphere on earth which can lift a mercury column of 760 mm in a vacuum tube.

One atmospheric pressure is 760 mm Hg
- It is equivalent to *1 kg/cm²* or *14.7 (15) lbs/sq inch* or *1030 cm of H_2O* or *1 bar* or *100 kPa* or *1000 millibar.*
- Atmospheric pressure at sea level will support a column of mercury to 760 mm height.
- Hence, 760 mm Hg is referred to as one atmospheric pressure.
- The partial pressure of oxygen in air is 21% of 760 mm Hg= 160 mm Hg.
- The exact partial pressures of atmospheric air are illustrated in **Figure 1.10**.
- The total is 752 mm Hg as the remaining 8 mm Hg is constituted by carbon dioxide and other trace gases.

Atmospheric pressure in high altitude
- At heights above sea level the weight of the overlying air is less. The molecules are less closely packed so that they exert less pressure.
- At 6000 feet above sea level the atmospheric pressure is 600 mm Hg; hence partial pressure of oxygen is 126 mm Hg.
- At 10,000 feet, the pressure sufficient to support a column of mercury is only 520 mm Hg.

Interesting aspects of partial pressures, atmospheric pressure and breathing in high altitude
- Carbon dioxide is excreted from the bloodstream into the alveoli and the partial pressure it exerts in the alveoli remains practically constant at 40 mm Hg.
- Another gas inevitably present in the alveoli is water vapor. Since the body temperature remains is constant, the partial pressure of water vapor in the alveoli remains constant at 47 mm Hg.
- Therefore, these two gases exert a combined pressure of about 90 mm Hg under all conditions.

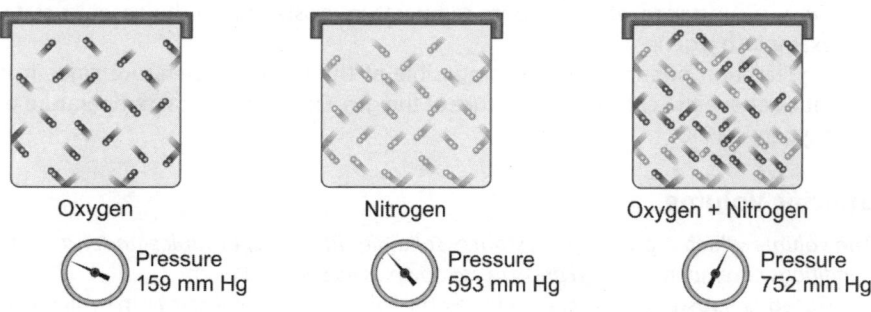

Fig. 1.10: The partial pressures of oxygen and nitrogen in atmospheric air

- Hence, at sea level the pressure of other gases (nitrogen and oxygen) in the lungs is 760 – 90 = 670 mm Hg.
- The percentage of oxygen in atmospheric air is unaffected by altitude and remains constant at 21.
- The percentage of oxygen in the alveolar gas is only 15%.
- At sea level, the partial pressure of oxygen in alveolar air is 15% of (760 – 90 = 670 mm Hg) = 100 mm Hg.
- At 6000 feet (1800 m) atmospheric pressure is 610 mm Hg and the partial pressure of oxygen in alveoli is 15% = 78 mm Hg. If the venous oxygen tension is 40 mm Hg, there is still a pressure difference (gradient) 78 – 40 = 38 mm Hg for adequate oxygenation of the blood.
- At 14000 feet (4200 m) the atmospheric pressure is 540 mm Hg. Partial pressure of carbon dioxide and water vapor remain constant in the alveoli as 90 mm Hg. So, combined pressure of nitrogen and oxygen is 540–90 = 450 mm Hg. Therefore, the pressure of oxygen in the alveoli is 15% of 360–54 mm Hg. Now the gradient of pressure between the alveoli and venous blood is reduced to 14 mm Hg. Oxygenation of blood resulting from this is sufficient to support life, though it leaves many of the body functions considerably impaired. Saturation of oxygen in hemoglobin will be about 80%.
- At 30000 feet (9100 m) the atmospheric pressure is 225 mm Hg. Alveolar oxygen pressure would be 15% of (225–90) = 20 mm Hg. This pressure is less than the tension of oxygen in the venous blood. Diffusion of oxygen occurs in reverse direction into the alveoli.
- It has been shown in experiments simulating conditions of 40000 feet, had shown that the alveolar oxygen pressure was 15 mm Hg and after a few breaths the pressure fell to 6 mm Hg, consciousness was lost. (reverse diffusion and sever hypoxia).
- At 50000 feet the total atmospheric pressure is only 90 mm Hg. So, in theory, the alveolar space is filled with CO_2 and water vapor only.

GAS LAWS

Vapor and Gas

- *Vapor* is the gaseous state of a substance which at room temperature and pressure is a liquid. Example: *water vapor, halothane vapor*.
- More scientifically, the vapor is gaseous state of the substance above its 'critical temperature' as above the 'critical temperature' it could not be liquefied.
- *Gas* is a substance which at room temperature exists only in the gaseous state. Example: oxygen.
- Liquefaction of such a gas is impossible at the room temperature since it is much above the critical temperature of the gas. Example: Critical temperature of oxygen –118°C.

Specific Volume

The volume which 1 g of any substance, solid, liquid or gas, occupies under a given conditions of temperature and pressure is known as its Specific Volume.
- Gaseous substance always occupies the whole of the container in which it is held.

- Thus, the molecule of the gas thin out to suit the size of the container.
- The specific volume is inversely proportional to the density.

Specific Volume = 1/density

- When a given weight of a gas is allowed to expand, its specific volume increases.
- There are fewer molecules in a cm³ and so less number of molecules bombard on unit are of the walls. Therefore, the pressure falls. Thus, the pressure is inversely proportional to the increase in the specific volume.

Boyle's Law (1662)

When the temperature is kept constant, the pressure of a gas is inversely proportional to the specific volume.

Pressure $\propto$ 1/Specific Volume

Since the density of a gas is inversely proportional to its specific volume, it can be defined as;

When the temperature is kept constant, the pressure of a gas is directly proportional to the density.

Pressure $\propto$ Density

The Boyle's Law is explained in **Figure 1.11**.

Practical Applications

If the O_2 cylinder is full, pressure is 120 (137) atm (2000 lbs/sq inch or 150 kg/sq cm). If the contents are reduced to half, in the process of use, the pressure is also reduced to half. The *specific volume* is doubled. The pressure gauge will be showing half of the original pressure—say 1000 lbs/sq inch. So if the total content of the cylinder is known in measures of liters then, by looking at the pressure gauge one can calculate the amount of gas remaining in the cylinder **(Fig. 1.12)**.

Pressure gauge is rarely used for N_2O, cyclopropane, CO_2 or any liquefied gases.
The cylinders when full contain a small amount of gaseous N_2O above the liquid N_2O at room temperature and the saturated vapor pressure is 51 atm. This continues to be the same although with the fall of temperature of the cylinder; the saturated vapor

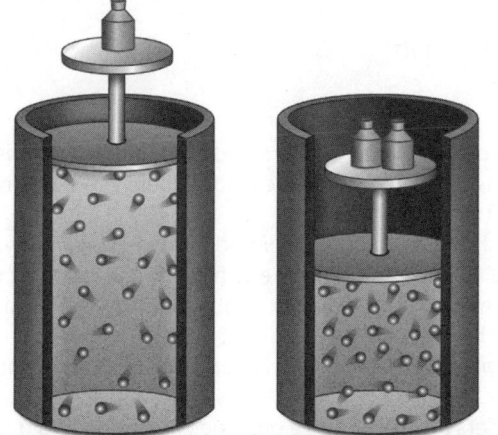

Fig. 1.11: Boyle's Law explained. • The pressure is inversely proportional to the volume;
• As the pressure applied is increased the volume gets reduced

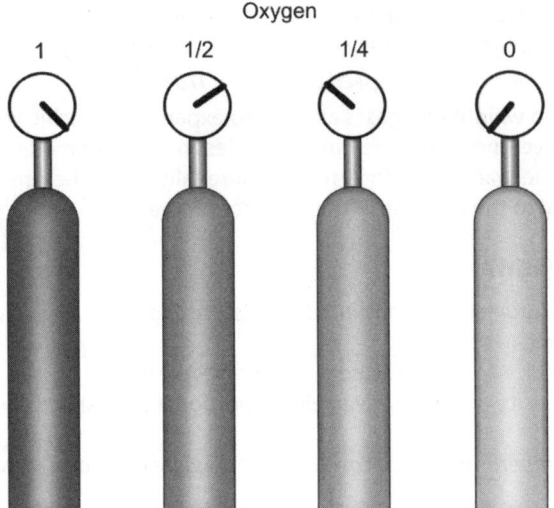

Fig. 1.12: Application of Boyle's Law in oxygen cylinder

pressure may be a little reduced, depending upon the temperature of the cylinder. But with the cylinder at 21°C, the pressure is always at 51 atm, which shows that there is some liquid in the cylinder, but gives no idea of how much liquid. When the last drop of liquid is vaporized the vapor pressure is still 51 atm. After that the vapor pressure falls rapidly (depending upon the flow rate) to zero. So, the pressure gauge does not serve any useful purpose in such cylinders of liquefied gases. In the modern anesthetic machines there are pressure gauges fitted and they indicate the pipeline pressure as 60 psi (4 bar).

But if the cylinder is used it serve to know whether all the liquid has been used up and the cylinder nearing to be empty **(Fig. 1.13)**.

- The amount of N_2O remaining in the cylinder can be ascertained only by weight.
- The weight of empty cylinder is seen stamped on it, i.e. Tare weight.
- The difference in weight is converted into the amount of liters of gas present in the cylinder.
- 455 L of N_2O weighs 850 g (1 L = 1.87 g).

Filling Ratio

The degree of filling of a nitrous oxide cylinder is expressed as *the mass of nitrous oxide* in a cylinder divided by *the mass of water* that the cylinder could hold. Normally, a cylinder of nitrous oxide is filled to a ratio of 0.67.

This should not be confused with the volume of liquid nitrous oxide in a cylinder. A full cylinder of nitrous oxide at room temperature is filled to the point at which approximately 90% of the interior of the cylinder is occupied by the liquid, the remaining 10% being occupied by gaseous nitrous oxide.

Simply, filling ratio is the weight of the fluid in the cylinder divided by the weight of the water required to fill it.

- Usually, nitrous oxide cylinders are filled from a pipeline containing liquid nitrous oxide under a pressure well above the saturation pressure of the temperature in the room.

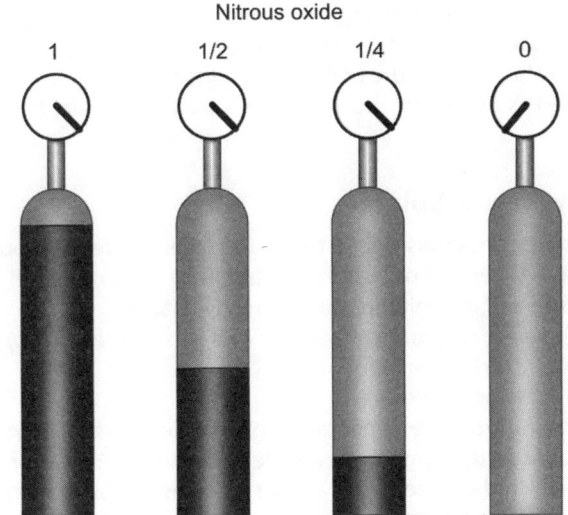

Fig. 1.13: Pressure gauge in N_2O cylinder. • The gauge shows full pressure until it is nearing exhaustion

- The cylinders are filled with a little gas above the liquid N_2O. When the specific volume is 1.5 cm³/g the cylinder is said to be full.
- The cylinder can be filled beyond this stage to when the cylinder is full of liquid.
- As the liquid is virtually incompressible, even an addition of even a minute amount of gas will result in enormous increase in pressure.
- Since the density of water is 1, the ratio is;

    Weight of N_2O in the cylinder/weight of water the cylinder could hold
    A 455 L cylinder has an internal volume of 1.3 L (1300 mL)
    The volume of water it can hold is 46 oz or 1300 mL   = 1300 g
    The volume of liquid N_2O in 'full' cylinder is 30 oz   = 850 g
    Therefore the filling ratio   = 30/46 or 850/1300 = 0.65

This gives the average density of the contents and the figure is known as the 'filling ratio'.
- N_2O cylinders are normally filled to a ratio of 0.67.
- This is suitable for temperate and tropical climates (0.75 is acceptable for temperate climates).

How this Filling Ratio is Practically Very Important?

The filling ratio of *0.65* corresponds to specific volume of *1.5*.
This cylinder;
    At 20°C   has a pressure of   *51 atm*
    At 40°C   has a pressure of   *90 atm*
    At 60°C   has a pressure of   *160 atm* (2400 lbs/sq inch)

This is possible in tropics and the pressure is similar to a full oxygen cylinder at the same temperature.

The filling ratio of *0.77* corresponds to specific volume of *1.3*.
This cylinder;
    At 20°C   has a pressure of   51 atm
    At 40°C   has a pressure of   125 atm
    At 60°C   has a pressure of   190 atm (2850 lbs/sq inch)

This is almost closer to the testing pressure of the cylinder.
When the cylinder is *completely filled* with liquid N_2O;
At 20°C, it may have a pressure of 51 atm or a little more.

But, if warmed as described above, will *cross the test pressure to reach dangerous values.*

Charles's Law (Law of Volumes)

Charles's law describes how gases tend to expand when heated. A modern statement of Charles's law is—When the pressure on a sample of a dry gas is held constant, the Kelvin temperature and the volume will be directly related.

If the pressure remains constant the volume of a gas is directly proportional to its absolute temperature (Kelvin temperature).

Figure 1.14 explains Charles' Law.

Absolute temperature is the temperature of an object on a scale where 0 is taken as absolute zero. Absolute temperature scale is Kelvin. Absolute zero is the lowest temperature at which the system is in a state of lowest possible (minimum) energy. No electronic device can operate at this temperature.

Common temperatures in the absolute scale are:
- 0°C (freezing point of water)   = 273.15 K
- 25°C (room temperature)   = 298.15 K
- 100°C (boiling point of water)   = 373.15 K
- 0 K (absolute zero)   = –273.15°C

To convert from the Celsius scale into the absolute temperature, add 273.15 and change °C to K. To get a temperature on the absolute scale to the Celsius scale, subtract 273.15 and change K to °C.

Conversion

Kelvin to Celsius: K = C + 273
Celsius to Kelvin: C = K – 273

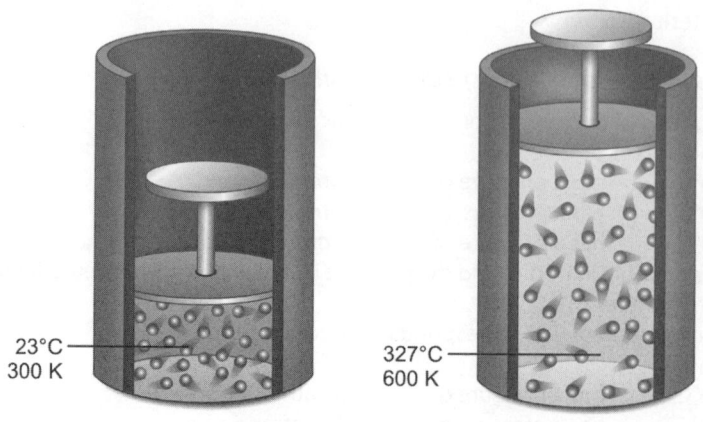

Fig. 1.14: Charles' Law

Note:
- The pressure applied on the gas is constant, but temperature is increased from 23°C = 300 K to 327°C = 600 K.
- Therefore, when the K (Absolute temperature) 300 K is doubled as 600 K the volume of the gas is doubled.
- *If the temperature remains constant, the volume of the gas varies inversely with its pressure.* (Therefore halving the pressure doubles its volume and doubling its pressure halves its volume.)
- The volume decreases by 1/273 for every degree it is cooled below 0°C and increases by 1/273 for every degree it is heated above 0°C.
- In this *absolute scale of temperature* is used (Kelvin temperature).
- 0° Absolute is equivalent to −273°C.
- 273 Absolute is equivalent to 0°C.
- Absolute temperature is mentioned as *K* (after Lord Kelvin).

Gay-Lussac's Law

If the volume remains constant, the pressure of a gas is directly proportional to its absolute temperature.

If the volume is kept constant, for each degree Celsius (°C) rise in temperature, the pressure of the gas raises by 1/273 of its pressure at 0°C.

Diffusion

Gaseous molecules tend to distribute themselves evenly in any given space.
- When two different gases are allowed to mix in a container, there is a rapid intermingling of molecules among the two gases and both the gases are uniformly distributed in the container.
  Example: In the alveoli the inspired air diffuses readily into the residual air.
- Liquids also have the same process of diffusion of intermingling of molecules, but at an extremely slow rate.
  Example: In spinal anesthesia diffusion of local analgesic is so slow that the upward spread is not a common problem by diffusion. There are other factors that cause the spread.

This happens with all gases and vapors whether it is monoatomic, diatomic, triatomic or multiatomic.

Example:

Monoatomic	Diatomic	Triatomic	Multiatomic
Helium (He)	O_2, N_2	O_3	C_3H_6 (Cyclopropane)
Xenon (Xe)	H_2	N_2O	C_2H_4 (Ethylene)

POYNTING EFFECT

- This is also known as *'overpressure effect'*
- The critical temperature and critical pressure of one gas may be affected by its admixture with another gas.
- When a cylinder is partially filled with liquid nitrous oxide is inverted and further filled with oxygen from a high pressure source, an unexpected phenomenon occurs. The oxygen gets dissolved in liquid nitrous oxide and subsequently nitrous oxide liquid evaporates and mixes with oxygen.

- At one point of time the cylinder contains a mixture of nitrous oxide and oxygen in gaseous form at a pressure of 2000 psi (137 atm) at room temperature.
- In this process, the critical temperature of nitrous oxide 36.5°C changes to a pseudocritical temperature of –6°C.
- This effect of modifying the critical pressure of one gas by mixing with other gas is called "Poynting effect".
- *Entonox* is a 50: 50 mixture of nitrous oxide and oxygen in gaseous form used in obstetrics analgesia.

Bernoulli's Principle (1738)

Daniel Bernoulli (1700–1782) in 1738 demonstrated that when a fluid passes through a tube of varying cross sectional areas (diameter) the pressure is least where the velocity (speed) is greatest. This is *Bernoulli's Effect*.

Bernoulli's theorem, or Bernoulli's Law states that when a fluid is passing through a tube of varying cross sectional areas, the velocity is highest in the narrowest portion and the pressure is lowest; whereas in the widest portion the velocity is low and the pressure is high.

Simply, when a fluid passes through a tube of varying diameters, the pressure is low at the point of maximum velocity.

Figures 1.15 and 1.16 explain the Bernoulli's principle.

The diameter of a tube is smoothly reduced to half to form a constriction and the again it is widened to the original diameter smoothly. When fluid is allowed to flow through this tube of varying diameters the speed is greatest in the area of constriction which can be measured by connecting a narrow tube vertically perpendicular to the tube where fluid flows. The pressure is highest in the proximal end lowest in the constriction and again raises to a higher level that is a little lower than that at the proximal end.

It is necessary to recall that Pressure = Force ÷ Area (Force acting on unit of surface area). In low velocity more molecules bombard the walls of the tube to exert pressure. In high velocity the time available for such bombardment is minimal and so exerts minimal pressure.

The pressure drop seen in the constriction is *due to the temporary conversion of pressure energy into increased kinetic energy.*

When the velocity (speed) of the flow is increased, the pressure drops further and may become negative (subatmospheric). Similarly if the constriction of the tube is

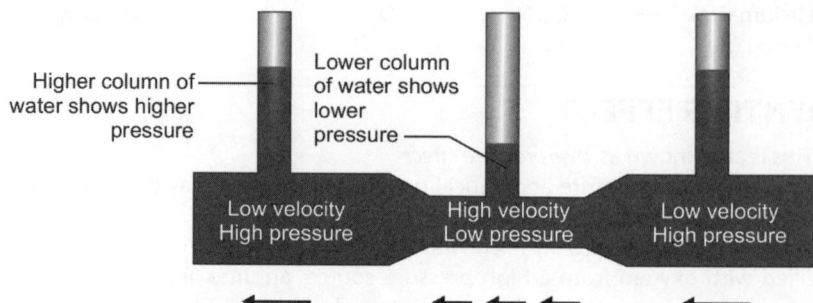

Fig. 1.15: Bernoulli's principle. • Fast moving fluid exerts low pressure and slow moving fluid exerts high pressure; • The velocity is highest and the pressure is lowest in the constriction of the tube; • Shown by attaching a narrow vertical tube where fluid level is seen as pressure

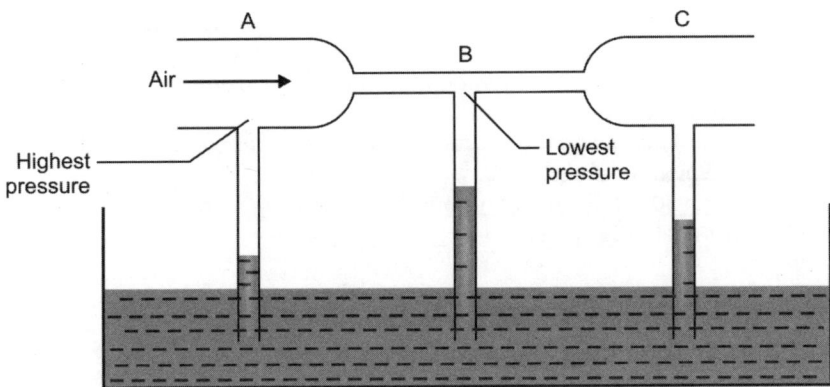

Fig. 1.16: Bernoulli's principle. • When air is the driving fluid the tubes are dipped in a container of water—water level being sucked show the pressure. • In the narrow portion of the tube 'B' the driving fluid has highest velocity and the pressure is lowest at that point. So the water level is sucked higher

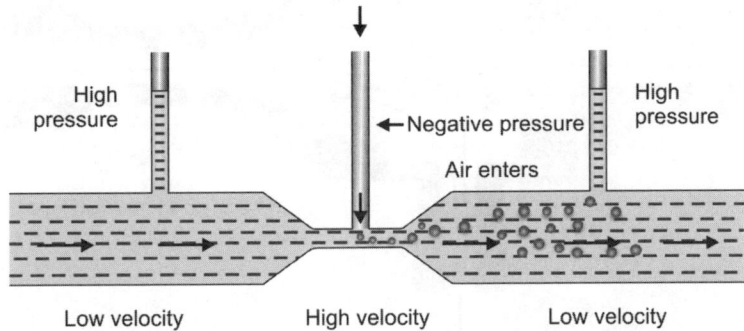

Fig. 1.17: Subatmospheric pressure caused by Bernoulli's principle. • The very high velocity of fluid at the very narrow tube causes drop in pressure; • The velocity is so high that the drop of pressure becomes subatmospheric; • The subatmospheric pressure causes entrainment of air bubbles through the side tube

made narrower, naturally the velocity increases and the same effect of developing subatmospheric pressure are caused **(Fig. 1.17)**.

Venturi

In 1797—about 60 years later, *Giovanni Battista Venturi* (1746–1822) an Italian physicist developed an appliance known as Ventury based on Bernoulli's principle. With suitable flow in the cone shaped *'venturi tube'* subatmospheric pressure can be easily produced.

Where the cross sectional area of the tube (Main driving fluid) is very much reduced like a 'Jet' and allowed become larger by gradual widening, or called 'swaying', there is a negative pressure created at the point of maximum narrowing. If a side port is attached at this point (Entrainment port), this will allow suctioning of fluid (Entraining fluid) connected to the entrainment port. This device is known as 'Venturi device' or 'Jet' **(Fig. 1.18)**.

The device is actually known as *'Injector'* where the smooth constriction of the venturi tube is replaced with *a nozzle through which fluid is injected at great velocity*. This is known as *'driving fluid'.* Subatmospheric pressure created around the nozzle.

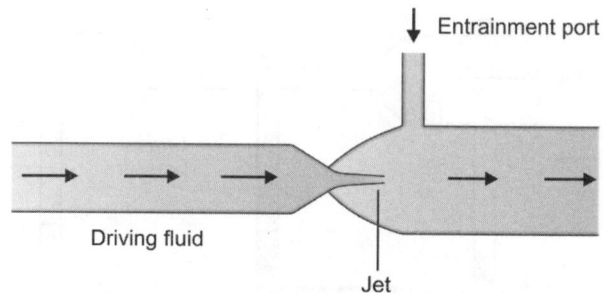

Fig. 1.18: Construction of Venturi device or Jet

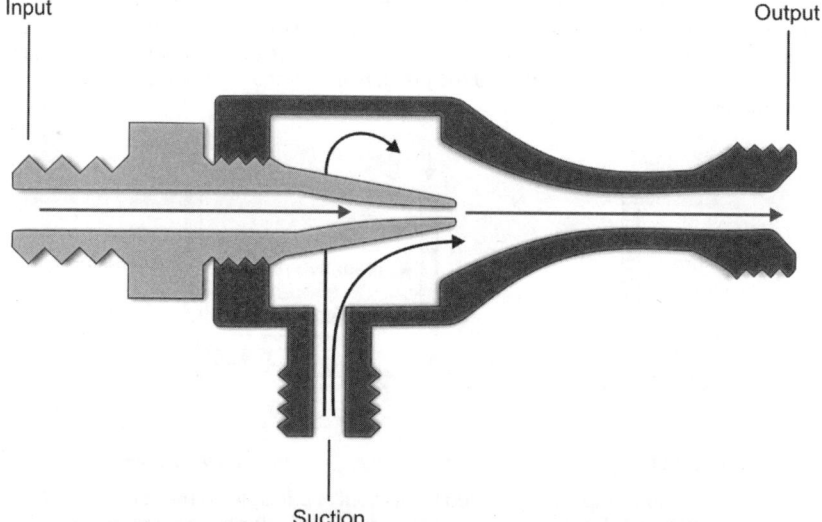

Fig. 1.19: Venturi device. • Input is driving fluid; • The constriction is replaced with a jet; • Suction is entrainment port; • The tube widens very smoothly; • The special funnel shaped downstream tube is called 'diffuser'

A tube that is known as *'entrainment port'* is connected to the main tube near nozzle that can allow the desired fluid—*'entrained fluid'* (Gas or liquid) in to the main stream by suction effect **(Fig. 1.19)**.

In a properly designed ventury device the driving gas may entrain as much as twenty times it own volume.

The appliances based on this device:
- Venturi suction
- Oxygen therapy mask—Ventimask **(Fig. 1.20)**
- Jet ventilator
- Macintosh laryngeal spray **(Fig. 1.21)**.

Ventimask

- The 'Ventimask' works on this 'Venturi Principle'
- It gives a predetermined concentration of oxygen to the patient and it can be set as needed.

Applied Physics   25

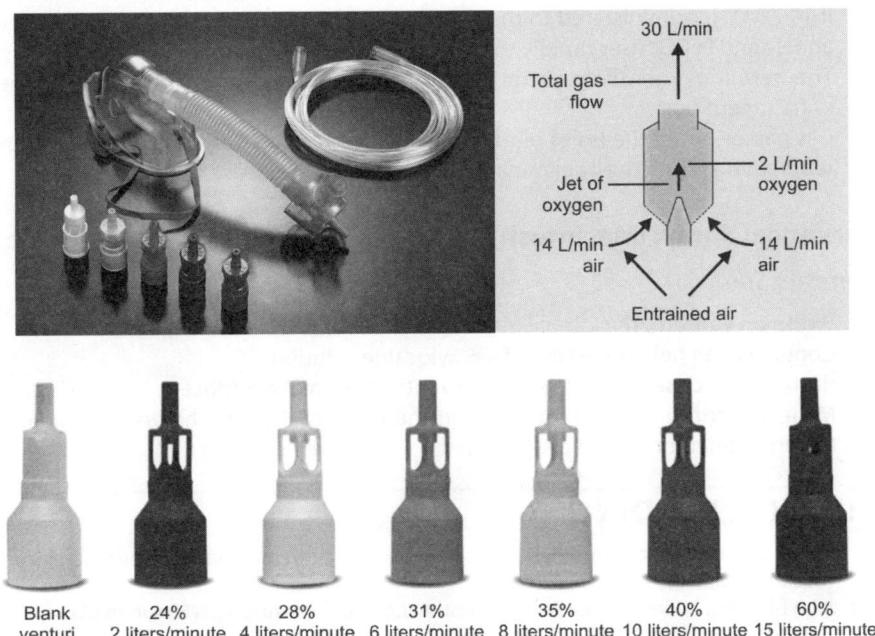

Fig. 1.20: Ventimask working with Venturi device. • Used for oxygen therapy with regulated percentage of oxygen; • Very large volume of air is entrained to maintain the percentage; • In addition the flow rate of oxygen controls the percentage; • Color coded ventury adapters for desired percentage of oxygen and the flow rate of oxygen needed are shown; • Oxygen tubing is attached to the adapter

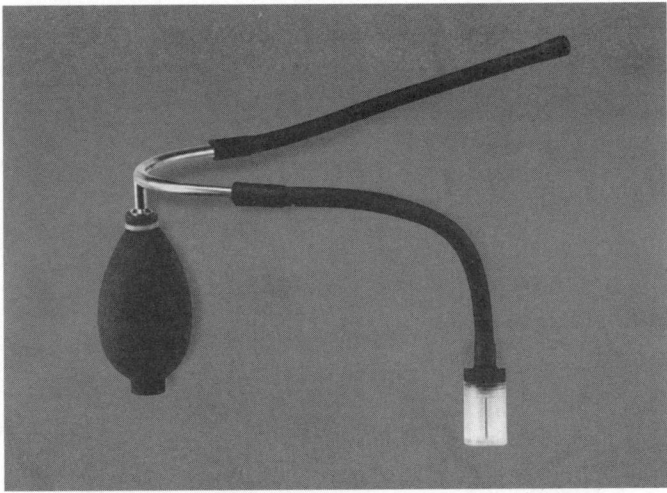

Fig. 1.21: Macintosh spray working on ventury principle

- It is used for guarded, calculated percentage of oxygen in air delivered to the patients who maintain their ventilation by the *hypoxic drive* and not by CO_2 drive. e.g. patients with COPD.

- If 100% O_2 is administered to them, it abolishes this hypoxic drive, they become apneic and $PaCO_2$ rises rapidly to make them unconscious, (CO_2 Narcosis)
- The actual oxygen concentration is determined by varying the size of the entrainment port.
- Gas passes out of the holes of mask mostly due to high fresh gas flow rate. Thus rebreathing is practically eliminated and there is no increase in dead space.

Laryngeal Spray: (Macintosh)

Forrester Spray

- Works on Venturi principle
- Container can hold only 4 mL of 4% xylocaine solution.
- Restricts the dose to 160 mg: this prevents accidental overdose
- Malleable sprout is used for spraying the nasal cavity, oropharynx, larynx and laryngeal inlet for topical analgesia.

FURTHER READING

1. Jerry A Dorsch, Susan E Dorsch. Understanding anesthesia equipment, 5th edn. Lippincott Willaims & Wilkins, Philadelphia; 2008.
2. John TB Moyle, Andrew Davey. Ward's anaesthetic equipment, 4th edn. WB Saunders Company Limited, Philadelphia; 1998.
3. Atkinson RS, Rushman GB, Davies NJH, Lee's synopsis of anaesthesia, 11th edn. Butterworth-Heinemann Limited London; 1993.
4. Sir Robert Macintosh, William W Mushin, Epstein HG. Physics for the anaesthetist, 4th edn. Blackwell Scientific Publications, Oxford; 1963.

chapter 2

Anesthesia Machine

INTRODUCTION

Anesthesia machine being the vital equipment for the safe conduct of anesthesia, it is mandatory that every beginner is well informed about it. Before operating any machine, one must know about its components and the principle on which each component works with the emphasis as to how it contributes for the effective functioning of the machine.

So also, regarding anesthesia machine, knowing the details starting from the origin, development, essential components and the principle on which each component works are all necessary for safe use of the machine.

Here it is planned to discuss a brief history of anesthesia machine to show how it had undergone the metamorphosis from the primitive form to the modern structure and function. Its essential components would be briefed in this chapter for the reader to have an overall view of the machine and to know how it functions. The details of each component would be dealt with elaborately in different chapters to have more details and better understanding. It would be easier to learn about the subsequent developments made on them one by one and understand them step by step.

The machine incorporates various devices each one individually capable of performing a specific function that are integrated as a single unit. This makes the functioning of the machine complete and safe for administration of anesthesia.

The purpose of anesthesia gas machine is to prepare a precisely known but variable gas mixture including life sustaining and anesthetizing gases. Depending upon the need a precise concentration of a volatile anesthetic agent may also be added in the anesthetic gas mixture.

Oxygen is the life sustaining gas and nitrous oxide is the anesthetic gas used in the mixture. Vapor of a volatile anesthetic agent such as halothane, isoflurane, and sevoflurane, etc. is also added in precise concentrations as needed.

The anesthetic mixture prepared in the machine is then delivered to the patient through the breathing system. Though breathing system is a part of anesthetic machine, it is discussed in a separate chapter because of its vast nature.

The aim and the design of the machine are only for fulfilling this fundamental purpose. Further changes were made in this basic design mainly with the view of improving the patient safety.

The modern anesthesia machines or 'Work Stations' are equipped with too many sophisticated additional gadgets than what is basically needed. These gadgets may be for monitoring the function of the machine or for monitoring patient's vital parameters with the ultimate aim of enhancing patient safety. Incidentally these improvements have added user convenience as well.

The striking point is, though many modifications have been brought out in the structure and safety features over the past many decades, the concept of the basic design has not changed much.

Hence, a clear knowledge of the basic design is a must for all the practicing anesthesiologists to understand the modern anesthesia workstation.

Anyone who has the thorough understanding of the design and purpose will be able to use the anesthetic machines safely. Every additional safety features in the newer machines only ensure added safety.

Why do we need anesthetic machine?
- Use gases from source of compressed gases (e.g. cylinders)
- Measure flow of gases
- Add vapors in known concentrations
- Deliver vapors and gases to patient via a breathing system
- Scavenge waste gases
- Monitor the machine and patient.

HISTORY

The anesthetic machines were made as early as 1860.

During First World War, in 1914 and *Captain Geoffrey Marshall*, a physician from Guy's Hospital, working as medical officer of Casualty Clearing Station in France, experimented with various anesthetic techniques and settled on nitrous oxide gas and oxygen. Marshall did not publish this till 1920. Finally *Coxeter* developed a machine for delivering the gas with oxygen.

However, it was *Henry Edmund Gaskin Boyle* who took up this and that was the origin of Boyle's apparatus, which he modified afterwards.

The machine, which incorporated a *water sight-feed flow meter* for nitrous oxide, was manufactured for the British Army for the remainder of the war.

Henry Edmund Gaskin Boyle was also commissioned during the war but served at the 1st London General Hospital. He imported a Gwathmey machine in 1916 and had discovered that with prolonged use the machine developed leaks, chiefly due to incompatibilities with the American cylinder connections. In 1917, crediting Gwathmey with the design of the machine he was using at that time, he got *Coxeter*, the instrument maker to copy James Tayloe Gwathmey's gas-oxygen machine, which became the first *Boyle's apparatus.*

This first version of the Boyle apparatus was made by Lord George Wellesley who later became managing director of Coxeter's, and the name *Boyle's machine* is a registered trademark of this company, later known as the British Oxygen Company (BOC).

This original machine had two nitrous oxide and two oxygen cylinders housed in a wooden box. This had a 'water sight feed' flow meter (a wet flow meter) and ether vaporizer. It had a pressure gauge on oxygen cylinder and fine adjustment valves. A Cattlin bag, a three way stopcock and a face mask completed the apparatus.

Boyle's anesthetic machine modified in every respect was in use in most British hospitals and elsewhere in the world.

Since its introduction by Boyle in 1917, the subsequent important modifications made in the machine were;
- *1920*: Vaporizer bottles were added
- *1926*: The second vaporizer bottle and by-pass control were added
- *1927*: Flow meter for carbon dioxide was included, the lever type controls for vaporizer and the familiar back bar were introduced.
- *1930*: Plunger device in vaporizer bottle was added

- *1933*: Dry bobbin type of flow meter added instead of 'Water-sight feed' type
- *1937*: The dry bobbin type flow meters were replaced by 'Rotameters'
- *1952*: Pin index safety system was introduced by Dr Philip Woodbridge
- *1958*: Bodok seal was introduced.

Five primitive models of Boyle's anesthetic machines with additional features added in each new model are shown in **Figures 2.1 to 2.3**.

Supplements Added

- *1921*: Waters to and fro absorption apparatus was introduced.
- *1930*: Circle absorption system was introduced by Brian Sword.

The modern anesthetic machine has no resemblance to the original model as it had undergone total modification over these decades.

Despite numerous modifications the modern machine retains many of the features of the original Boyle's machine, a British Oxygen Company trade name in honour of the British anesthetist HEG Boyle (1875–1941).

In India till 1960s the 'Boyle F' model originally manufactured by British Oxygen Company (BOC) and later by Indian Oxygen Limited (IOL) was in use throughout the country. Later in 1970s a bigger version with additional features known as 'Boyle Major' was introduced. This machine was known as 'BOC International Continuous Flow Anesthetic Machine' in other countries **(Figs 2.4A and B)**.

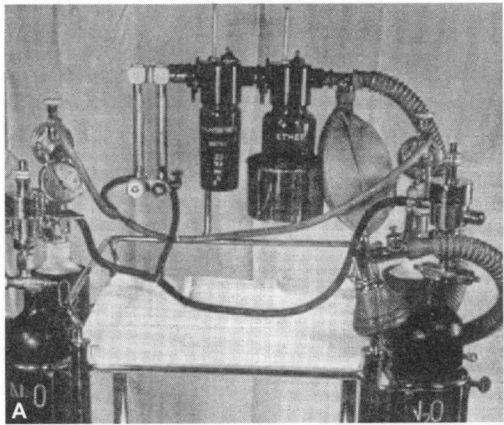
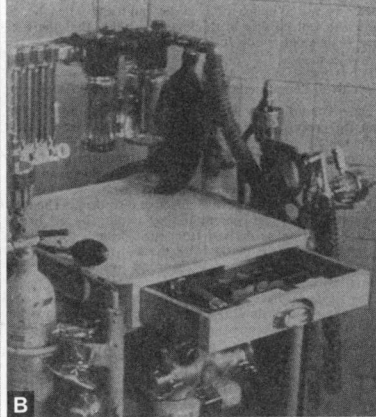

Figs 2.1A and B: Two primitive versions of Boyle's machines. • (A) 1940 model machine; • Baskets support the cylinders–no yokes; • 'Adams' pressure reducing valves are seen in all cylinders with a pressure gauge for oxygen cylinder; • Flexible hoses deliver the gases to the respective flow meters; • The back bar to which the flow meters and vaporizer bottles are fixed is supported by a vertical rod; • Two Boyle bottle vaporizers, one for chloroform and the other for ether; • Ether bottle is surrounded by a warm water jacket to improve vaporization; • Common gas outlet points to the right side not to the front to which Magill's breathing system is attached; (B) Model belonging to a few years later; • Baskets support all cylinders except cyclopropane cylinder for which yoke is provided; • 'Adams' valves are used for pressure reduction; • 'Adams' pressure reducing valve for nitrous oxide shows 'fins' to transfer heat whereas that for oxygen has no 'Fins'; • There is a back bar that support three flow meters and two vaporizer bottles, one for chloroform and the other for ether. No hot water jacket for ether vaporizer bottle; • Common gas outlet is facing forward to which the 'Magill's breathing system is attached; • There is a work top to keep essential items like endotracheal tube, connectors, laryngoscope, syringes loaded with drugs, etc.

30 Anesthetic Equipment Made Easy

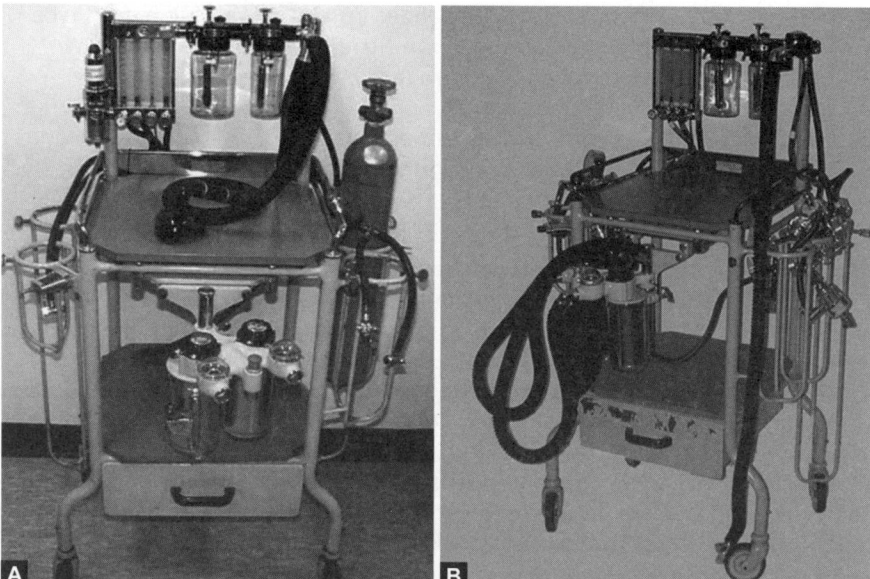

Figs 2.2A and B: One of the early 'Boyle's machine' belonging to 1940s (A) Note that there is only one 'yoke' for cyclopropane cylinder on the left side; • No 'yoke' for holding the other cylinders, but there are metal 'baskets'; • There are two baskets on left side for oxygen; • There are three baskets on the right side, the rear two are for nitrous oxide and the one in front is for carbon dioxide; • The outlet of pressure reducing valve is connected by flexible hoses to the back of flow meters with clipping devices as in cycle pumps; • There are four flow meters in the 'Flow meter block' on the back bar of the machine; oxygen, carbon dioxide, cyclopropane and nitrous oxide from left to right; • On the right of 'Flow meter block' there are two 'Boyle bottle vaporizers', one for ether and the other for trilene; • At the right end of the back bar there is the 'common gas outlet' and above that the 'emergency oxygen flush' button is seen; • Just below the work top (platform), there is the 'Boyle Circle absorber Mk II' unit seen. There are two metal canisters seen. One on the left is an ether vaporizer used as 'vaporizer inside the circuit' (VIC). The one on the right side is a 'one pound soda lime canister' for carbon dioxide absorption. The whole unit can be drawn out or pushed in through a sliding device; (B) Shows the circle breathing system with the corrugated breathing hoses attached to it; • Just behind the common gas outlet there is a flow diverting device. By turning it to 'Open' position, gas mixture enters the Magills breathing system. By turning it to 'Closed' position, the gas flow is diverted backwards and is carried through a rubber hose to enter the 'Circle breathing system'

These two models are still in use in many smaller institutions of our country and in many developing countries. The construction of these machines is so simple and all the components could be easily seen and reached for a beginner to observe and learn.

These olden days' machines are shown only to understand the evolution of the present day anesthesia machines.

The present day anesthetic machines retain the 'Boyle concept' but are fully modernized.

Components of an Anesthetic Machine

A basic anesthetic machine, for example 'Boyle F' or 'Boyle Major' incorporates the most of the components that are essential for delivering the anesthetic gas mixture

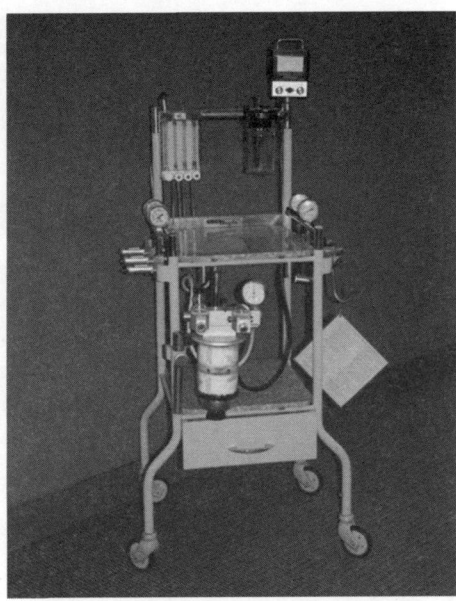

Fig. 2.3: A Boyle's machine belonging to later years 1960s. • There are three 'yokes' on either side; • Left side, rear two are for oxygen and the front yoke is for cyclopropane; • Right side, the rear two are for nitrous oxide and the front one is for carbon dioxide; • Pressure gauges seen for oxygen as well as nitrous oxide cylinders; • There is a back bar that supports 'Flow meter block' which contains four flow meters—oxygen, cyclopropane, carbon dioxide and nitrous oxide from left to right; • Chloroform vaporizer has been removed and replaced with a dummy tube; Just above the *'common gas outlet'* is the *'flow diverting device'* to change *'open'* or *'closed'*; • At the right extreme end of the back bar the 'emergency oxygen flush' is provided. By turning it on, oxygen flows into the breathing system at a rate of about 35 L/minute; • The working pressure of the Boyle F' model was 14 psi so the flow rate is 35 L/minute; • *In modern machines universally it is 60 psi (4 bar) so the emergency oxygen flow rate is about 75 L/minute*; • There is 'Boyle Circle absorber Mk III' without the breathing hoses; • There is a pressure gauge for monitoring the airway pressure in the circle system

to the patient as an integrated unit. These machines lack modern sophistications and are commonly known as *Anesthetic Machines*.

Two versions of the original 'Boyle's Machine' namely *'Boyle F'* and *'Boyle Major'* were in extensive use in India and many developing countries for many decades. Large numbers of those machines are still very much in use **(Figs 2.4A and B)**.

The features like oxygen failure alarm, hypoxia prevention devices, ventilators, monitors, etc. could be discussed separately.

MODERN WORKSTATIONS

Modern machines are different from traditional basic anesthetic machine which incorporate only the essential components. Manufactured by various firms the newer machines incorporate various features for safety and sophisticated monitoring devices. These are known as *'Anesthesia Workstations'* **(Figs 2.5A and B)**.

- Modern anesthetic machines retain the essential elements of the original Boyle's concept.
- They do not have many external connections and so chances of disconnections are limited.

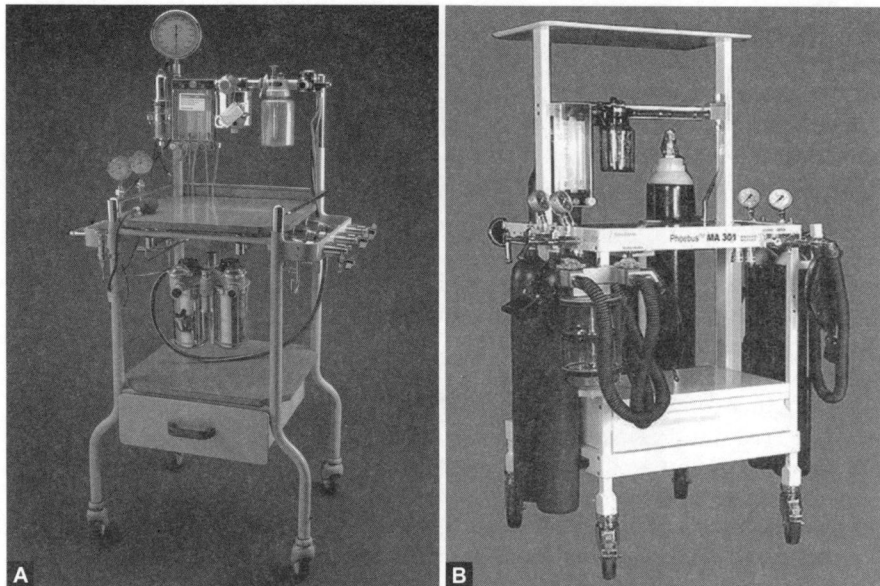

Figs 2.4A and B: (A) Boyle F; (B) Boyle Major; • Boyle Major is similar to 'BOC International continuous flow anesthetic machine' but the oxygen cylinder is on the right side; • Noticeably the nitrous oxide cylinder and the flow meters are on the left side

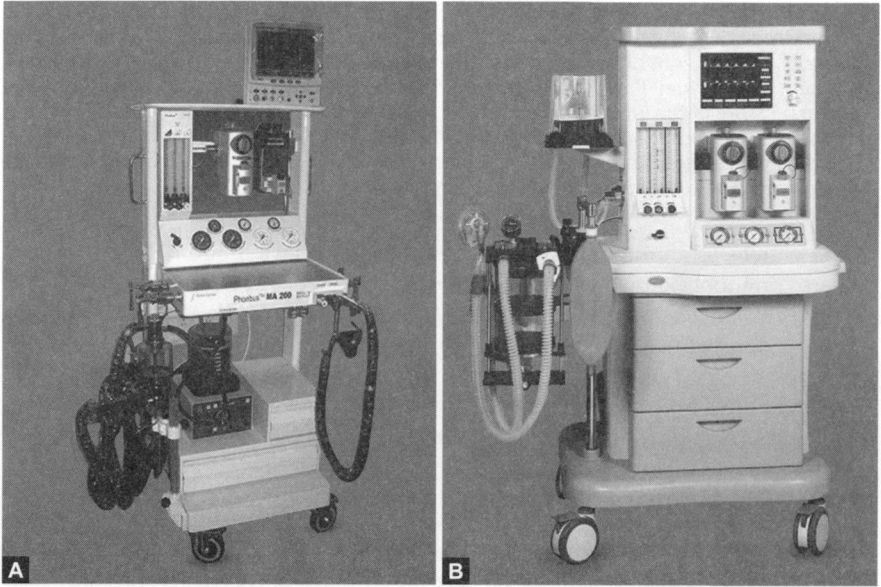

Figs 2.5A and B: Modern anesthesia machine and anesthesia workstation; (A) Modern anesthesia machine where the basic structure is somewhat retained and it has some resemblance of the older machines; • Improvements such as the pressure gauges in the front panel for easy visibility are seen; Back bar with 'Selectatec' provision for fixing modern calibrated vaporizers; Anesthesia ventilator is provided; Vital parameter monitor is provided on the top; • Safety devices oxygen failure alarm, hypoxic guard, etc. are incorporated; (B) Anesthesia workstation incorporating most of the available sophistications and safety features and has no resemblance to the older machines

- Most of the machines incorporate sophisticated electronic devices and gadgets to control every function of the machine with built in monitors for monitoring the function.
- Highly sensitive safety devices to prevent disaster due to malfunctioning machine with audible and visual alarms are regular feature.
- Every machine is provided with anesthetic ventilators to deliver the anesthetic mixture and ventilate the patient during anesthesia.
- All vital parameters of the patient could be monitored with the monitors provided in the machine.
- Gas analyzers particularly for oxygen and analyzers for the concentration of volatile anesthetic agents in breathing systems are also features of some machines.
- Safety specifications have ensured standardization of features between different makes of machines.
- Computer-controlled anesthesia systems are becoming more common.
- The 'Workstations' manufactured by various manufacturers have the standard specified by the American National Standard Institute (ANSI). But each one is different in its own structure and function.
- The Work Stations are powered by electricity; provided with a 'Master switch' that switches ON or OFF the function of the devices in the machine.
- Once the master switch is in OFF position, only battery charger and electrical outlets will be active.
- If an anesthesiologist is well versed with the use of one Work Station it does not ensure that he can use all makes of such machines. Hence, it is mandatory that one carefully reads and understands the features, safety devices, monitors, alarms, etc. of the particular machine before using it.

The last versions of the Boyles machine are considered for discussion of the components in this chapter **(Figs 2.4A and B)** as the components are assembled in an open and easily accessible way.

The components of conventional anesthetic machines:
- The frame structure with wheels
- The source of gas supply
- Yoke assembly
- Pin index system
- Bodok seal
- Pressure gauge
- Pressure reducing valve (Pressure regulator)
- Pressure relief valve
- Back bar
- Flow meters
- Vaporizers
- Common gas outlet
- Adjustable airway pressure limiting (APL) valve
- Emergency oxygen flush
- Anesthetic breathing systems (breathing circuits) for delivering the anesthetic mixture to the patient's respiratory system.

The Frame Structure

For housing all essential components:
- Any anesthetic machine must have a *frame structure* on which all the essential components are arranged suitably for effective functioning.

- The design and the arrangement may vary a little with different manufacturers, but the essential components are basically the same. Schematic representation of the essential components is seen in **Figure 2.6**.
- Box shaped sections (Hollow Square tubular structures) of welded steel or aluminum provide a rigid metal framework mounted on wheels is used for housing all the components of the machine.
- The wheels and brakes are for easy mobility and stabilizing the machine for use.
- The wheels have *antistatic rubber tyres* that dissipate static electric charges to the ground and prevent accumulation of charges in the machine.
- Accumulated charges of static electricity may cause malfunctioning of the flow meters and there is a risk of fires and explosions if a flammable anesthetic agent like ether is used. Though ether is rarely used in modern anesthesia, still the entity of fires and explosions in operating room is a matter of concern.
- In olden days machines the components were assembled compactly but in an open fashion for easy accessibility.
- Usually, a drawer is provided below the lower platform for storing customized accessories.
- The lower platform is used for keeping additional items like a second laryngoscope, endotracheal tube, etc. which can be easily reached during times of need.
- The top platform is known as *'Worktop'* or *'Work surface'* which is used for keeping items for immediate use such as laryngoscope, endotracheal tubes, connector, catheter mount, syringes loaded with drugs, etc.

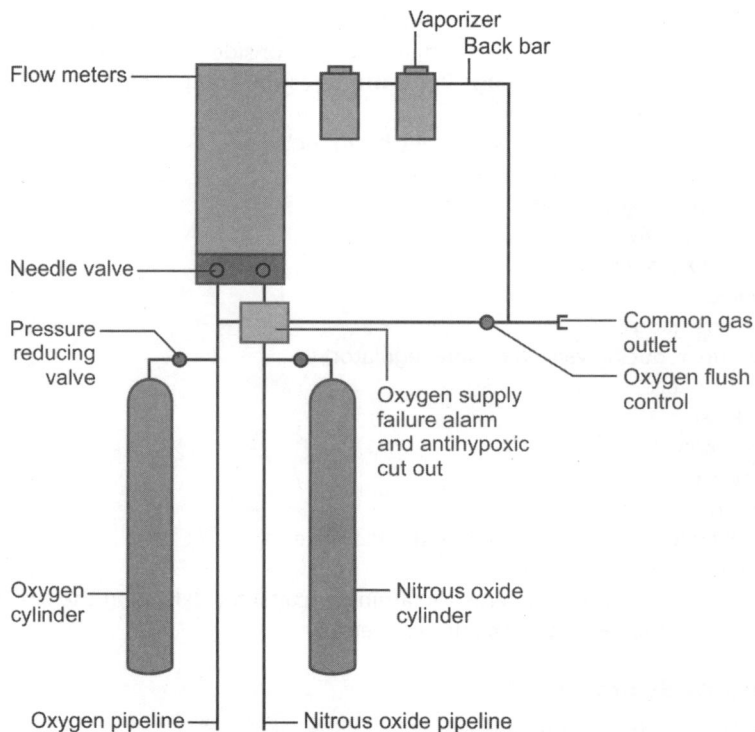

Fig. 2.6: Schematic representation of essential components

- In modern workstations, the frame and structures are very compact. The cylinder yokes and the central pipeline connectors provides on the back of the machine.
- The pressure gauges are provided on the front panel on an inclined surface for easy visibility.
- The architecture is very compact where the components are well covered.
- There is provision of drawers and shelves for storing customized accessories.
- The work surface and the machine can be kept very clean easily.

Gas Supply to the Machine—Source of Gases

The source of gases may be either cylinders or pipeline supply:
- The anesthesia machines usually incorporate *cylinders of appropriate gases* attached to it.
- In the machine, the point where cylinders are fixed is called *yoke, yoke assembly* or *yoke hanger*.
- Commonly oxygen (O_2) and nitrous oxide (N_2O) cylinders are fixed to yoke of the machine.
- In modern machines compressed air also is used as a carrier gas.
- The cylinders which can be fixed to the yoke of the machine are known as *A-Type* or *20 Cu ft* or *10 LWC* (Liters Water Capacity) cylinders **(Fig. 2.7)**.
- It has to be noted that in India these cylinders are known as *'A-Type'* cylinders whereas in some other countries it is named as *'E-Type'*.
- The *A-Type* cylinders are fitted with a special outlet valve known as *Flush valve*. **(Figs 2.7 and 2.9)** (A-Type cylinders and Flush valve will be discussed in detail under the chapter gas cylinders used in anesthesia).
- These cylinders can be opened by using a special cylinder key that turns the spindle of the valve anticlockwise **(Fig. 2.8)**.
- *Central pipeline* is commonly the main source of gases. In pipeline, the gas is fed into the pipeline from 'bulk cylinders' (cylinders of 50 L water capacity or D-Type) kept in manifold room from where the supply ends up in wall outlets of operating room.

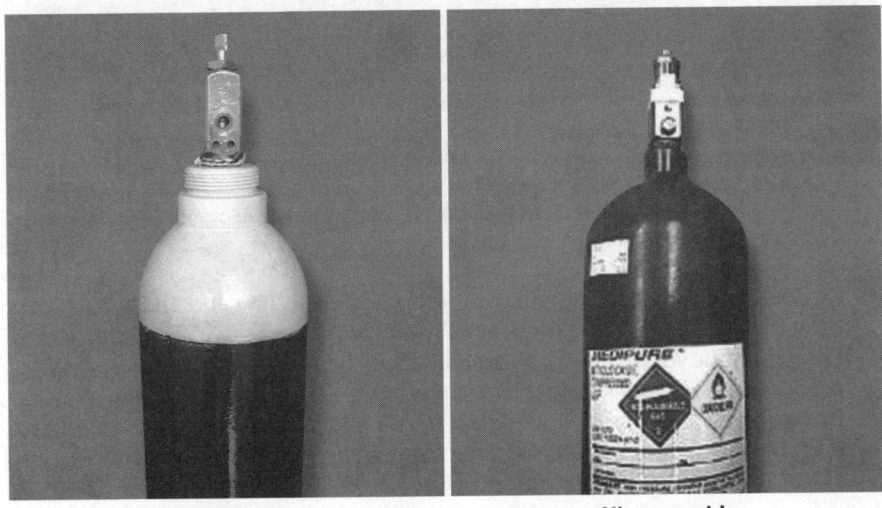

Oxygen   **Nitrous oxide**

Fig. 2.7: 'A-Type' cylinders with 'Flush valve' for fixing to the 'Yoke'

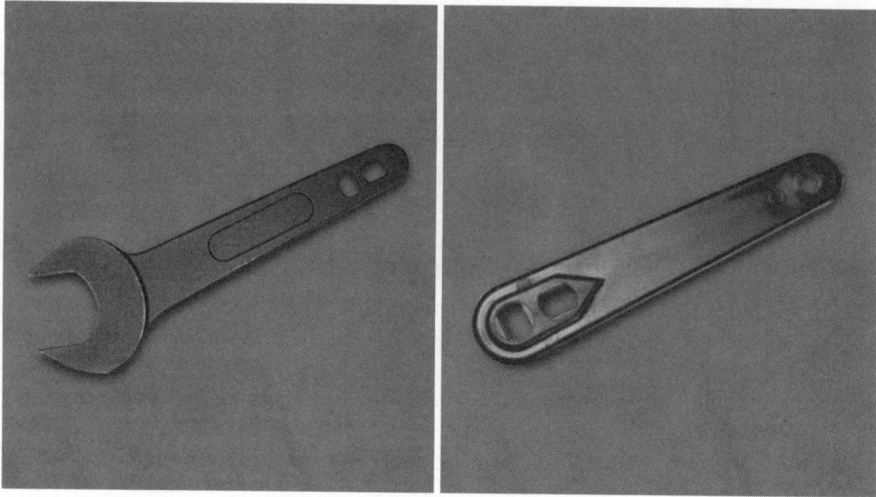

Fig. 2.8: Cylinder spanners for A-Type cylinders. There are two types: • The one with a spanner at one end for tightening the gland nut of the valve; • The tail end is used to open the spindle of the cylinder; • The other key is only for opening the spindle

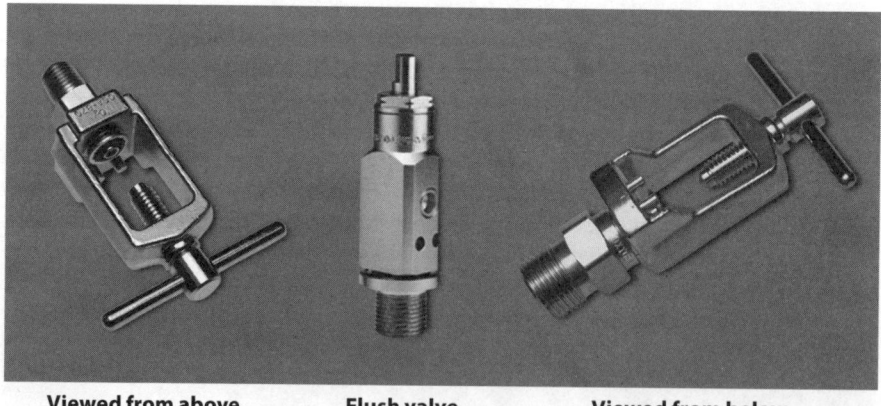

Viewed from above   **Flush valve**   **Viewed from below**

Fig. 2.9: The 'Yoke' hanger assembly of Boyle's machine; Note the nipple for entry of gas into the machine; • The Bodok seal is seen around the nipple; • Just below the nipple are seen two stout 'pins' of the 'Pin index system'; • The 'Flush valve' of 'A-Type' cylinder is seen with gas outlet for accepting the 'Nipple' and the two holes below to accept the pins of 'Pin index system'

- Flexible hose with special quick connecting probe at one end and a *Yoke block* on at the other end can be used for delivering the gas to the yoke **(Fig. 2. 10)**.
- Commonly the yoke block is permanently fixed to the yoke and the quick coupling probe is used for connecting the machine to the wall outlet at the times of use.
- Even when a machine is working on pipeline supply of gases, the other yoke must have an A-Type full cylinder attached to it as a spare for emergency.

The gas cylinders and central pipeline are discussed in detail in Chapters 3 and 4.

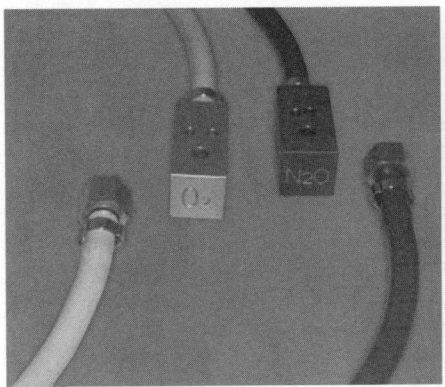 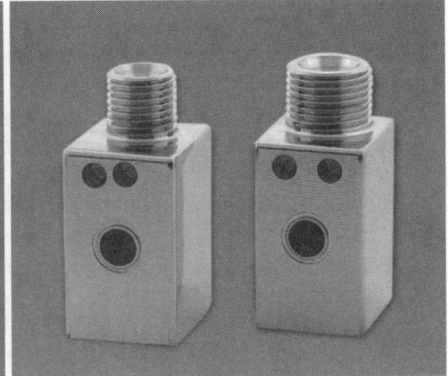

Fig. 2.10: The 'Yoke blocks' with 'Pin index' for O_2 and N_2O. • Note, the blocks and the hoses are color coded with the symbol of the gas engraved on them; • The yoke blocks have the pin index safety system to prevent connecting wrong gas; • The yoke block could be fixed to the corresponding yoke for delivering the gas from pipeline supply to the machine

The Yoke

For Fixing cylinder or yoke block of the pipeline
- 'Yoke assembly' also known as 'Yoke hanger' is for fixing and supporting the cylinder and to give gas tight seal between the cylinder and the machine **(Fig. 2. 9)**.
- 'Yoke assembly' usually consists of four components—*Pin index, filter, non-return valve, Bourdon gauge*.
- In any anesthetic machine, 'Flush valve' of 'A-Type' cylinder can be fixed to the yoke.
- Alternatively, the 'Yoke block' of pipeline is fixed to the 'Yoke' provided for that purpose **(Fig. 2.10)**.
- In 'Boyle's machine' the yokes are provided on the sides of the machine whereas in modern 'Anesthesia workstations' it is on the rear side of the machine for accepting cylinders.
- In modern machines, usually pipeline supply is received by *'Noninterchangeable Screw Threads'* (NIST) connectors at the machine end of the hose.
- The yoke has a stout frame and a screw handle to fix the cylinder by means of the flush valve.
- There is a 'nipple' projecting from the machine end into the yoke. If the nipple is damaged, it may be impossible to obtain gas tight seal with the cylinder valve.
- When the flush valve of the cylinder is fixed, the nipple enters into the gas outlet of the valve.
- As the gas outlet of the valve is flat (flushed with the surface of the body of the valve), and has no connections or screws provided, there will be large leak of gas around the nipple.
- A special washer known as *Bodok seal* is placed around the nipple and the valve is tightened with the screw. This makes an airtight seal and prevents any gas leak when the cylinder is opened.
- The screw must be tightened only with the power of fingers and hand. No other instrument is used to tighten the screw; otherwise it may cause serious damage to the gas outlet and body of the valve.

Bodok Seal

For preventing leak around the nipple of machine
- It was introduced in 1958
- When the flush valve is fixed on the yoke assembly of the anesthetic machine, the 'nipple' of the yoke enters the gas outlet of the flush valve.
- As this attachment does not provide a gas tight fit and when the cylinder valve is opened, there will be significant leak and loss of gas.
- To make an airtight fit between the cylinder outlet and the nipple, a especially designed washer known as 'Bodok seal' is fixed around the nipple **(Fig. 2.9)**.
- It has a dimension of 1.5 cm diameter and 1.5 mm thickness **(Fig. 2.11)**. Bodok seal has been discussed in detail in Chapter 3.

Pin Index Safety System

For preventing fixing wrong cylinder on the yoke
- The pin index system was introduced in 1952.
- Just below the inlet nipple, there are two short stout pins projecting from the yoke. These are known as pins of *'Pin index'* system. These pins are gas specific.
- There will be corresponding holes in the Flush valve of the cylinder of the specific gas.
- The pin index is specific for each gas. It is a safety device that it will not accept a flush valve of another gas with different pin index **(Figs 2.9 and 2.10)**.
  Pin index safety system (PISS) will be discussed in the Chapter 3 on cylinders.

Pressure Gauge

For measuring the pressure in the source of gas cylinder or pipeline
- This device is placed just beyond the yoke hanger, in-between the pressure reducing valve and nipple (gas inlet) of the yoke.
- In traditional machines it is fixed on the body of the yoke on the path of the gas from the flush valve to pressure reducing valve.

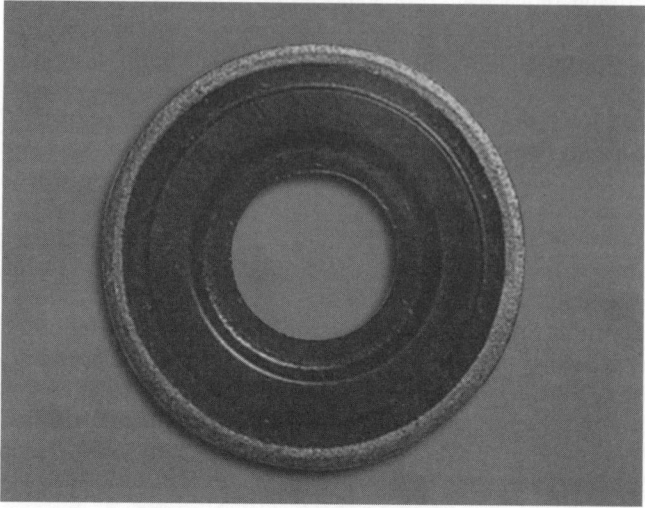

Fig. 2.11: Bodok seal

Anesthesia Machine

- It will measure the pressure of gas in the cylinder attached to the yoke, when the cylinder is opened and is read on the dial as lbs/sq inch (psi) or kg/sq cm.
- The dial is color-coded; Oxygen—white, Nitrous oxide—French blue, Medical air—Grey **(Figs 2.12C and D)**.
- The name of the gas is written on the dial.
- *'Use no oil'* and *'Open valve slowly'* are the warnings usually seen on the dial.
- In most of the machines, it is found fixed with an angle for easy observation of the dial on the top of yoke assembly.
- There are pressure gauges for oxygen, nitrous oxide and compressed air (if used) in the machine.
- The pressure gauge works on the principle of 'Bourdon tube' and is known as 'Bourdon Gauge' **(Figs 2.12A to D)**.

Bourdon Gauge

- Bourdon tube is a 'C" shaped tube with *oval cross section* closed at one end. When pressure is applied to the other end, it tends to straighten as the pressure tries to make the oval cross section into round cross section.
- When pressure is withdrawn, it is restored to its original shape.

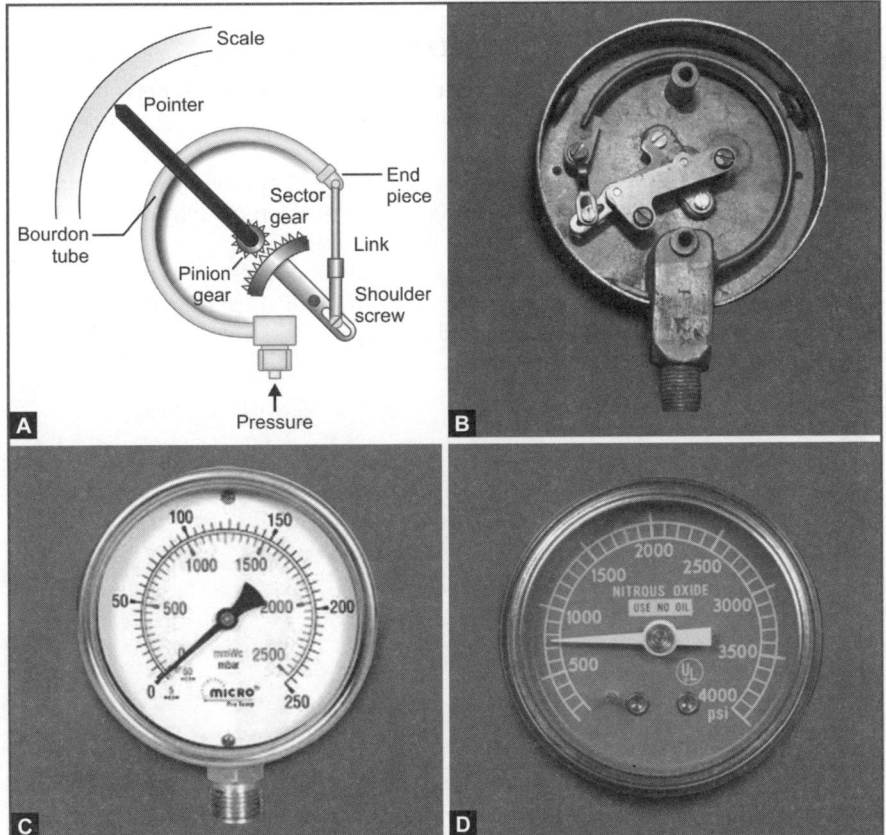

Figs 2.12A to D Pressure gauge for oxygen and nitrous oxide cylinders.
- Pressure gauges with color-coded dials

- By connecting a link and pinion a needle can be moved on the dial to read the pressure **(Fig. 2.12A)**.
- The actual Bourdon tube with the link and pinion mechanism inside a pressure gauge is shown in **(Fig. 2.12B)**.
- If the Bourdon tube ruptures, the gas is vented through a hole provided on the back cover.

Practical significance of pressure gauge
- Oxygen in a cylinder is in gaseous state under normal conditions, (not a liquefied gas as N_2O).
- The gauge will show the pressure which will indicate the amount of gas present in the cylinder (Refer to Boyle's Law).
- For example, if the full cylinder capacity is 600 L and the full cylinder pressure is 150 kg/sq cm (2000 psi) when the gauge shows 100 kg/sq cm, it means that 2/3 of the gas still remains in the cylinder. In other words, 400 L of gas is remaining in the cylinder.
- Thus, for oxygen cylinder a pressure gauge is essential to warn about the quantity of gas available in the partially used cylinder **(Fig. 2.13)**.
- For liquefied gases like N_2O the pressure gauges may not have a very significant use; however modern machines incorporate pressure gauges for N_2O.

Assessing the Contents of the Nitrous Oxide Cylinders

- Pressure gauge is not useful to find out the contents of N_2O cylinders.
- When full, the cylinder contains a small amount of gaseous nitrous oxide above the liquid.
- At room temperature this saturated vapor pressure of nitrous oxide 51 atm.
- This continues to be the same although with the fall of temperature of the cylinder, the saturated vapor pressure may be a little reduced.
- But with the cylinder temperature as 21°C, the vapor pressure is always 51 atm which indicates that there is a little of liquid nitrous oxide present in the cylinder, but give no idea as to how much liquid is present.

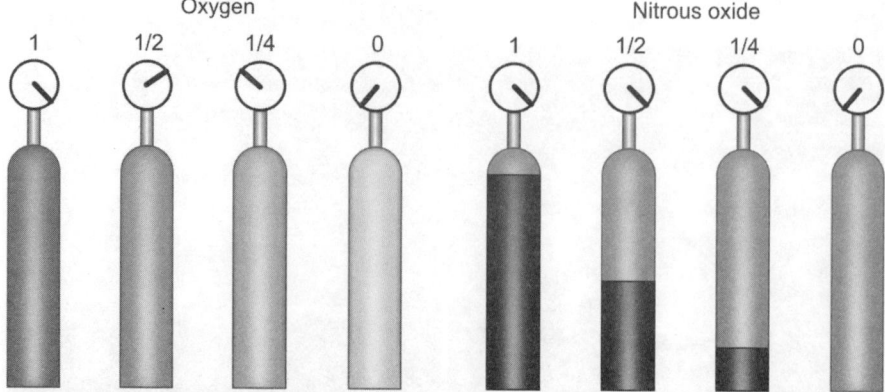

Fig. 2.13: Pressure gauge in oxygen cylinder and in nitrous oxide cylinder. • In oxygen cylinder the contents of the gas corresponds to the pressure; • In nitrous oxide cylinder the pressure remains constant (Full) till the last drop of liquid is evaporated and then drops as the vapor is used up

- When the last drop of liquid is evaporated the pressure is still 51 atm. After this vapor pressure falls rapidly (depending upon the flow rate) and touches zero.
- The amount of nitrous oxide in the cylinder can be ascertained by the weight.
  - Weight of empty cylinder is seen on it (Tare weight).
  - 455 L of nitrous oxide weighs 850 g.
  - The weight of liquid in the cylinder can be converted into number of liters of gas.

Pressure Reducing Valve (Pressure Regulator)

For reducing the high pressure of the source to the working pressure of the machine components: The pressure of the gases in the cylinders (oxygen at 2000 psi and nitrous oxide at 750 psi) will be at a relatively higher pressure that cannot be tolerated by the delicate instruments in the back bar of the machine. If such pressures are delivered directly to the patient's respiratory tract, it may lead to dangerous consequences like pressure damage to lung 'barotrauma'.

For that reason, whatever be the source of the gas, the pressure at which it is delivered to the instrument cluster within the machine has to be reduced to an acceptable low level. This is known as the 'operating pressure' of the machine.

- Pressure reducing valve (pressure regulator) provides safe, consistent, reduced working pressure inside the machine.
- The modern day anesthetic machines operate at 50–60 psi (4 bar or 420 kP) pressure.
- The older generation of machines, for example, 'Boyle F' was operating at 14 to 16 psi (1 bar) pressure–which is no longer in use.
- This low pressure of 50–60 psi is in use even when 'Boyle Major' was introduced.
- This change was made universally and obviously this allows having an outlet for oxygen in the machine for operating certain pneumatic devices which needed 60 psi pressure, e.g. anesthetic ventilator.
- Therefore, the gases from the cylinders pass through pressure reducing valves to bring down the high pressure to a constant low pressure of 50–60 psi.
- Once the cylinder is opened, the gas at high pressure flows into the reducing valve and the pressure gets reduced, as it is set (60 psi).
- The output pressure can be set as per the requirement in these valves and so it is set at 60 psi and fixed.
- The cylinder pressure will fall gradually as the gas is used. It may fall from 2000 psi to any low level. The valve is designed in such a way that even if the pressure in the cylinder falls very low as 200 psi, the outlet pressure is constantly maintained at 60 psi.
- The modern pressure reducing valves are efficiently designed that, when a pipeline with 60 psi pressure is connected to it, it behaves like a by-pass and allows the pressure to the outlet without alteration **(Fig. 2.14)**.
- Modern machines have secondary pressure regulators.
- The primary reducing valve has reduced the pressure from 2000 psi to 60 psi (4 bar).
- These secondary pressure reducing valves will level out the gas delivery. When the pipeline pressure is likely to get reduced during peak hours of use with maximum demand to about 20% than the set working pressure of the machine (4 bar).
- This fluctuation in the pressure is likely to cause changes in the flow meter performance.

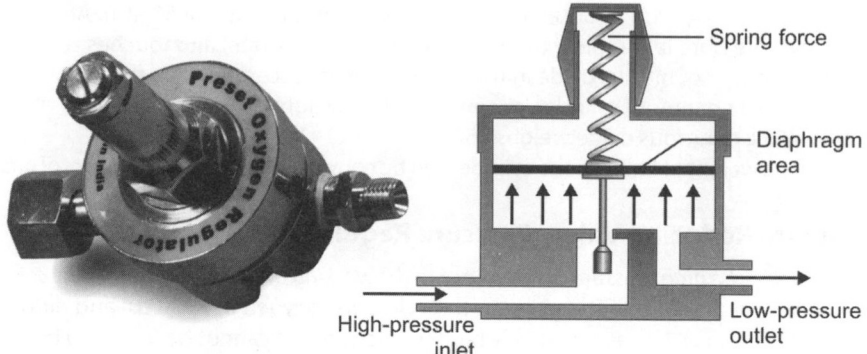

Fig. 2.14: Pressure reducing valve used in anesthetic machine

- The secondary pressure reducing valve set below the anticipated drop in pressure will make the emergent pressure more uniform.
- Some pressure reducing valves continuously allow gas to flow out when the cylinder is open (weeping their cylinder contents) even if pipeline pressure and flow is present.
- Some manufacturers keep the output pressure from the cylinder at a level a little lower than 420 kP (a little less than 4 bar) so that the machine will preferentially use pipeline supply which has higher pressure.

The pressure reducing valve is discussed in detail in Chapter 5.

Pressure Release Valve

For venting gas during any inadvertent pressure surge in the system

- The operating pressure of all the devices in the anesthetic machine such as flow meter, vaporizer, etc. is 50–60 psi (4 bar).
- The pressure reducing valve reduces the high pressure from the cylinder to safe pressure of 60 psi. There may be minimal fluctuations in the outlet pressure to a range of a few psi which is insignificant and is acceptable.
- In case, the valve becomes defective and malfunctions, the outlet pressure may rise very high and damage the equipment.
- This high pressure may accidentally be transmitted to the patient's airway through the breathing system and cause serious barotrauma.
- To prevent these dangers, just at the outlet of pressure reducing valve, a pressure release valve is provided which will release the excess pressure and vent the gases out into the atmosphere. **(Fig. 2.15)**.
- The valve is adjustable and the release pressure is adjusted as 70 psi and is set.
- In the event of the pressure going above 70 psi, the valve releases the pressure and protects the machine and patient's airway.
- When more than one cylinder outlets are joined in a single manifold as in Boyle's machine, one pressure release valve is provided in the manifold.

Back Bar

For supporting the flow meters, vaporizers, common gas outlet, APL valve, etc.

- This describes the horizontal part of the frame of the machine, which supports the flow meter block, vaporizers and some other components of the machine.

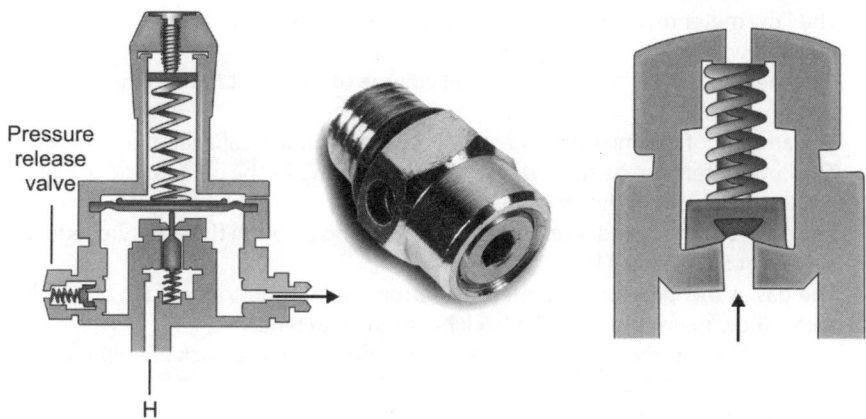

Fig. 2.15: Pressure release valve. • The pressure release valve is fixed in the low pressure chamber; • The second figure shows the release valve. The required pressure can be set with screw on the top which can be adjusted with an Allen key; • The section of the valve shows the rubber diaphragm at the outlet and the spring to retain it

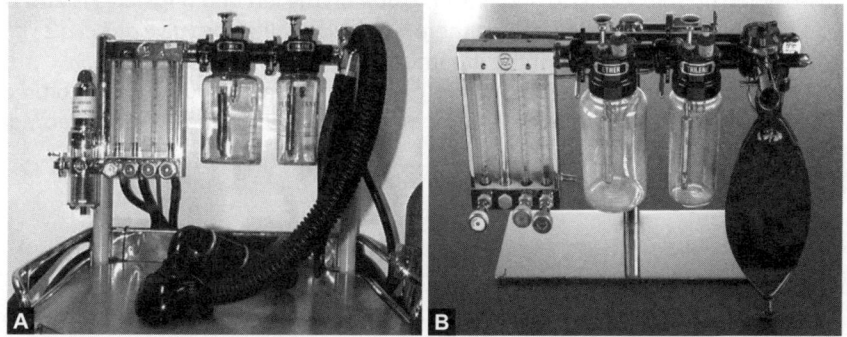

Figs 2.16A and B: (A) Back bar of the Boyle's machine; • The back bar supports flow meter block, ether bottle vaporizer, trilene bottle vaporizer, common gas outlet and emergency oxygen flush button; • The Magill's breathing system is attached to the common gas outlet; (B) Model of Back bar where the common gas outlet with changeover switch for open and closed breathing systems is seen on the top at the right end; • Bag mount of Magill's semi-closed breathing system is fixed on the common gas outlet; • Emergency oxygen flush is seen on the extreme right

- In Boyle's machine, the back bar supports the flow meter block, vaporizer bottle (Ether bottle), Tec vaporizer (Halothane, Isoflurane or Sevoflurane), adjustable airway pressure release valve (adjustable pressure limiting valve-APL), common gas outlet and emergency oxygen flush button **(Figs 2.16A and B)**.
- Most of the modern anesthetic machines may not have the traditional back bar described here.

From now onwards, the components on the back bar may be discussed one by one in the order of arrangement.

Flow Meters (Rotameters)

For measuring the flow rate of gases
- The flow meters in modern machines are 'Variable orifice—fixed pressure difference' type known as 'Rotameter'.

- The flow meter measures the flow of gases in L/min in general and in fractions of liter at low flow.
- They help to deliver the required total volume of gases in L/min to the breathing system.
- The amount of gas mixture necessary for each patient is calculated as L/min.
- The flow meters can be set to deliver the volume and fix the percentage of oxygen not less than 33% in the mixture.
- The gas from the cylinder or pipeline after passing through the pressure reducing valve is at 50–60 psi (4 bar).
- The gas at this pressure is carried by narrow metal tube to the back of the flow meter (flow meter block) in the back bar of the machine.
- These tubes carrying different gases are connected to the back of flow meter by screw threaded hexagonal connectors.
- These connectors are agent specific, having different size of hexagonal nuts and the size of threads. A tube carrying another gas cannot be connected to the flow meter by mistake. This is a safety mechanism.
- In the older machines, the oxygen flow meter is on the left end and nitrous oxide flow meter is on the right end. In newer machines, for reasons of safety, it is reversed—oxygen on the right end and nitrous oxide on the left end **(Figs 2.17A and B)**.
- At the bottom of each flow meter, there is a device called *Pin valve* or *Needle valve* which allows slow release of the gas into the flow meter tube.
- The gas flow thorough the flow meters (oxygen and nitrous oxide) mix the common pathway at the top of the flow meter block and flow towards the common gas outlet of the machine.

Flow meters will be discussed in detail in Chapter 6.

Vaporizers

For vaporizing the volatile anesthetic agents to the required concentration
- All volatile anesthetic agents such as *ether, halothane, isoflurane, sevoflurane, or desflurane,* etc. as the name implies, are supplied as liquids.

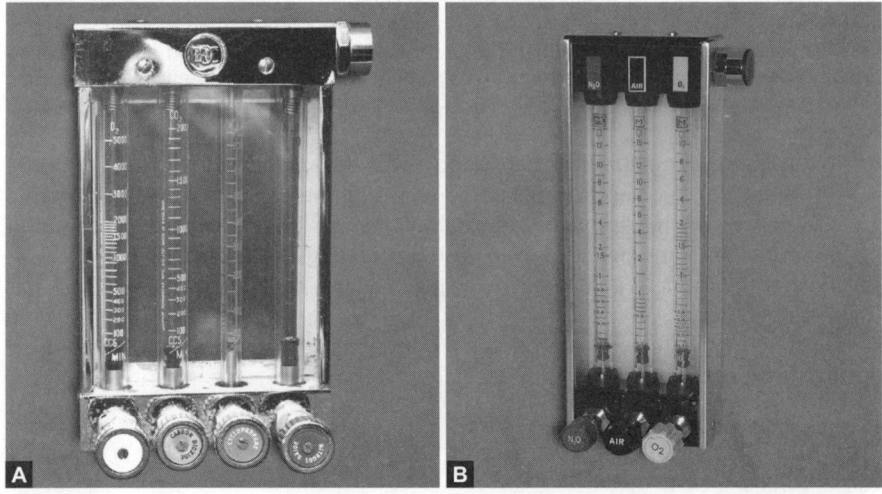

Figs 2.17A and B: Flow meter block: (A) Old machine—oxygen flow meter is at left end; (B) Newer machine—oxygen flow meter is at right end

Anesthesia Machine

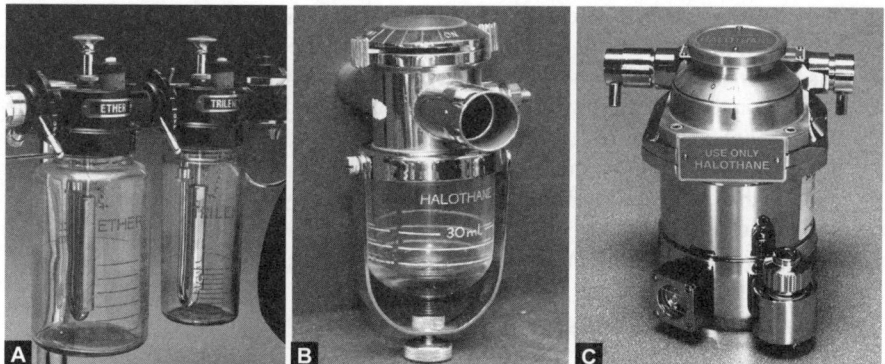

Figs 2.18A to C: Vaporizers: • Boyle bottle vaporizer, Goldman Halothane vaporizer and Fluotec Mark 3 vaporizer

- Vaporizer is a device that converts a volatile liquid into its vapour form **(Figs 2.18A to C)**.
- The vaporizers deliver the desired concentrations of the volatile agents to the gas mixture (usually O_2 and N_2O) to make the combination as the *anesthetic mixture*.
- Vaporizers are generally fitted on the back bar of the machine next to the flow meter block. Examples are Boyle bottle vaporizer for ether and Fluotec Mark 3 vaporizer for halothane.
- Boyle bottle vaporizer is a crude non-calibrated vaporizer.
- Goldman halothane vaporizer is a noncalibrated vaporizer but is a simple vaporizer with minimal resistance to flow and has the advantage of maximum 2.5% halothane with 8 L flow rate.
- Fluotec Mark 3 is a calibrated vaporizer.

Vaporizers will be discussed in detail in Chapter 7.

Adjustable Pressure Limiting Valve

For releasing inadvertent built up pressure in breathing system

- This valve is also known as *spill valve, expiratory valve, pop off valve* or *pressure relief valve*.
- It allows excess gas to escape when a preset pressure is exceeded, thus minimizing the risk of barotrauma to the patient.
- This is usually situated at the end the back bar near the common gas outlet of the machine where the breathing systems are attached.
- It is present in both semi- closed breathing systems as well as in closed breathing systems.
- Many adjustable pressure limiting (APL) valves do not have calibrations and are adjusted empirically to give a desired peak inspired pressure.
- Some breathing systems may include a pressure gauge for monitoring system pressure. The pressure required for opening the APL valve could be adjusted and set using the pressure gauge as a guide.
- It comprises of a light weight disc which rests on a 'knife edge' to minimize the area of contact and to reduce the risk of adhesion resulting from the surface tension of condensed water.
- The disc may have a stem which acts as a guide to position disc correctly.

- The valve disc is held in place by a weak spring, the tension of which can be adjusted by a screw mechanism thereby adjusting the pressure required to open the valve.
- It is a *'spring loaded disc on knife edge'* type of valve where, by using the screw, the pressure in the breathing system can be limited. Therefore, it is called as *Adjustable pressure limiting valve* (APL) **(Fig. 2.19)**.
- It is designed to relieve the excess pressure built up in the breathing system by venting the excess gas by lifting the disc. Or else, it may damage the vaporizer and patient's respiratory tract.
- Most valves are encased in a hood for gas scavenging.

Emergency Oxygen Flush

- The outlet from the pressure reducing valve has a low working pressure suited for feeding to the flow meter.
- A bypass from this is led to a suitable place near the common gas outlet of the machine controlled by a spring loaded switch.
- By opening this. O_2 at the working pressure will be fed into the breathing system.
- This is also known as "Emergency O_2 flush"
- Older machines—working pressure inside machine is 14 psi
- When opened it delivers O_2 at approximately 35 L/min flow rate.
- Modern Machine—working pressure inside machine is 60 psi
- Flow rate in emergency outlet is around 65 L/minute.
- If there is sudden loss of gas from the breathing system due to any reason, this control is pressed to fill the system with oxygen.
- A metal tube from the outlet manifold of the pressure reducing valves carries oxygen, which by-passes the flow meters and vaporizers and directly supplies the gas to this port.
- In old type of Boyle's machines, it is present on the right end of the Back bar and is activated by *a locking switch* (*See* **Fig. 2.16**).
- In modern machines, *a non-locking spring loaded button* **(Fig. 2.20)** usually activates this as locking switches accidentally activated may cause serious barotrauma to the lung.

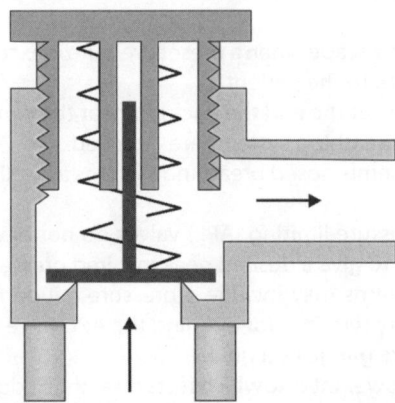

Fig. 2.19: Adjustable pressure limiting valve. • The disc is resting on an opening with 'knife edge'; • The disc has a stem to guide its movements; • The light spring retains the disc with an adjustable screw; • APL valves are used in both types of breathing circuit

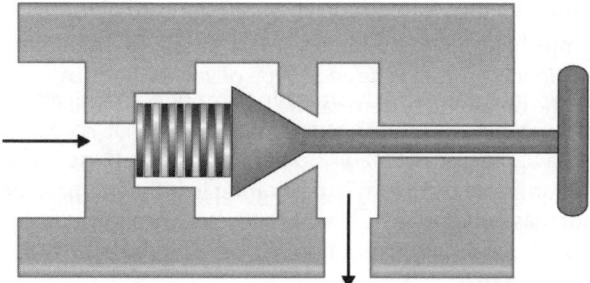

Fig. 2.20: Emergency oxygen flush. • Note the spring loaded nonlocking button to activate it

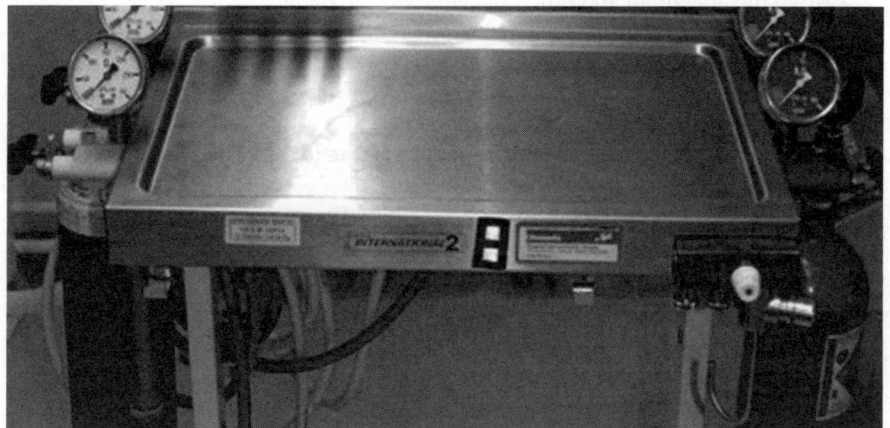

Fig. 2.21: Emergency oxygen flush button is seen at the right end of work surface. • The common gas outlet with swivel is seen just below that

- In newer machines it is situated just below the work top of the machine commonly on the right end near the common gas outlet **(Fig. 2.21)**.
- When the button is pressed, oxygen flows at a rate of about 35–75 L/min is delivered into the breathing system.
- Oxygen flush will work even if the machine is switched off—in modern workstations.

Common Gas Outlet

For Fixing the Breathing System

So far, all the components of anesthetic machine starting from gas cylinders, pressure reducing valve, pressure release valve, flow meters, back bar, vaporizers, adjustable pressure limiting valve (APL), emergency oxygen flush, have been discussed briefly.

From the above discussions, it is clearly understood that all these component devices in the machine are necessary for generating a suitable *anesthetic mixture* to be delivered to the patient's respiratory tract.
- The *anesthetic mixture* is usually, oxygen, nitrous oxide and the vapor of the chosen volatile anesthetic agent.
- In some machines air may also be used as a carrier gas.

- Anesthetic mixture thus formed travels along the conduit to reach the right end of back bar and comes out of the machine through the port known as *'Common gas outlet'*.
- The anesthetic mixture exits the machine through a conically tapered outlet. In traditional machines it is a 23 mm female outlet that accepts a 22 mm male connector of a bag mount of Magill's breathing system **(Figs 2.16A and B)**.
- It may be 22 mm male or 15 mm female outlet in different machines.
- This common gas outlet may be fixed or swiveled through at least 90° **(Fig. 2.20)** and should be strong enough to withstand a bending force, since heavy equipment are often attached to it.
- Some outlets include a male thread for securing heavy devices like a fuel cell oxygen analyzer.
- The breathing system is attached to the common gas outlet. Through the breathing system the anesthetic mixture is delivered to the patient.
- For reference it may be noted that in 'Boyle F' machine it is on the right end of back bar just in front of the emergency oxygen flush whereas in 'Boyle major' machine it is found in the front of table top tray (Work surface) on the right side adjacent to emergency oxygen flush **(Fig. 2.20)**.
- A changeover switch to divert the fresh gas mixture to the closed breathing system when needed is provided adjacent to this.
- In most of the modern anesthetic workstations, the common gas outlet is on the left side of the machine.
- In any anesthetic machine, only to this common gas outlet, a suitable *'Anesthetic breathing system'* is attached to deliver the anesthetic mixture to the patient's respiratory tract.

Breathing Systems

- The part of the anesthetic machine comprising of various components through which the patient breathes the anesthetic mixture is named as *Anesthetic breathing system*.
- The breathing system suitable for a patient will be attached to the common gas outlet of the anesthetic machine.

'Breathing systems' which deliver the anesthetic gas mixture to the patient are functionally integral part of anesthesia machine and are part of low pressure system. For the sake of convenience breathing systems, are discussed in detail separately in Chapter 8.

Worktop of Anesthetic Machine (Work Surface)

- There is a tabletop made of stainless steel, aluminum metal, wooden board or glass known as *worktop, work surface* or *tabletop tray*.
- The space on the worktop is for keeping essential equipment, drugs, syringes, etc. for use during the conduct of anesthesia *(See Fig. 2.21)*.

OXYGEN FAILURE ALARM

Features of an ideal device:
- It must depend on oxygen pressure only.
- Should not use battery or main power.

Anesthesia Machine

- Alarm must be audible for sufficient length of time and volume and character.
- Ideally a warning of impending failure followed by an alarm if failure occurs.
- When it starts functioning, the other gases must cease flowing and the breathing system opened to atmosphere.
- It should be impossible to resume anesthesia unless the oxygen supply is restored.

In spite of all vigilance, the risk of failure of oxygen supply and delivering hypoxic mixture to the patient is always imminent. Now oxygen failure warning devices are fitted in all anesthetic machines.

- Most of them are powered by oxygen pressure and *do not depend on electricity mains* or *battery power*.
- They are activated by a fall in oxygen pressure and produce a loud whistle. This sound will be reset only when the correct oxygen pressure returns.
- An earlier oxygen failure warning device was *Ritchie Whistle (1960)* and many modern devices are similar in principle. This is the device which does not depend on other source of power to activate it, but activated by the failing oxygen supply.
- It produces an audible alarm >60 db that can be heard at a distance of 1 meter from the machine for 7 seconds or more.
- Activated when the oxygen pressure falls to 260 kPa (38 psi), a spring causes the anesthetic gas cut-off valve to begin to close and oxygen failure whistle valve to open, permitting a flow of oxygen to operate the whistle.
- The whistle continues to sound until the oxygen pressure has fallen to 40.5 kPa (6 psi).
- The alarm cannot be switched off, silenced or reset until the oxygen supply is restored.
- The alarm is coupled with a cut-off valve that cuts-off anesthetic gases and opens the machine circuit to air.
- When the anesthetic gases cut-off valve is closed, the hypoxic gas mixture coming from the flow meter is vented to the atmosphere through the pressure relief valve on the back bar **(Fig. 2.22)**.

Safety Devices to Prevent Hypoxic Gas Mixtures

- Certain safety devices are incorporated in modern machines to prevent delivery of hypoxic mixtures.
- These devices may work on *pneumatic, mechanical or electronic mechanisms*.
- In some the flow controls of oxygen and nitrous oxide are interlocked in such a way that any time the concentration of oxygen in the mixture does not drop below 25%.

Fail-safe System

The newer machines have a safety as 'Fail-safe System.
- The *fail-safe device ensures that whenever oxygen pressure is reduced and until flow ceases, the set oxygen concentration will not decrease at the common gas outlet.*
- Fail-safe valve is fitted to all lines supplying flow meters *except oxygen*.
- Controlled by O_2 supply pressure. Shuts off or proportionately decrease the flow if O_2 supply pressure decreases.
- The loss of oxygen pressure results in *alarms*, audible and visible, at 30 psi pipeline pressure.

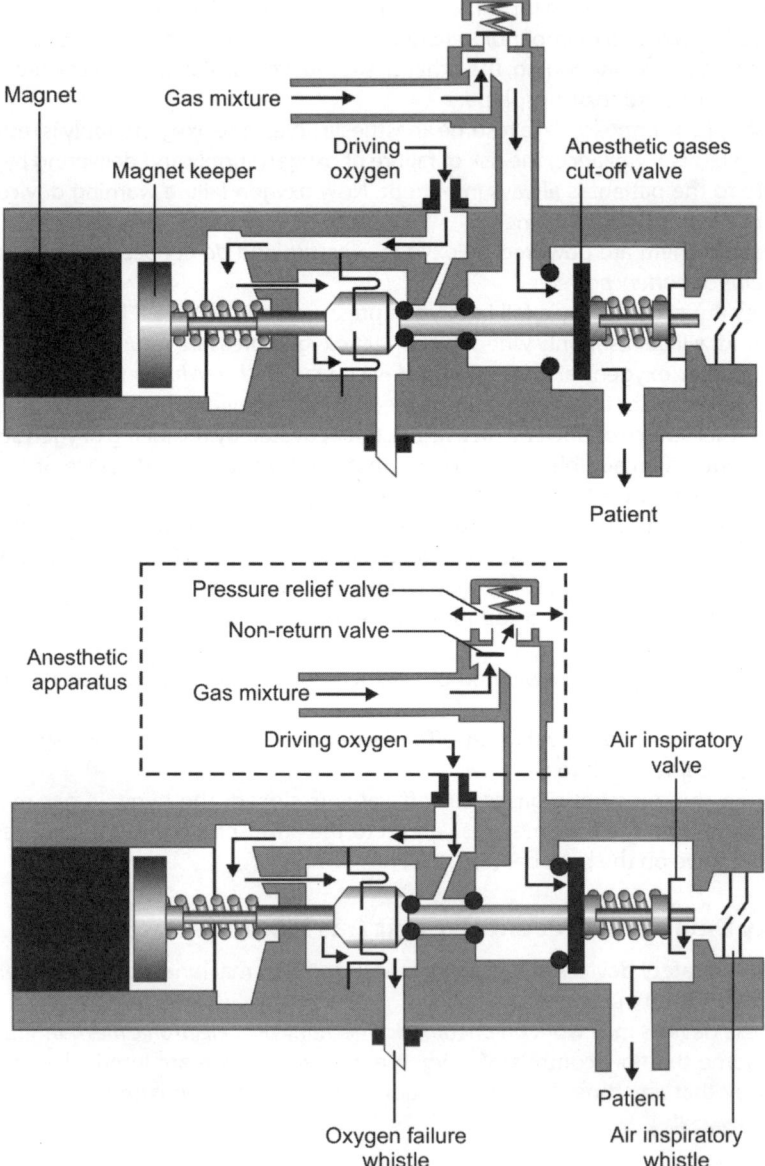

Fig. 2.22: Principle of oxygen failure alarm. • Oxygen pressure is keeping the gas mixture flow through the port to patient; • Oxygen pressure failure moves the piston backwards to occlude gas mixture and the port is opened to the atmosphere

Limitations

- Fail-safe systems *do not* prevent hypoxic mixtures.
- If there is adequate pressure in the oxygen line, nothing in the fail-safe system prevents turning on a gas mixture of 100% nitrous oxide (This could be prevented by the hypoxic guard system).

- Similarly, it could not prevent turning on 100% helium if used (Which would not be prevented by the hypoxic guard also, since the hypoxic guard *only* connects oxygen and nitrous oxide flow meters).

Hypoxic Guard (Minimum Ratio Gas System)
- It is a safety device present in modern machines, which does not allow delivering hypoxic mixture to the patient. This is a safety device working on pneumatic principle **(Fig. 2.23)**.
- In this, it is not possible to open N_2O when O_2 is not on flow. But when O_2 is on flow N_2O can be opened, even then it will allow a flow at a rate sufficient to maintain at least 25% of O_2 in the inspired mixture.
- If the O_2 supply fails N_2O flow is automatically stopped thereby preventing the patient from breathing N_2O alone.
- It uses a ratio mixer valve.
- Oxygen supplied to this valve exerts a pressure on one side of the diaphragm, which is opposed by the pressure of nitrous oxide on the opposite side.
- The construction ensures an increase in oxygen flow rate by a ratio of 25% of any increase in the nitrous oxide flow rate.
- When O_2 is not on flow, N_2O flow will be stopped even if the N_2O flow meter is open.
- If there is flow in O_2 flow meter, N_2O flow will be allowed in the flow meter. But even then it will allow a flow of N_2O at a rate sufficient to maintain at least 25% of O_2 in the mixture.
- During use if O_2 supply fails, N_2O flow is automatically stopped thereby preventing the patient breathing N_2O alone.

Device with a 'Slave Control Valve' for N_2O
In another system there is a 'slave control valve' for nitrous oxide which is acted upon by the oxygen pressure **(Fig. 2.24)**.
- The pressure exerted on the oxygen diaphragm is greater than that exerted by N_2O diaphragm.

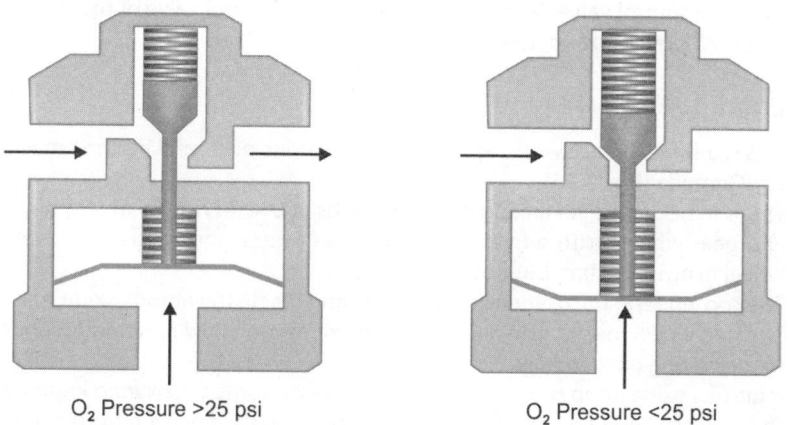

O_2 Pressure >25 psi O_2 Pressure <25 psi

Fig. 2.23: Hypoxic guard device (Minimum ratio gas system). • When the oxygen supply pressure is above 25 psi the valve is open to allow flow of nitrous oxide; • When the pressure drops below 25 psi there is a gradual reduction of flow of N_2O and it stops

52 Anesthetic Equipment Made Easy

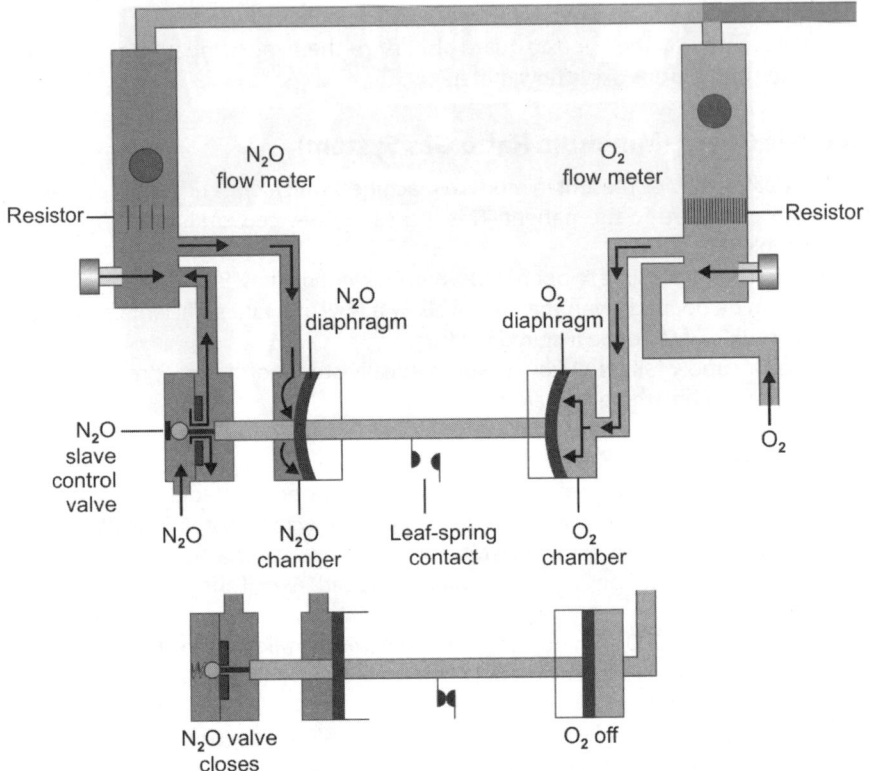

Fig. 2.24: The N_2O from the flow meter flows through the conduit at the top which joins the conduit from the top of O_2 flow meter

- This causes the shaft to move to the left opening the 'slave control valve'. Now nitrous oxide flows towards the pin valve (flow control valve) of the flow meter.
- When the oxygen pressure is inadequate, the shaft moves to the right and closes the slave control valve. Now, even when the flow control valve of the flow meter is open there will be no flow of nitrous oxide.

Link 25

- This is a safety device working on mechanical principle found in some machines, e.g. Ohmeda **(Fig. 2.25)**.
- This is a mechanism of linking both the knobs of O_2 and N_2O by means of a chain and gear wheels with a freewheel device (as present in bicycles—activate the wheel in one direction but not in reverse).
- The cog wheel in the oxygen knob is larger and that in the nitrous oxide is smaller.
- The free wheel mechanism allows opening of oxygen flow meter independently for delivering oxygen only.
- If nitrous oxide knob is opened, simultaneously it turns the oxygen knob also so that at least 25% of oxygen flows corresponding to the flow of nitrous oxide.
- If nitrous oxide is flowing, oxygen flow cannot be closed completely below a set level.

Anesthesia Machine

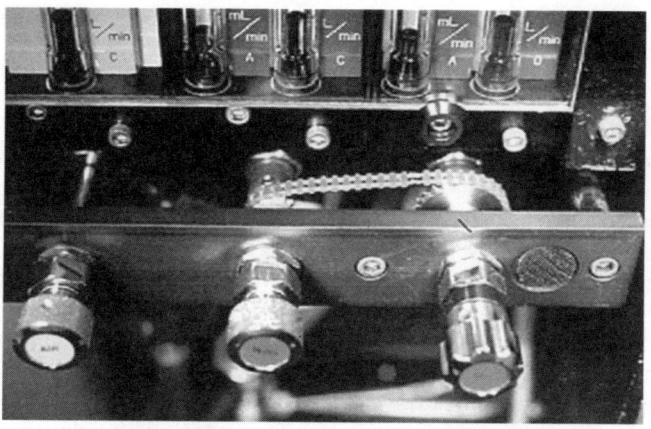

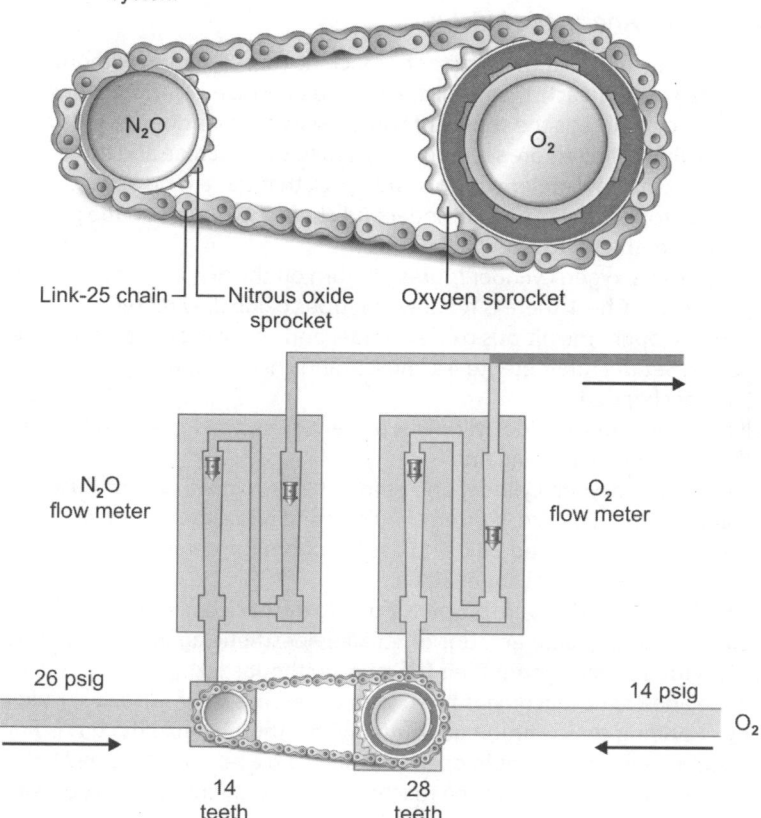

Fig. 2.25: Link 25 safety device

Limitations
- It does not consider other flow meters of other gases like Air or CO_2. Hence, may cause serious dilution of oxygen and result in hypoxic mixture.

- It cannot compensate for the variations in gas supply which may affect the flow meter performance.

Electronic Device

- It uses a paramagnetic oxygen analyzer to continuously sample the gas mixtures from the flow meters.
- If inspired oxygen fraction drops below 25%, the nitrous oxide flow is temporarily cut-off.
- An increase in inspired oxygen fraction will temporarily restore nitrous oxide flow.
- A stop fitted to the oxygen flow meter control valve ensures a minimum flow of oxygen at 175–250 mL minute, even with the valve apparently closed.
- More advanced machines have linked the flow of nitrous oxide to that of oxygen to ensure that a minimum of 25% oxygen will be always delivered to the patient.

Checking the Anesthetic Machine

It has to be ensured that the anesthetic machine must function without fault.

Before starting each theater list, *checking anesthetic machine (Boyle's machine)*, which uses cylinders as the source of compressed gases is done as follow:
- Check that cylinders are securely attached to the machine and turned off (closed).
- Open all the flow meter controls and check that there is no flow.
- Turn on (open) the oxygen cylinder and check its content on the pressure gauge. Set the rotameter to read 4 L/minute.
- If a second oxygen cylinder is present, turn off the first and check the contents of the second. Check there is no flow in nitrous oxide flow meter.
- Turn on (open) the nitrous oxide cylinder and check the contents on the pressure gauge. Set the rotameter to 4 L/minute and check that oxygen rotameter setting has not changed.
- If a second nitrous oxide cylinder is present, turn it on (open) to check its contents then turn it off (close) again.
- Turn off the oxygen cylinder and empty the system via oxygen flush. The oxygen failure-warning device, if fitted should sound and should vent all the gases from the machine. There should be no gas flow from the common gas outlet.
- Turn on the oxygen cylinder again.
- Check that vaporizers are properly fitted to the back bar, without leak. They should contain an adequate amount of volatile anesthetic agent and controls operate (dials rotate) throughout their full range without sticking.
- If the anesthetic machine is fitted with a pressure relief valve, it should be tested by occluding the common gas outlet with a thumb while the gas is flowing. The pressure relief valve should open with an audible release of the gas. If the pressure relief valve is not fitted in the machine, this test should not be done as this may damage the vaporizers.
- Check the breathing circuit to ensure that it has been assembled correctly, close the valve, fill with gas and squeeze the reservoir bag to ensure there are no leaks. Open the valve following this check and ensure the circuit empties.

- Check the function of other equipment such as suction apparatus and laryngoscopes and ensure that all the drugs, facemasks, endotracheal tubes, connectors, catheter mounts and airways required are present.
- If the machine is attached to the pipeline, then, do the check attaching and detaching the pipelines and as well as checking the cylinders.

The 'Three Pressure' Systems

The gases required for anesthetic machine are derived from the common sources available in high pressure as cylinders. The pressure has to be reduced to a safer level fit to be delivered to the patient's airway.

Hence, an anesthetic machine is functionally subdivided into three pressure systems **(Fig. 2.26)**:
1. *High pressure system*—from cylinders to pressure reducing valves.
2. *Intermediate pressure system*—from the pressure reducing valves to the flow meters and emergency oxygen flush.
3. *Low pressure system*—from flow meters to the common gas outlet.

For the sake of better understanding, based on the pressure acting on various components, the components come under three pressure systems are classified as follow.

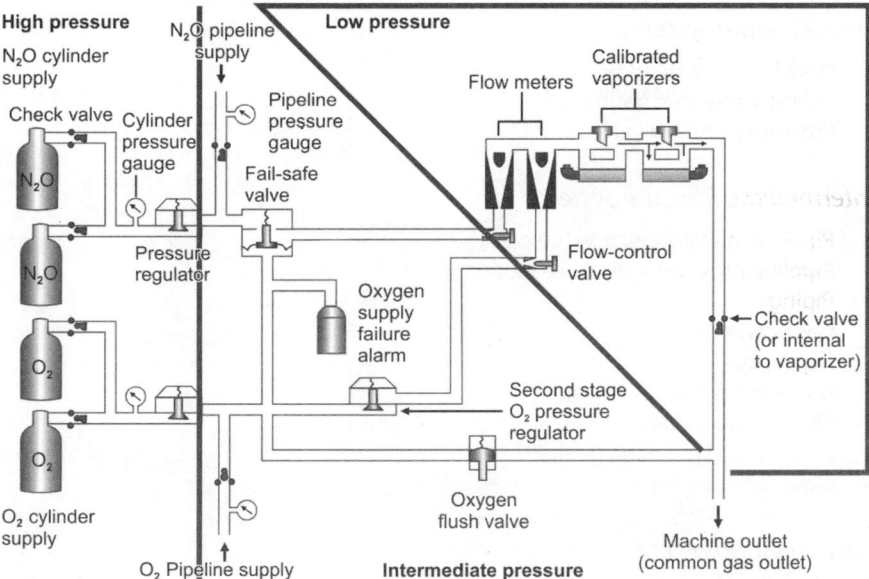

Fig. 2.26: The schematic diagram of the 'three pressure system'. • The portions within the vertical line—yoke, cylinder pressure gauge and pressure reducing valve—form high pressure system (O_2—2000 psi and N_2O—750 psi); • The outlet of pressure reducing valve, oxygen failure alarm, tubing up to the flow meter block and emergency oxygen flush form the intermediate pressure system (54–55 psi); The portion from the flow meter to the common gas outlet forms the low pressure system (12–16 psi)

In *older type of machine* the components coming under each system are:

High Pressure System

- Yoke hanger assembly
- Pressure gauge
- Pressure reducing valve.

Intermediate Pressure System

- Pipeline inlet connection (60 psi)
- Pipeline pressure indicator (Gauge) (if present)
- Piping up to flow meter
- Emergency oxygen flush.

Low Pressure System

- Flow meter
- Pressure relief device (APL)
- Vaporizer mounting device
- Common fresh gas outlet.

Most of the modern machines (*Anesthesia workstations*) have three distinct groups of components coming under the three pressure systems:

High Pressure System

- Yoke hanger assembly
- Cylinder pressure gauge
- Pressure reducing valve.

Intermediate Pressure System

- Pipeline inlet connection (60 psi)
- Pipeline pressure indicator (Gauge)
- Piping
- Gas power outlet
- Master switch
- Oxygen pressure failure alarm
- Oxygen flush valve
- Second step reducing device
- Flow control valve.

Low Pressure System

- Flow meter
- Unidirectional check valves
- Pressure relief device (APL)
- Vaporizer mounting device
- Common fresh gas outlet.

At this point of time, it is essential to briefly discuss how the modern anesthetic machines are different from the older ones.

Modern Anesthetic Machine—Work Stations (What is Different?)

These machines incorporate the basic components compactly arranged with well covered and smooth exterior. Apart from this, drawers and shelves for storing customized accessories are also provided. In addition, various safety devices and monitors are incorporated which varies with every manufacturer.

Seven groups of basic component are:
- *Gas supplies*: Pipelines and cylinders
- Gas flow measurement and control (flow meters)
- Vaporizers
- *Gas delivery*: Breathing system and ventilator
- Scavenging
- Safety devices
- Monitoring devices to monitor the function of the machine as well as the vital parameters of the patient.

Various manufactures offer modifications of the standard machine to suit the need of working situations.
- Compact or wall-rail mounted designs may be suitable for areas where space is restricted. These may have a single position back bar.
- Larger models may be trolley or ceiling-mounted (pendant).
- MRI—compatible models are made from non-ferrous metals and can be used safely up to the 1000 Gauss line. Gauss—(German physicist Carl Friedrich Gauss) is the unit of measurement of a magnetic field which is also known as the 'magnetic flux density' or the 'magnetic induction'.
- Workstations have been developed for total IV anesthesia. In these, syringe drivers are located on a 'back bar' or mounted onto tube and rail systems with integrated monitoring.
- A typical modern workstation has the architecture with easily cleaned work-surfaces.
- Machines are mains powered and a rechargeable battery provides up to 60 minutes of backup.

SCAVENGING SYSTEM

Anesthetic mixture exhaled by the patient that escape through the expiratory valve or release valve of the breathing system causes serious environmental pollution of the operating room.

The exhaled gases from the breathing system is collected by the 'Scavenging system' and diverted into the waste gas evacuation system that discharges the gases at a remote safe location. This also is considered a part of anesthesia machine.

Modern scavenging has four components namely *collecting, transferring, receiving and disposal* systems **(Fig. 2.27)**.

Collecting System
- Collects the waste gases from the breathing system and conveys to the transfer system.
- This usually comprises of a gas-tight shroud enclosing the APL valve of the breathing circuit or expiratory port of the ventilator utilizing 30 mm conical connections.

58 Anesthetic Equipment Made Easy

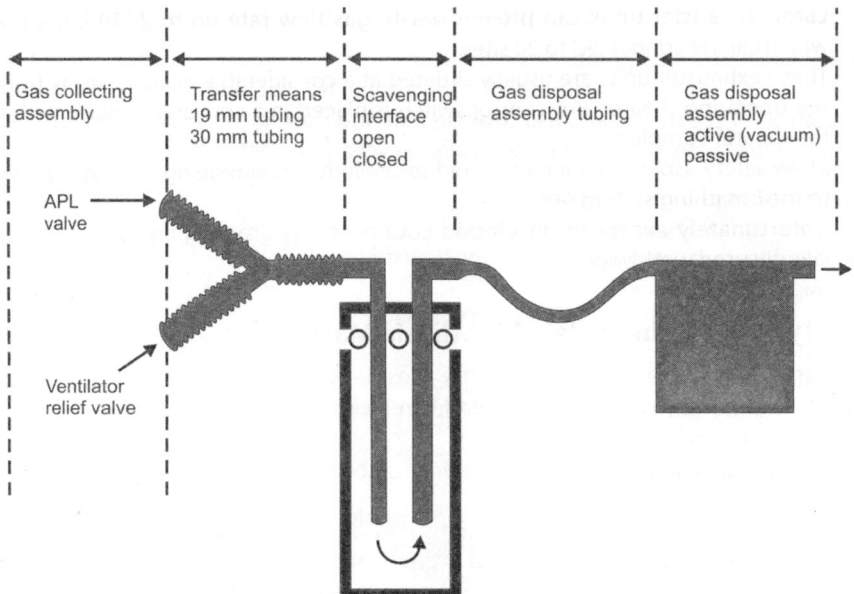

Fig. 2.27: Anesthetic waste gas scavenging system. • Waste gas collecting system, transfer system, collecting system and the disposal system are schematically represented

Transfer System

This comprises of flexible wide bore tubing leading from the collecting systems to the receiving system.

Receiving System

This system has the following components:
- A *reservoir* of rigid material that temporarily stores the outflow of waste gases.
- An *air brake*. The reservoir is open at the bottom to allow air entrainment when there is less flow of expired gases. This prevents subatmospheric pressure of the system being transferred to the patient's airway.
- A *flow indicator*. There is a clear window at the top of the reservoir with a colored float. When the active system works and the rate of extraction is normal (120 L/minute) the float appears and if the rate of extraction is low (80 L/minute) it disappears.
- A *filter*. It is placed at the bottom of the unit that prevents fluff entering the system and blocking.
- An entry port on the side and an exit port on the top of the reservoir.
- A wide bore, noncollapsing tube connects the exit port to the wall socket of the disposal system.

Disposal System

- The subatmospheric pressure required is generated by an exhauster unit, which uses a fan to generate a low pressure.
- The unique nature of the system is the small pressure gradient and large flow rates.

- Large exhauster units can provide waste gas flow rate up to 2400 L/minute which can be connected to 20 sites.
- These exhauster units are usually situated at a considerable distance away from the operating theater. But control switch is placed in a convenient place within the theater complex.
- Many safety aspects are incorporated to prevent vacuum being directly applied to the breathing system.

Unfortunately except in developed countries, the scavenging system is not prevalently used worldwide.

Safety Features in Boyle's Anesthesia Machine

The various safety features present in the anesthetic machine that protects both the machine and the patient are enumerated here below:

Antistatic Rubber Wheels

Wheels are made of conductive rubber (Antistatic), so that static charges if present will be dissipated and conducted to the ground.

Cylinders

- Color coding for visual identification
- Label stating the name of the gas and symbol
- Pin index safety system (PISS) for preventing wrong cylinder being attaché to the yoke
- Pressure release safety plug (Not found in all cylinders).

Yoke

- Pin index system does not accept wrong cylinder in the yoke
- Bodok seal for airtight fit
- Check valve (Non–return valve).

Pressure Gauge

- Color coded dial
- Name of the gas is written on the dial
- Gas vent provided at the back for venting the gas if the bourdon tube ruptures
- Positioned with an angle for easy viewing
- Cautions—"Use no oil" and "Open the valve slowly" are written on the dial
- Particularly for oxygen, the pressure gauge gives an idea of the amount of gas present in the cylinder and approximate duration for which it can be used.

Pressure Reducing Valve (Pressure Regulator)

- Reduced the cylinder pressure of 2000 psi (O_2), 750 psi (N_2O) to a safe lower pressure of 55–60 psi.
- This pressure is acceptable for all the instruments within the anesthesia machine.
- This will offer safety against the possible damage of 'barotrauma' caused by a sudden surge of high pressure into the airway.

Pressure Relief Valve (Safety Valve or Pop off Valve)

- Situated at the outlet of the pressure reducing valve. Usually, one valve for the manifold of outlets from two reducing valves.
- This valve is set to open at a slightly higher pressure than the outlet pressure of the reducing valve. Safety valve opens or blows off at 70 psi (525 kPa).
- In case of inadvertent sudden rise in working pressure due to faulty pressure reducing valve, this valve will open and release the pressure to the atmosphere.
- The high pressure is neither allowed into the instruments nor the patient's airway.

Gas Specific Feeding Connectors to the Flow Meters (Pin Valve)

- These are metal tubes leading from the outlets of the reducing valves to the back of the concerned flow meters.
- They have *non-interchangeable hexagonal connecting nuts with non-interchangeable screw threads*.
- As the size of the nut and the screw threads have marked difference in sizes for different gases, it is impossible to connect the wrong gas to the flow meter.

Pin Valve

- Pin valve works as a fine pressure reducing valve. Pressure surge is not possible.
- The screw threads are so fine that counter clockwise rotation of the knob once can move the pin to a very small distance and allow small flow in to the flow meter tube.

Knob of Oxygen Flow Meter

- Control knobs of all gases are color coded.
- Control knob of oxygen flow meter is especially profiled—'fluted' that it is identified by touch.
- It projects out than the other knobs.

Flow Meter

- Rotation of bobbin and antistatic spray in the flow meter tube prevent bobbin sticking to the wall.
- Bobbin stop at the top of flow meter tube prevents bobbin getting stuck.
- Fluorescent plate behind the flow meter bank that emits fluorescence in dark environment which make the bobbins of flow meter easily visible to ensure the flow of gases.

Position Oxygen Flow Meter

- It is positioned in the downstream in the flow meter bank.
- In case of any leak in the flow meter bank, this arrangement helps in preventing hypoxic mixture of gases being delivered to the patient to some extent.

Adjustable Pressure Limiting (APL) Valve

- This is meant for limiting the airway pressure that can be adjusted using a spring loaded screw.
- It is usually positioned near the common gas outlet of the machine.

- Usually, it incorporates a device that prevents 'back pressure' during IPPV.
- Such a valve is present in the closed circle breathing system where it is placed on the expiratory limb. The gas lost into the atmosphere is the exhaled gas containing CO_2.

Emergency Oxygen Flush

- This is the provision for filling the reservoir bag and breathing system with oxygen when there is a sudden loss of gas during work.
- This is supplied by the outlet from the reducing valve at 55–60 psi and has a non-locking push button to activate the flow.
- Flow rate of about 65 L/minute.
- Antistatic Rubber The reservoir bag, corrugated rubber tube and the face mask are all made of antistatic rubber.
- Antistatic rubber conducts the static charges and does not allow charges to accumulate to cause static sparks.

Oxygen Supply Failure Alarm

- This is available in all modern Boyle's machines.
- Whenever oxygen supply pressure falls to a specified level (30 psi) an audible alarm is activated for at least 5 seconds.
- This has limitations as it depends on pressure, not flow. It does not prevent other gases flowing when there is no oxygen.

SAFETY FEATURES IN WORKSTATIONS

Apart from these the common safety features, the modern Anesthesia Workstations have some specialized safety features. These are based on the following American standards.

1979: American National Standard Institute (ANSI)
1988: American Society for Testing and Material (ASTM) F 1161–883
1994: ASTM 1161–944 (Reapproved in 1994 and discontinued in 2000)
2000: ASTM 1850–005.

This insists on monitoring the following:
- Continuous breathing system pressure
- Exhaled tidal volume, end tidal CO_2 concentration
- Inspired oxygen concentration (FiO_2), anesthetic vapor concentration
- Oxygen supply pressure, oxygen saturation of hemoglobin (SpO_2)
- Arterial blood pressure (NIBP), Continuous ECG

Hence, the modern workstations are provided with these monitors with small variations.

Electrical system has the following safety features:
- Master switch
- Power failure indicator
- Reserve power (Battery Backup)
- Electrical outlets
- Circuit breakers
- Data communication ports.

Pipeline Wall Outlets

- Color coded labeled
- Primary valve or automatic shut off valve
- Secondary valve or isolation valve
- Schraeder probes or quick connectors have diameter index system–non-interchangeable
- Color coded pipeline hoses.

Fail-safe Valve

- Located downstream from the nitrous oxide supply source
- This valve shuts off or proportionately decreases the supply of nitrous oxide (and other gases) if the oxygen supply pressure falls.

Pressure Sensor Shut-off Valve

This valve shuts-off nitrous oxide supply if the oxygen pressure drops below 20 psi.

Oxygen Failure Protection Device

- It works on proportioning principle.
- The device consists of a *seat nozzle connected to a spring loaded piston*
- The pressure of all other gases controlled by oxygen failure protection device (OFPD) decrease proportionately with oxygen pressure.
- When oxygen supply is 50 psi the nitrous oxide flow is permitted fully.
- When it drops to 25 psi the flow of nitrous oxide is halved.
- If the supply oxygen stops the device closes the nitrous oxide fully.

Flow Meter

- Apart from the other safety features, 'master' and 'slave' mechanisms of gas delivery between N_2O and O_2.
- Here for N_2O, there is an additional pressure reducing valve on the upstream to the flow meter. This valve works as a 'slave valve' to the oxygen pressure from the pressure reducing valve (55–60 psi).
- This 'slave control valve' for nitrous oxide controlled by the oxygen pressure **(Fig. 2.24)**.
- The pressure exerted on the oxygen diaphragm is greater than that exerted by N_2O diaphragm.
- This causes a shaft to move horizontally to the left opening the 'slave control valve'. Now nitrous oxide flows towards the pin valve (flow control valve) of the flow meter.
- When the oxygen pressure is inadequate, the shaft moves to the right and closes the slave control valve.
- Now, even when the flow control valve of the flow meter is open there will be no flow of nitrous oxide.

Hypoxia Preventing Devices

- All are proportioning devices. May work on mechanical, pneumatic or electronic control).

- In Datex Ohmeda 'Link 25' is the mechanical device.
- In Dragger, oxygen ratio monitor controller (ORMC). This uses a slave control valve for N_2O. A pneumatic device.
- All these provide at least 25% oxygen in the mixture and minimum mandatory flow of 250 mL.

Vaporizers

- Interlocking 'Selectatec' mounting device.
- When one vaporizer is in use, the 'interlock' locks the other vaporizer mounted by a mechanical device.
- Prevents accidental uses of two vaporizers simultaneously.
- Back pressure compensation by a check valve (non-return valve).

Oxygen Analyzer

- This evaluates the integrity of the low pressure system to ensure that there is no leak.
- Concentration element is exposed to room air to calibrate 21%.

Ventilators

Pressure sensors to detect excessive airway pressure due to ventilator malfunctioning.

Scavenging System

Removes the anesthetic waste gases and delivers at remote place outside the theater.

CHECKING THE ANESTHESIA MACHINE

- Make sure that a *'self-inflating resuscitator bag'* is available.
- Perform the self-check by the machine (automatic) designed by the manufacturer.

Power Supply

- Plugged in
- Switched on
- Back up battery charged.

Gas Supply and Suction

- Gas and vacuum pipeline—'tug test'
- Check cylinder 'full' and turned off
- Flow meters functioning
- Hypoxic guard working
- Oxygen flush working
- Suction working.

Breathing System

- Check the whole system is patent and leak free using "two bag test"
- Vaporizers fitted correctly, filled, leak free

- Soda lime color checked
- Alternative system—Bain's, T Piece checked
- Correct gas outlet selected.

Ventilator
In working condition and configured correctly.

Scavenging
In working condition and configured correctly.

Monitors
- Correctly calibrated and in working condition.
- Alarm limits and volume set.

Airway Equipment
Full range required with spares.

Two Bag Test
A two bag test must be performed after the breathing system, vaporizer and ventilator have been checked individually.
- Attach the patient end of the breathing system (including angle piece and filter) to a test lung or bag.
- Set the fresh gas flow to 5 L/minute and ventilate manually. Check the whole breathing system is patent and unidirectional valves are moving. Check the function of the APL valve by squeezing the bag.
- Turn on the ventilator to ventilate the test lung. Turn off the fresh gas flow or reduce to the minimum. Open and close each vaporizer in turn. There should be no loss of volume in the system.

SELF-INFLATING RESUSCITATOR BAG (BAG VALVE MASK)

History
- The 'bag-valve mask' (BVM) concept was developed in 1953 by the German engineer Holger Hesse and a Danish anesthetist Henning Ruben and they named it as 'Ambu bag'.
- Later the company that started manufacturing this device in 1956 was also called 'Ambu'
- This was the first brand of resuscitator bag came into market and 'Ambu bag' is the Trade mark of the company. But it became synonymous with resuscitator bag and any brand of resuscitator bag is referred to as 'Ambu bag'.

The resuscitator bag in anesthesia machine is essential additional equipment as that will be handy in needs when there is unexpected machine malfunction.

- The resuscitator bag is a lifesaving equipment that is used to establish artificial respiration to anyone who is in respiratory arrest due to any cause including paralyzed anesthetized patient.
- Different varieties of such bags are available in the market, but the most common type in extensive use worldwide is the one which is made of silicon rubber **(Fig. 2.28)**.
- It must be available any place where there is a first aid rescue service is available such as an ambulance or emergency centers in a factory, etc.

The four basic components of a resuscitator bag are:
1. A self-inflating bag
2. A unidirectional inlet valve at the tail end
3. A unidirectional non-rebreathing valve at the patient end
4. A connector with a face mask that can accept endotracheal tube connector also.

This basic structure is meant for *resuscitation with atmospheric air* in an emergency situation.

Apart from that there are other accessories provided for O_2 *enrichment*, or reservoirs at the tail end for *providing 100% O_2*.

- Maximum volume of the bag is *1600 mL* and it has an adjustable pressure limiting valve that prevents the pressure rising above *70 cm* of H_2O.
- Oxygen concentration can be approximately increased to 50% with an oxygen flow rate of 4–6 L/minute.
- Similar bags for use for children and for neonates with smaller capacities are available.

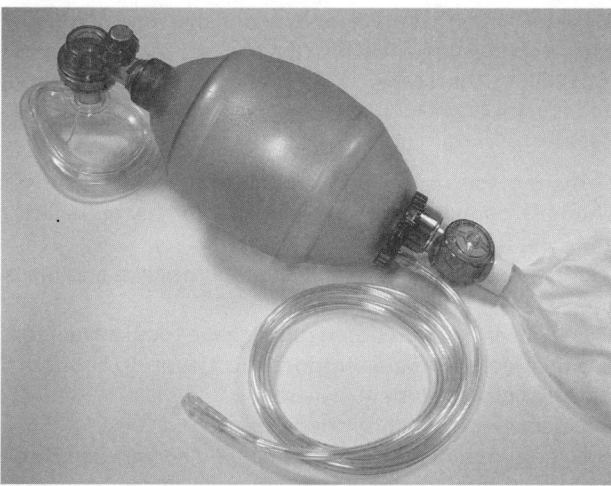

Fig. 2.28: Self-inflating resuscitator bag with unidirectional valve and mask. • For patients above 30 kg; • Bag 1600 mL-foldable for easy transportation; • Unidirectional valve is flap type; • Mask is made of transparent polycarbonate with flap rim for better fit; • Provision for oxygen enrichment with a reservoir of 2600 mL and a release valve; • The whole system can be dismantled; cleaned if needed could be autoclaved

Self-Inflating Bag
- This is made of soft rubber with resilience and that retains the shape once the compression is released so that is refilled with air entering through the unidirectional valve in the tail end.
- Some bags are made of soft rubber and are filled with foam, so that it refills by the expansion of the foam.
- The modern resuscitator bags are made of *silicon rubber* and are autoclavable.

Unidirectional Inlet Valve
- It is situated at the tail end of the bag. Usually, it is a flap valve. There is a provision for connecting an oxygen source to the inlet to enrich the air with O_2.
- Many newer bags have an attachment of *a reservoir of O_2* at the tail end with a capacity equal to that of the resuscitator bag, so as to feed 100% O_2 each time the bag is refilled. O_2 source (tube) with adequate flow is connected to this reservoir.
- The modern inlet valves are available with the body made of transparent *Polycarbonate* and the flaps made of *silicon rubber*.

Nonrebreathing Unidirectional Valve
- This valve is situated in the mouth of the bag. This allows the air from the bag, when compressed, to enter the lungs and during passive expiration the expired air is directed to atmosphere. Thus, rebreathing is prevented. Various types of valves are available.
- The modern valves have their body made with transparent *Polycarbonate* and silicon rubber flaps.
- Usually, an *adjustable pressure limiting valve* is provided at the proximal portion of the body of the valve that prevents hyperinflation and barotrauma.
- This valve has a connecting end which fits to a face mask or to a 15 mm universal connector of endotracheal tube.

Face Mask
- The mask is made of transparent polycarbonate body with silicon rubber flap brim.
- Transparent mask permits to observe and look for any secretions in the mouth and nose.

All these components are autoclavable in modern valves and the bag is foldable for easy storage.

The resuscitator bags made of silicon rubber have some advantages.
- These are available in India as import substitution products (Rao's Silicon Resuscitators manufactured by *M/s Anesthetics, Mumbai*).
- The bag is foldable for easy transport in a bag.
- If needed, all the components can be dismantled and reassembled easily.
- The bag is made of food grade silicon rubber which can be autoclaved to 136°C for about five minutes.
- The transparent parts of unidirectional valves and clear hood mask are made of polycarbonate. These are also autoclavable.
- The nonrebreathing valve has very low resistance and low dead space (7 mL).
- The valve and mask connection has 360° swivel that is comfortable for the user.
- The patient end is fitting to all 22 mm or 15 mm facemasks and endotracheal connectors.

- The oxygen reservoir bags for enriching the air with oxygen are available.
- The child size resuscitators are provided with pressure limiting (release) valve which limits the inflation pressure to 40 cm H_2O.
- 500 mL resuscitator bag is available with pressure limiting valve to prevent high pressure inflation in children from 7 to 30 kg **(Fig. 2.29)**.
- 240 mL resuscitator bag with pressure limiting valve is available for children up to 7 kg **(Fig. 2.30)**.
- Unidirectional valves with or without pressure limiting valve are shown in **Figures 2.31A to C** with its mechanism.
- Reservoir bag for oxygen enrichment is attached to the back of the resuscitator bag through a release valve which vents excess oxygen to the atmosphere **(Figs 2.32A and B)**.
- All the features of the three sizes of resuscitator bags are shown in **Figure 2.33**.

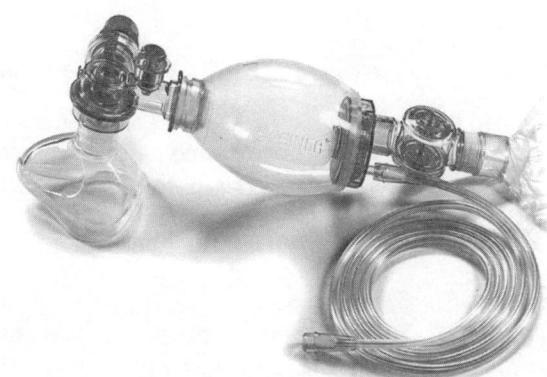

Fig. 2.29: Resuscitator bag child size. • For children from 7 to 30 kg; • Bag 500 mL; • It has a pressure limiting valve (40 cm H_2O) for safety; • Oxygen enrichment reservoir 2600 mL with release valve

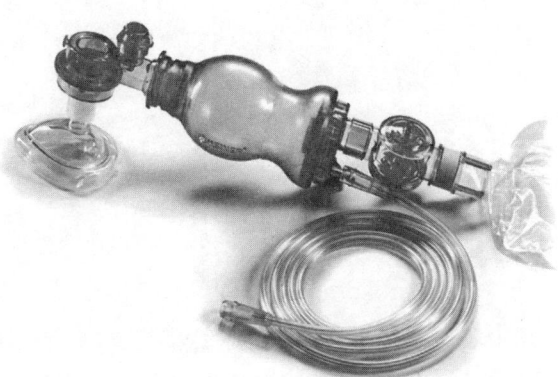

Fig. 2.30: Resuscitator bag infant size. • For babies up to 7 kg; • Bag 240 mL; • Pressure limiting valve (40 cm H_2O); • Oxygen enrichment reservoir with release valve 600 mL

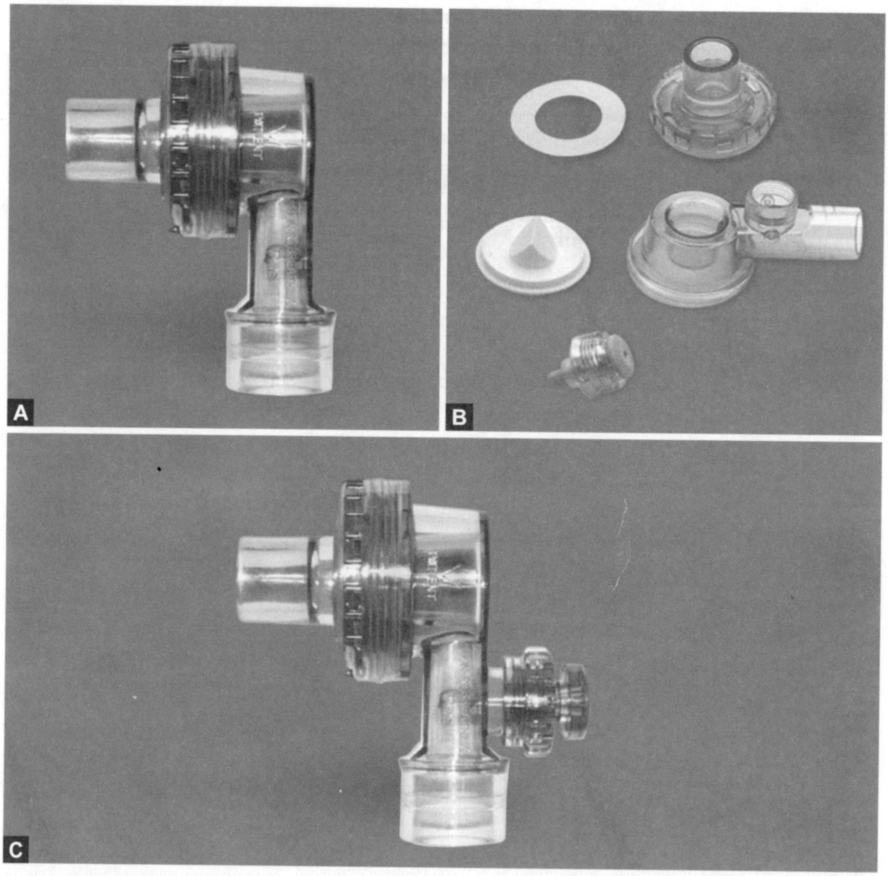

68 Anesthetic Equipment Made Easy

Figs 2.31A to C: Unidirectional valve. (A) Without pressure limiting valve; (B) Mechanism dismantled to show the 'Fish mouth valve', 'Flap valve and 'Pressure limiting valve; (C) With pressure limiting valve

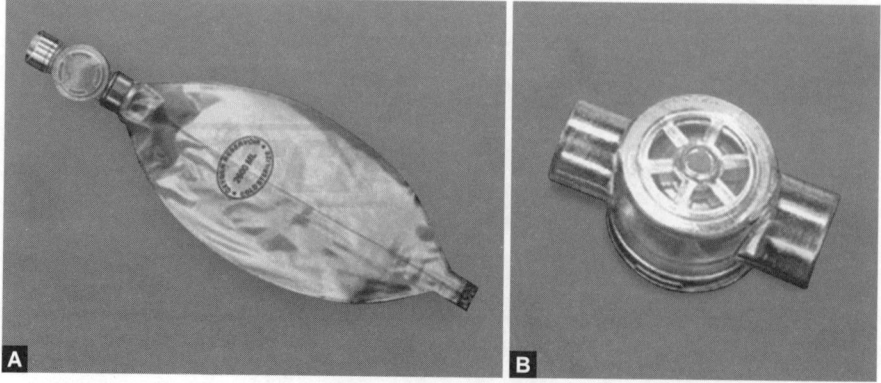

Figs 2.32A and B: (A) Oxygen reservoir bag with release valve; (B) Release valve

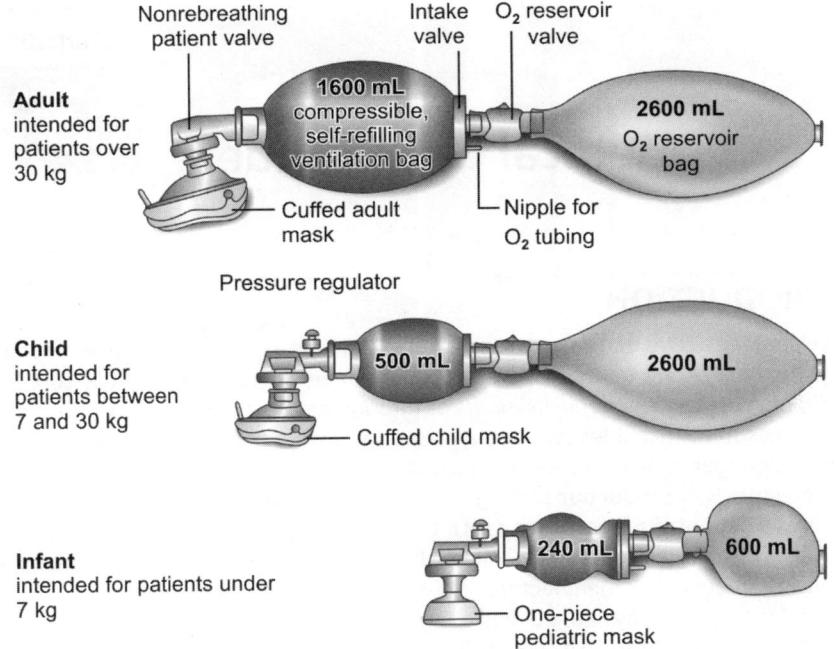

Fig. 2.33: All the features of the three sizes of resuscitator bags

FURTHER READING

1. Gurudatt CL. The Basic Anesthesia Machine. N Indian J Anaesth. 2013;57(5):438-45.
2. Jerry A Dorsch, Susan E Dorsch. Understanding Anesthesia Equipment, 4th edn. London. Lippincott Williams and Wilkins, 1999.
3. Jerry A Dorsch, Susan E Dorsch. Understanding Anesthesia Equipment, 5th edn. London. Lippincott Williams and Wilkins, 2008.

chapter 3

Medical Gas Cylinders

INTRODUCTION

Gas cylinder is a term that is commonly used to describe a pressurized container of gas used for storage and transport. The gases used in anesthesia are generally supplied under high pressure, either in cylinders or through pipeline from large cylinders.

In anesthesia machines cylinders are used routinely or if pipeline is used cylinders are for emergency backup. Air is supplied either as pressurized cylinders or from compressors. Bulk production of oxygen is usually by fractional distillation of liquid air.

In every country there are a series of regulations and standards for manufacture and the use of medical gas cylinders. In spite of these regulatory measures that are designed to ensure safety in the manufacture and distribution of medical gases, accidents do occur. If it occurs, it may cause devastating damage to all the personnel in the scene. Therefore, it is mandatory to have clear knowledge of medical gas cylinders considering safety as the highest priority.

HISTORY

In the history oxygen and other gases were compressed and stored at high pressure in seamless hand-forged steel containers in 1880.

Until 1946, medical gas cylinders were made of either *low carbon steel alloy* or *high carbon steel alloy*.

Present day medical gas cylinders are commonly made of steel alloys like Molybdenum steel. Now aluminum cylinders covered with carbon-steel fibers, glass fibers (fiber glass material) and covered with epoxy gel coating are used with the advantage of light weight, high tensile strength and more capacity are available. MRI compatible aluminum cylinders have also come to use.

Oxygen, nitrous oxide, and medical air are usually supplied from pipeline.

Low Carbon Steel Alloy

These cylinders were used to store liquid gases, i.e. carbon dioxide, *nitrous* oxide, cyclopropane, ethylene, ammonia, etc.

High Carbon Steel Alloy

These cylinders were used to store oxygen, nitrogen, hydrogen, air, etc.

Composition	High carbon steel	Low carbon steel
• Carbon	0.4–0.48%	0.15–0.25%
• Manganese	0.5–0.9%	0.45–0.75%
• Silicon	0.3%	0.3%
• Sulfur	0.045%	0.045%
• Iron	same	same

The main disadvantages were their heavy weight and high wall thickness.
After 1946, alloys with light weight were used in place of carbon steel.
1. *Manganese steel* — for liquefied gases
2. *Molybdenum steel* — for high pressure gases

Modern cylinders are all made of *Molybdenum steel* alloy only.

Advantages

- Light weight
- Thin wall
- High tensile strength

	Composition	*Manganese steel*	*Molybdenum steel*
•	Carbon	0.4%	0.3–0.4%
•	Manganese	1.3–1.7%	0.4–0.9%
•	Silica	0.3%	0.3%
•	Sulfur	0.04%	0.35%
•	Phosphorous	0.04%	0.35%
•	*Molybdenum*	–	0.15%–0.25%
•	Chromium	–	0.8–1.1%

Features of Ideal Cylinders

- Cylinders are 'solid drawn' from molten alloy or made of seamless tubes **(Figs 3.1A and B)**.
- No welding or any other metal is used.
- Strict formula of composition is adhered to during manufacture.
- Molybdenum 0.15%–0.25%
- Chromium 0.8%–1.1%
- The wall thickness must be uniform.
- Wall thickness is very small, usually one-fourth of an inch (4.2–6.25 mm).

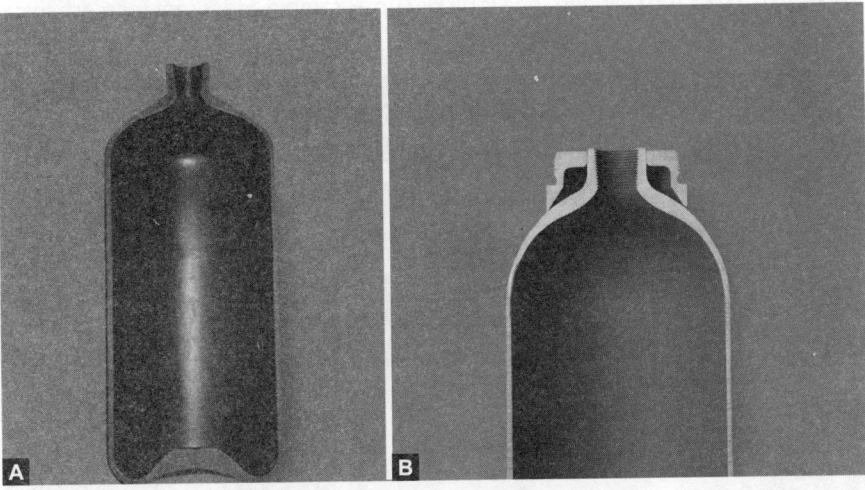

Figs 3.1A and B: The 'solid drawn' cylinders without joints or welding (A) The whole cylinder is 'solid drawn' from molten alloy without joint or weld; (B) An attachment is screwed on to the outer side of neck for fixing the protective cap for the valve

- Before closing the cylinder, it is carefully checked for uniform wall thickness and for any surface defect both internally and externally.
- Then the cylinders are put in a furnace at 860–890°C and heated till the whole cylinder reaches the temperature and then they are carefully removed and cooled to room temperature. This is known as *'Heat Treatment'*.
- Then they are cleaned and dried.
- After this stage, no oil or grease should come in contact with the cylinders.
- Any cylinder having a diameter of 100 mm or more which is used for storing a poisonous gas, flammable gas or gas that supports combustion, needs a protective screw cap or metal cap with vent hole for the valve end.
- The valve must be completely inside this cap and is protected from injury **(Figs 3.2A and B)**.

In a batch of 100 cylinders, one sample cylinder is taken and is subjected to the following tests. Because the cylinders are subjected very high pressure and rough use, they are subjected for mechanical tests as well as hydraulic tests.

Tests

Mechanical Tests

- Tensile test
- Impact test
- Flattening test
- Bend test.

Hydraulic Test

Tested for withstanding a pressure of 232 kg/sq cm (Approximate 3000 psi)
- All the cylinders are subjected to hydraulic test—repeated every six years

Mechanical Testing

In every batch of 100 cylinders, one is picked up as sample and is sent for mechanical testing.

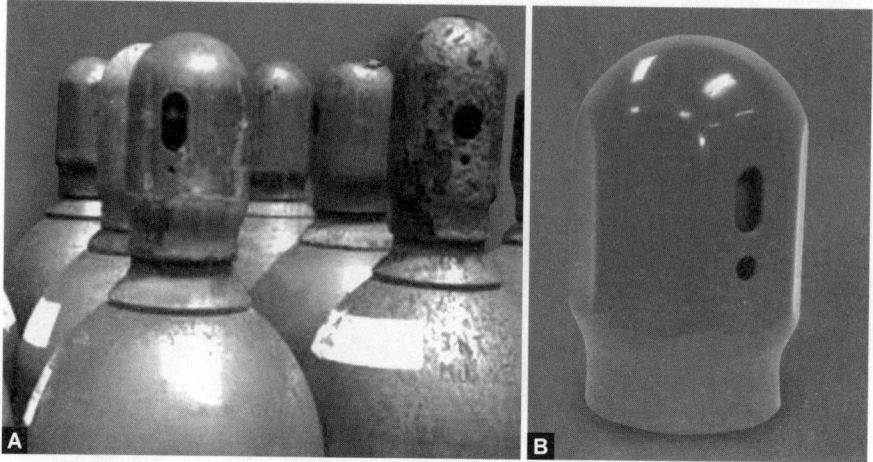

Figs 3.2A and B: Cylinders with protective cover with vent holes for valve end

Tensile test
- Strips of standard size are cut longitudinally and stretched until they elongate.
- The 'yielding point' should not be less than 15 tons/sq inch.

Flattening test
- Middle part of the empty cylinder is kept between two compression blocks, similar to the carpenter's vice.
- Then pressure is applied to compress it and the flattening is watched.
- The cylinder gets flattened slowly. The compression is stopped when the distance between the blocks is equal to 6 times the thickness of the wall of cylinder.
- Now without removing the load, the cylinder is examined.
- If no cracks are seen, both externally and internally, it is considered as satisfactory. These two tests were done before 1946.

Now the common tests done are:

Impact test
- Six pieces are cut from the sample cylinder for testing (Three longitudinal pieces and three transverse pieces are taken). These are struck by a mechanical hammer.
- The mean energy required for causing a fracture should not be less than
  5 feet lbs   for transverse pieces
  10 feet lbs   for longitudinal pieces

Bend test
- A ring of 25 mm width is cut across the cylinder and that is divided into 4 quarters (strips) of equal length.
- Each strip is then bent inwards. Each strip has to remain without cracks, when fully bent inward.

Hydraulic Test

- Cylinders in use are periodically tested with *hydraulic test alone—every 6 years*.
- There will be a mark impressed on the body of the valve with a round having the No 1, 2 or 3 indicating how many times the cylinder has gone for test thereby indicating the age of the cylinder.
- Each time on the neck of cylinder a different colored ring with date of testing will be placed. This indicates the year in which it was tested and the batch to which it belongs.

Water Jacket Method

- The cylinder is enclosed in a water jacket with a gauge.
- Then a hydraulic pressure of 232 kg/sq cm is applied into the cylinder.
- The change of volume on applying and after removal of internal hydraulic pressure is assessed. 0.02% of total stretch is acceptable.
- Tested for 3000 psi (232 kg/sq cm). This is the testing pressure of the cylinder.
- When the cylinder is subjected to the first hydraulic test a hexagonal metal ring is placed between the neck and valve.
- The color of the ring indicates the year of manufacture.
- Cylinders undergo hydraulic test every 6 years and a round metal ring of different color is replaced. The number of test is engraved on the shoulder.

- This helps to assess the age of the cylinder.
  The various pressures of cylinders
- Working pressure : 2000 psi
- Testing pressure : 3000 psi (approximately 50% more than working pressure)
- Bursting pressure : 6000 psi (Double the testing pressure).

PARTS OF A CYLINDER

Any cylinder has the following parts; Body, shoulder and valve **(Figs 3.3A and B)**
- A 'neck' or 'stem' to which the outlet valve is fixed
- The neck widens out as a 'shoulder'
- The shoulder continues as an uniform cylindrical 'body'
- The bottom of the body or base may be flat or concave (like a bottle) so that it can stand on a smooth floor. Some A-type cylinders have hemispherical base which need a supporting rack to store
- Wall thickness ranges from 4.2 mm to 6.25 mm
- Transporting the cylinder must be done by manually carrying or by using a cylinder trolley
- The dangerous practice of holding the cylinder valve and dragging the cylinder along the floor will make the corners of the base thinned out and make the cylinder weak.

The cylinder outlet valve will be discussed in detail later.

The Shoulder of the Cylinder

It is the smoothly tapering upper end of the body that ends up as the neck onto which the cylinder outlet valve is fixed by the screw threads.

There are some details of the cylinder engraved on the shoulder.
The basic details to be engraved are the following;
- Manufacturer's name, serial number, working pressure, testing pressure, month and year of first hydraulic test and subsequent tests done.
- Additional information may be added as per the rules of the country where it is used **(Figs 3.3A and B)**.

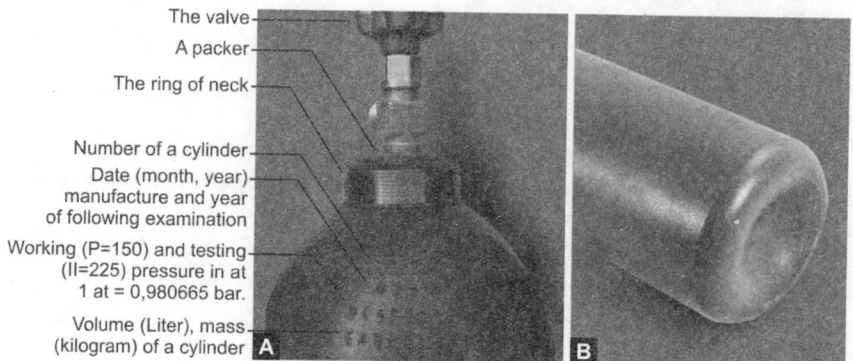

Figs 3.3A and B: The parts of a gas cylinder. • Valve, neck, shoulder and body of the cylinder are seen; • The base with concavity is shown (solid drawn)

Steel-Carbon Fibers Cylinders

In the recent years there is a move to change from traditional steel cylinders to steel-carbon fiber cylinders. These are aluminum cylinders wrapped with carbon-steel fibers in Epoxy resin matrix. Overwrap with fiberglass with epoxy gel coating on this makes the cylinder ultralight weight and highly durable. These cylinders hold more gas **(Fig. 3.4)**.

MRI compatible cylinders are made of *Aluminum*.

Types of Cylinders and their Capacities

There is no uniform nomenclature for different sizes of cylinders universally. Different countries have different coding for capacities of cylinders. This may cause confusion regarding the capacities of cylinders.

In India the following system is in use. AA, A, B, and D cylinders are in medical use. These are also

What is called 'A–Type' in India is called 'E–Type' in USA **(Fig. 3.5)**.

AA - 12 Cubic feet (presently not in common use)
A - 20 Cubic feet - 5 L Water capacity
B - 40 Cubic feet - 10 L Water capacity
C - 100 Cubic feet - (Not for medical use)
D - 200 Cubic feet - 50 L Water capacity

- AA and A-Type cylinders are supplied with 'Flush valve' that can be attached to the 'Yoke' of anesthetic machine. 'AA' cylinders are too small and are seldom used.
- The standard 'A' size oxygen cylinders are supplied at 134 bar (2000 psi) pressure and contain 680 L of oxygen (approximate value).
- B-Type and D-Type are provided with 'Bullnose' valves.
- D-Type is used in manifold room of central pipeline supply of oxygen.

Now oxygen cylinder pressure is standardized to 150 bar (150 atm)—approximately 2200 psi pressure.

- In a cylinder with *1 L water* capacity *150 bar* pressure will compress 150 L of O_2 into it.
- Hence, multiplying the water capacity of the cylinder by 150 (bar) will give the number of liters of gas in the cylinder.

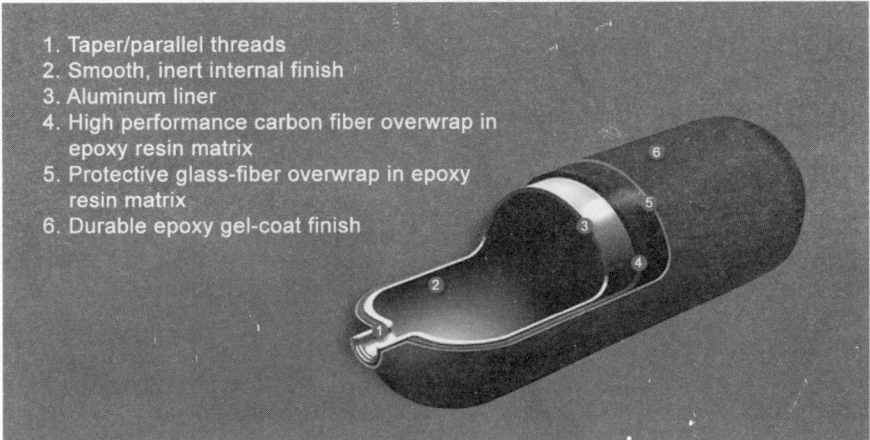

1. Taper/parallel threads
2. Smooth, inert internal finish
3. Aluminum liner
4. High performance carbon fiber overwrap in epoxy resin matrix
5. Protective glass-fiber overwrap in epoxy resin matrix
6. Durable epoxy gel-coat finish

Fig. 3.4: Steel-carbon fiber cylinder

- The exact water capacity of each cylinder minimally vary and is printed on the cylinder.
- It is an approximate value. For example 50 L water capacity cylinder may have actual capacity as 48 or 49 L.
- *20 cu ft = 5 L* Water capacity = A-Type—contains—5 L × 150 = 750 L O_2
- *40 cu ft = 10 L* Water capacity = B-Type—contains—10 × 150 = 1500 L O_2
- *200 cu ft = 50 L* Water capacity = D-Type—contains—50 × 150 = 7500 L O_2

Oxygen and nitrous oxide cylinders of A- and B-Type are used inside the operation theater. A-Type is fixed to the yoke assembly whereas; *B-Type* is used with a conversion kit consisting of a pressure reducing valve, flexible hose and a Yoke block **(Fig. 3.6)**.

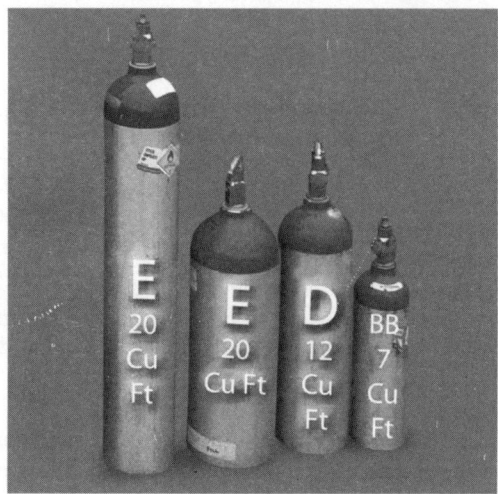

Fig. 3.5: The 20 cu ft cylinder known as 'A- Type' is called 'E–size' in USA

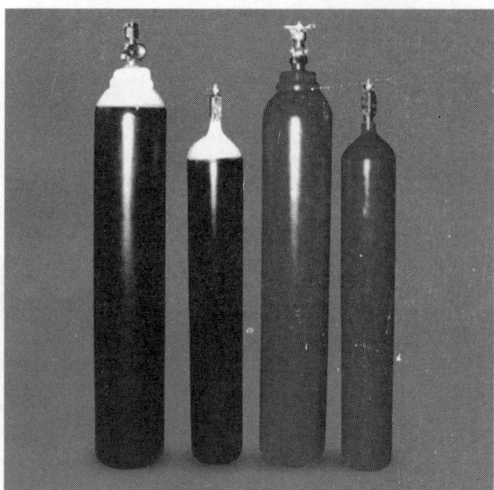

Fig. 3.6: A- and B-Type cylinders of oxygen and nitrous oxide; A-Type cylinder has 'Flush' valve and B-Type has 'Bullnose' valve

Identification

1. Visual (Universal color coding)
2. Label (Either stuck on the shoulder or tied on the neck of the cylinder)
3. Embossed on the cylinders (name of the gas, quantity, etc.).

Color Coding (Visual)

Unfortunately there is no international color coding system for the contents of anesthetic gas cylinders (or pipelines). In the USA oxygen is supplied in green cylinders, in the UK the cylinders are black with white shoulders and in Germany they are blue. However, it is easier to identify the cylinder by color (in the country of use) even for those who cannot read the label.

In India the following color coding is used:

Gas	Shoulder	Body	Pressure
N_2O	Blue	Blue	750 psi
C_3H_6	Orange	Orange	75 psi
CO_2	Gray	Gray	720 psi
N_2	Black	Gray	2000 psi
Air	White and Black	Gray	2000 psi
Oxygen	White	Black	2000 psi

It has to be remembered that the visual color coding is not universal. For example, oxygen cylinder in India and UK is colored black body with white shoulder (**Fig. 3.7**) but in USA it is uniform green color or aluminum colored body and green shoulder (*See* **Fig. 3.5**).

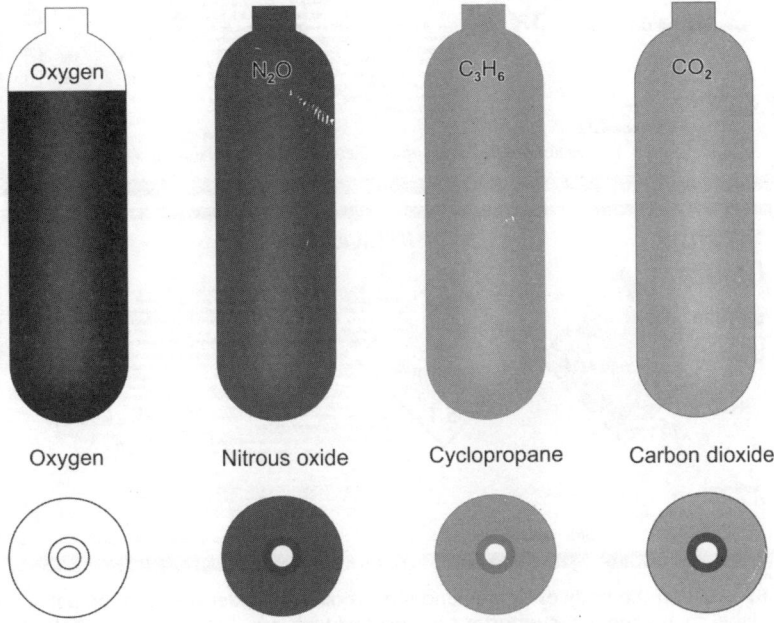

Fig. 3.7: Color coding of cylinders in anesthesia machine

78 Anesthetic Equipment Made Easy

In UK all medical gas cylinders will be changed to a white cylinder body; the shoulder colors that identify the gas and the product specific valve will remain unchanged. It is to make medical gas cylinders easily distinguishable from non-medical gas cylinders. The changes would be completed by 2025.

Label

Each cylinder has a label on the shoulder or body. It should not be covered with any cloth or cover. The following information is found on it **(Fig. 3.8)**:
- Name of the gas and chemical symbol of gas
- Name of the manufacturer
- Red stripes : If the gas is explosive
- Yellow stripes : If the gas is poisonous
- A diamond shaped symbol to denote the hazard and quality of the gas (flammable, non-flammable, supporting combustion, explosive, poisonous, etc.).
- Quantity of the gas when it is full

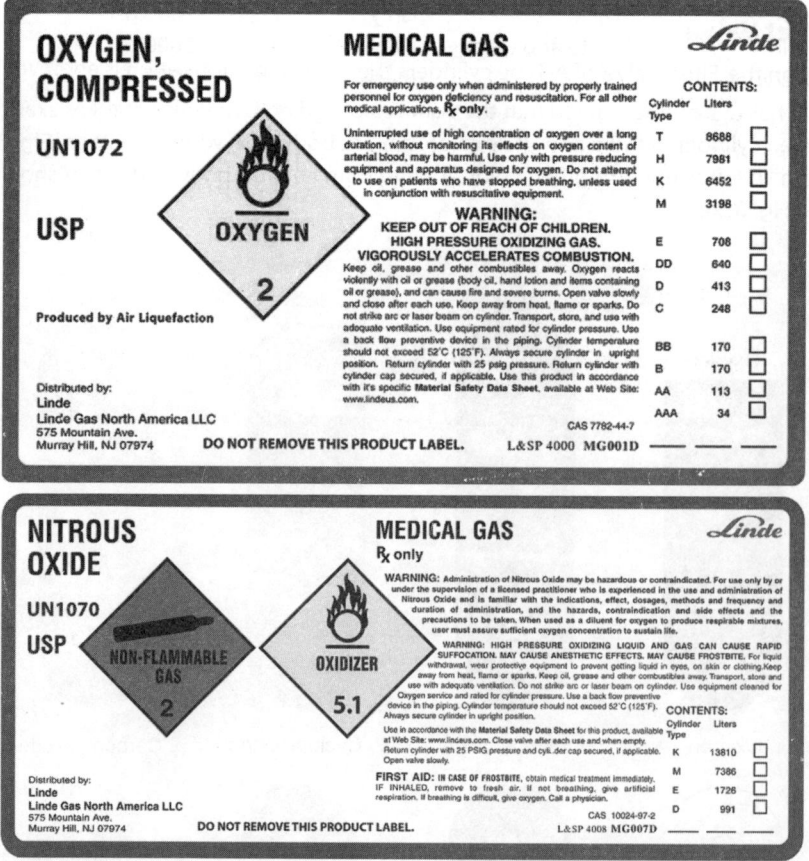

Fig. 3.8: Label on the body of oxygen and nitrous oxide cylinder showing the details. • The oxygen label shows one sign-supporter combustion (oxidizer); • The nitrous oxide label shows two signs—Nonflammable gas and supporter of combustion (oxidizer)

- Maximum cylinder pressure
- Cylinder size
- Directions for use.

Other common signs are shown in **Figure 3.9**.

Cyclopropane is a highly potent anesthetic gas. It is not in use now because it is an explosive in any concentration with oxygen. It was supplied in light aluminum alloy cylinders colored orange to indicate that it is an explosive gas.

Ethylene oxide is not an anesthetic gas. It is very commonly used for sterilizing delicate instruments, implants, etc. It is worth remembering that it is an explosive gas as well as poisonous—neurotoxic gas. Hence, the cylinders containing the gas will have orange shoulder with a yellow stripe below. Orange denotes it is explosive and yellow stripe denotes it is poisonous.

Usually, ethylene oxide is dispensed with CO_2 to minimize the risk of explosion. Ethylene oxide 15% and carbon-dioxide 85%.

Information Engraved on the Shoulder

The information engraved on the shoulder of the cylinder is shown in **Figure 3.10**.

Outlet Valve

Only on the 'Flush valve' of A-Type cylinders the following information is engraved.

Fig. 3.9: Some of the signs seen in the labels of gas cylinders

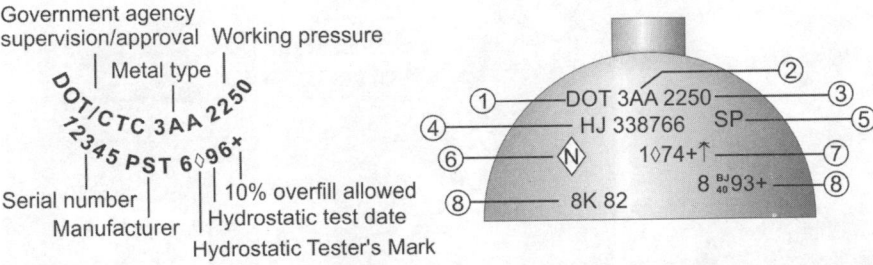

Fig. 3.10: The details engraved on the shoulder of a cylinder. 1. Agency; 2. Material specification —3AA Made of steel; 3 AL or 3 ALM made of aluminum; 3. Working pressure; 4. Serial number; 5. Distributor; 6. Manufacturer; 7. First hydraulic test with month and year separated by manufacturer's mark. The + mark indicates permission for 10% excess filling; 8. Next hydraulic tests with month and year separated by tester's mark

All these information are engraved on it
- Name of gas   - N$_2$O
- Manufacturer   - BOC (Manufacturer's name)
- Tare weight   - Empty weight
- Cylinder size   - 20 cubic feet (A)
- Year of manufacture   - 1992

There will be a colored washer on the neck, made of either plastic or aluminum.
- Hexagonal washer   -   New cylinder (Less than 6 years old)
- Round washer   -   Old cylinder (More than 6 years old)

Every 6 years cylinders are subjected for test and then the washer is changed to a round metal washer of different color for every 6 years.

Cylinder Outlet Valves

Flush Valve

- *Flush valve* are especially designed outlet valves fitted in 'A-Type' cylinders. This valve can be fixed to the Yoke of the anesthetic machine **(Figs 3.11A to C)**.
- This valve is different from the valves of other bigger cylinders like B-Type cylinders (used in the wards for oxygen therapy for patient) that the outlet has no provision such as screw threads for connecting.
- The body of the valve is made of brass metal plated with chromium.
- The 'spindle' is made of hard steel. The lower end of spindle may be convex or cone shaped and sits tightly on a seat of similar shape to close the cylinder.
- On the top of the valve there is hexagonal nut, also known as 'gland nut' through which the outer end of the 'Spindle,' protrudes out.
- Below the gland nut, around the spindle a tight packing of noncombustible material such as 'Teflon' is provided to prevent leak around it. The gland nut is used for tightening the packing around the spindle if there is any leak **(Fig. 3.13)**.
- The 'spindle' is used for opening and closing the cylinder with the help of a special spanner (Cylinder key) **(Figs 3.12A to C)**.

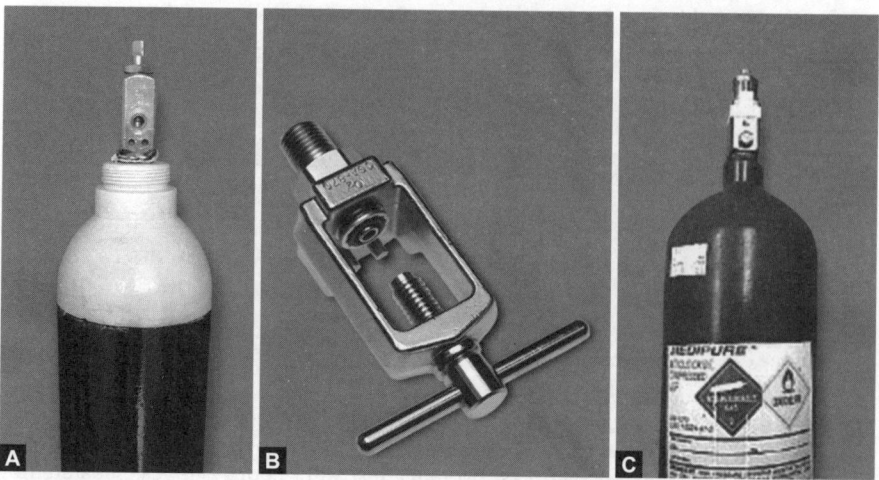

Figs 3.11A to C: Yoke assembly and 'A-Type' cylinders of O$_2$ and N$_2$O with flush valve.
- The Yoke hanger assembly of an anesthetic machine with pin index, nipple and Bodok seal

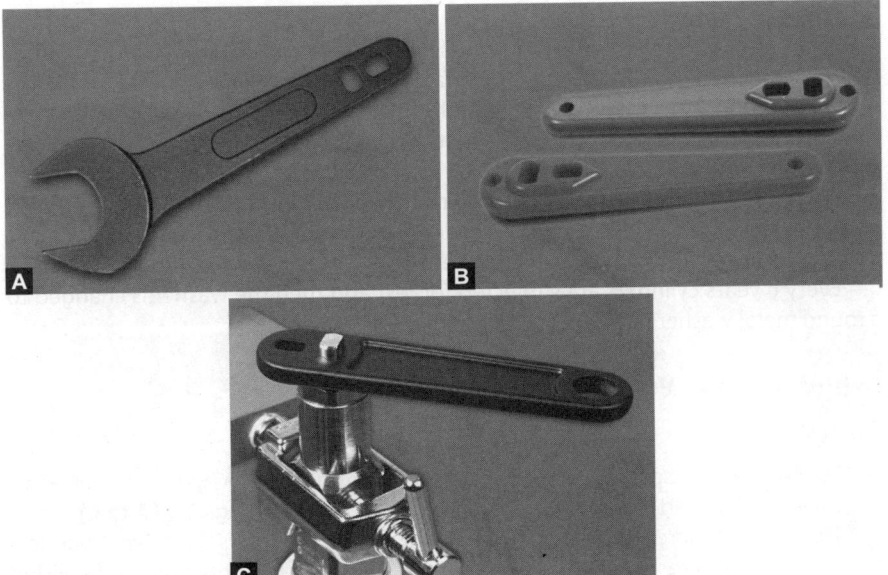

Figs 3.12A to C: Two types of cylinder spanner or key. • The key A at one end has the key for opening the spindle and on the other end a spanner fir tightening the gland nut to stop the leak around the spindle; • The key B has the provision for opening the spindle at one end and at the other end a hole to tie a chain to attach it to the machine; • The figure C shows a cylinder fixed on the yoke with the key on the spindle

- This key must always be kept tied to the machine with a strong thread or chain of sufficient length. This is for emergency use.
- The flush valve has 4 faces; one of the faces has a 7 mm diameter outlet port in the middle.
- Just below that are two holes of 4.75 mm diameter and 6 mm deep for accepting the pins of pin index system.
- The gas outlet of the valve must be closed with a stopper (plastic cover) provided for that purpose, which is removed just before fixing the cylinder to the machine **(Fig. 3.13)**.
- If the stopper is not present, before fixing the cylinder to the yoke of the machine, the spindle is opened and closed rapidly to allow a short burst of gases to escape.
- This is known as *'Cracking'* the cylinder. This will blow off any dirt in the outlet valve. Otherwise, the dirt may get into the pressure-reducing valve and cause malfunctioning.
- On the opposite face of the valve there is a shallow conical depression to fix and tighten the screw of 'T' handle to secure the cylinder on the yoke.
- Just below this, there is a safety plug which melts at a particular temperature and lets out the contents (Wood's metal). This plug is not provided in all valves.
- The external appearance and internal structures of flush valve as seen in longitudinal section are shown in **Figure 3.13**.
- The safety plug is made of 'Wood's metal'.

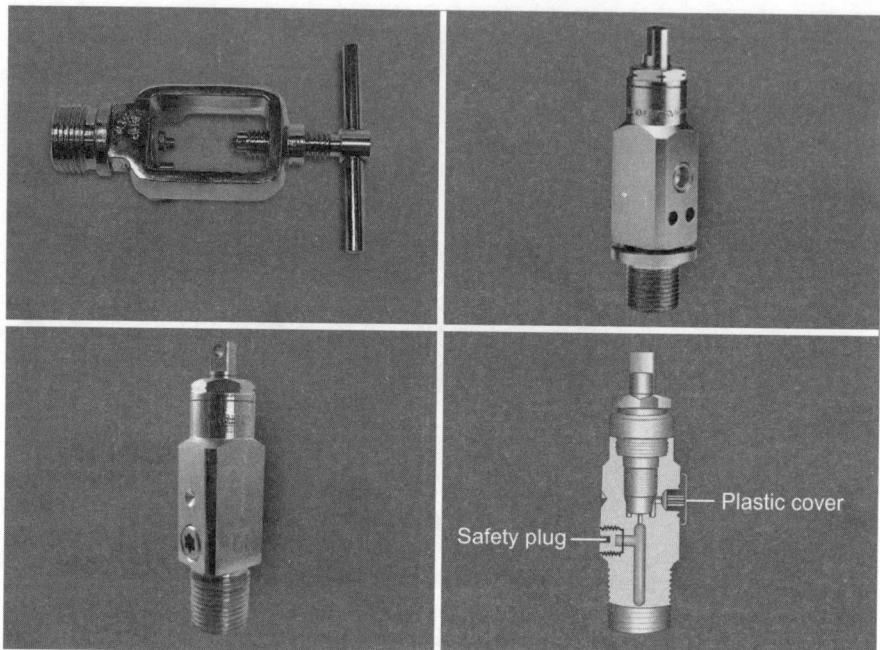

Fig. 3.13: Yoke of anesthetic machine, flush valve as seen outside and inside. • Yoke assembly shows the nipple and Bodok seal around it. The screw for fixing the cylinder valve is seen; • The gas outlet with pin index holes seen on one side; • On the opposite side, a conical depression to tighten the screw and just below that the safety plug is seen. (Safety plug is not provided in all valves); • The safety plug will melt and release the contents of the cylinder if dangerous pressure builds up in the cylinder due to high temperature. It is not pressure sensitive but temperature sensitive

Wood's Metal

- It is a eutectic fusible alloy that contains 50% bismuth, 25% lead, 12.5% tin and 12.5% cadmium. It is also known as Lipowitz alloy and named after Barnabas Wood.
- It has a melting point of approximately 70–72°C (158°F)
- Medical *gas cylinders* in the United Kingdom have a Wood's metal seal which melts in fire, allowing the gas to escape and reducing the risk of *gas explosion*.
  The information provided on the valve is given below **(Fig. 3.14)**:
- The name of the gas
- The empty weight of the cylinder
- The working pressure (2,000 psi)
- Serial number and the manufacturer's name (BOC)
- On one side, the gas outlet and the pin index holes are present.
- On the opposite side there is a small conical depression that allows tightening of the tip of the screw that secures the valve in the yoke.

Bodok Seal

- It was introduced in 1958.
- The Bodok seal is a specialized washer that ensures a gas tight seal between the cylinder valve and the machine.

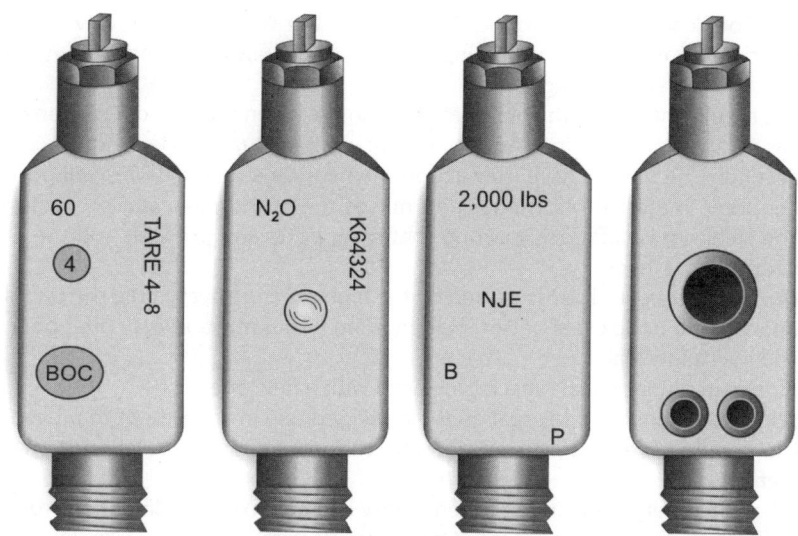

Fig. 3.14: The flush valve with the information on four faces. • On the top is the outer end of spindle to open or close the cylinder; • The hexagonal gland nut is seen below that; • Name of gas, empty weight, test pressure, serial number, and manufacturer's name are the information; • On one face the gas outlet and pin index holes are present; • On the opposite side a shallow conical depression for tightening the screw that secures the valve in the yoke

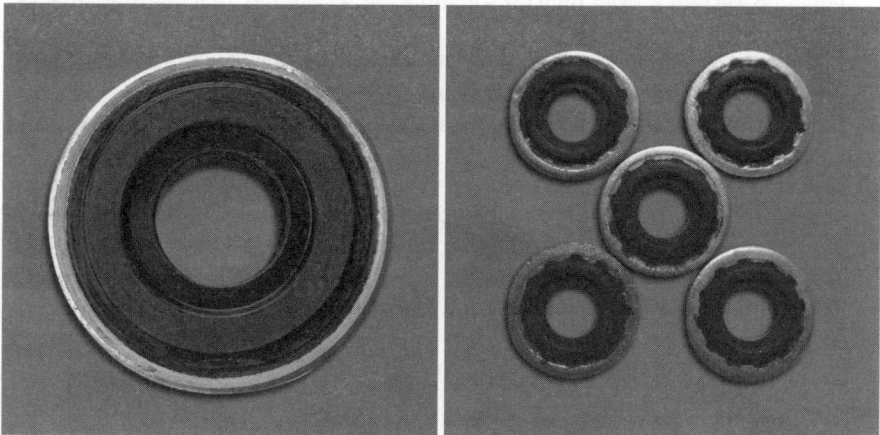

Fig. 3.15: Bodok seal. • Bodok seal is made of hard synthetic rubber material (neoprene) and is surrounded by a tough steel or aluminum rim to prevent rupture by the high pressure of gas coming out of the cylinder; • When the Bodok seal is placed around the nipple and the flush valve is tightened, by the screw, airtight fit will be achieved; • When the cylinder is opened, gas from the cylinder enters the machine through the nipple to enter into the pressure reducing valve of the machine

- The Bodok seal is a special washer made of a neoprene (noncombustible synthetic rubber) with a peripheral metal ring, which protects and prevents splaying of the washer **(Fig. 3.15)**.
- The metal ring may be steel or aluminum.
- The seal is incombustible and resistant to the high pressure imposed upon it by the gas in the cylinder. (A full cylinder of oxygen has a pressure of 2000 psi or 150 bar).

- The Bodok seal is fixed around the nipple of the Yoke, the flush valve outlet of the cylinder is fixed onto the nipple, and the screw is tightened. This in normal conditions gives an airtight fit.
- The nipple enters into the outlet of the cylinder. When the cylinder is opened, the gas escapes into the nipple and with tight washer usually no leak occurs.
- Secondly the gas pressure may act on the neoprene material. This will push the neoprene material that bulges and makes the seal tighter and prevents leak. The steel rim is sufficiently strong that it supports and prevents rupture of the neoprene washer.
- Due to the repeated stress caused by the high pressure every time the cylinder is opened, the Bodok seal gets damaged more frequently and may offer poor seal and may allow leak.
- A damaged Bodok seal must be replaced with a new one.
- Adding additional Bodok seal on the damaged one in an attempt to prevent the leak should never be practiced, as it may make the pin index safety system (PISS) ineffective.
- When the safety of pin index system is lost, it allows fixing a cylinder of wrong gas to the yoke causing danger resulting in serious damages.

Pin Index Safety System

- Pin index safety system (PISS) was introduced in 1952 to prevent connecting wrong cylinder on wrong yoke.
- Pin index system is used only for AA and A-Type cylinders that are used in anesthesia machines.
- Before the introduction of PISS, any cylinder with a flush valve can be attached to any yoke, which caused wrong gas cylinder fixed on the yokes.
- It is a non-interchangeable safety measure that it is not possible to fix a wrong cylinder in any yoke.
- Two stout short pins project from the yoke which fit into the holes of the same size drilled correspondingly on the body of the valve **(Figs 3.16 and 3.17)**.
- There is an imaginary 'V' shaped pattern on the body of the flush valve on which six points are marked from one to six.
- The points 123 are on the left limb and 456 on the right limb **(Fig. 3.16A)**.

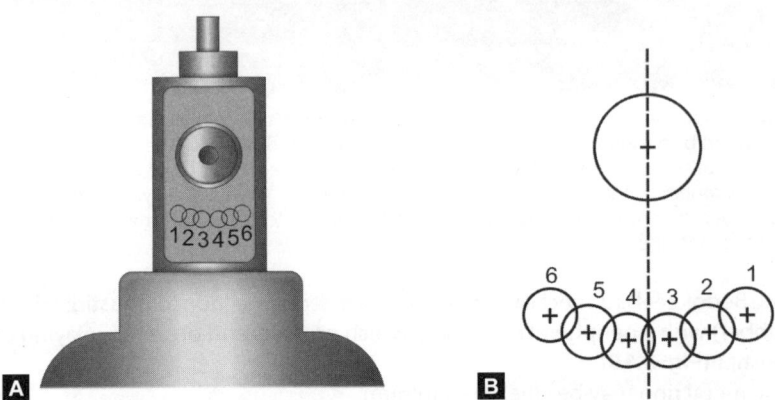

Figs 3.16A and B: The pin index: (A) The position of holes on a cylinder valve; (B) The position of pins in the yoke; • Note the "V" shaped positioning of the imaginary points one to six; • For Entonox (premixed 50% oxygen and 50% nitrous oxide), a central point numbered 7 is used

- The corresponding pins project from the yoke with the 'mirror image' numbers **(Fig. 3.16B)**.
- The pins are 4.75 mm in thick and 6 mm long. The pin for Entonox–7 is slightly thicker.
- A particular combination (configuration) of one from each side is used for a gas and is universally followed.
- For Entonox (50% N_2O + 50% O_2) a central point with the number 7 is used.
- The pin index for oxygen, nitrous oxide, Entonox, air and carbon-dioxide are shown in **(Figs 3.17A to D)**.

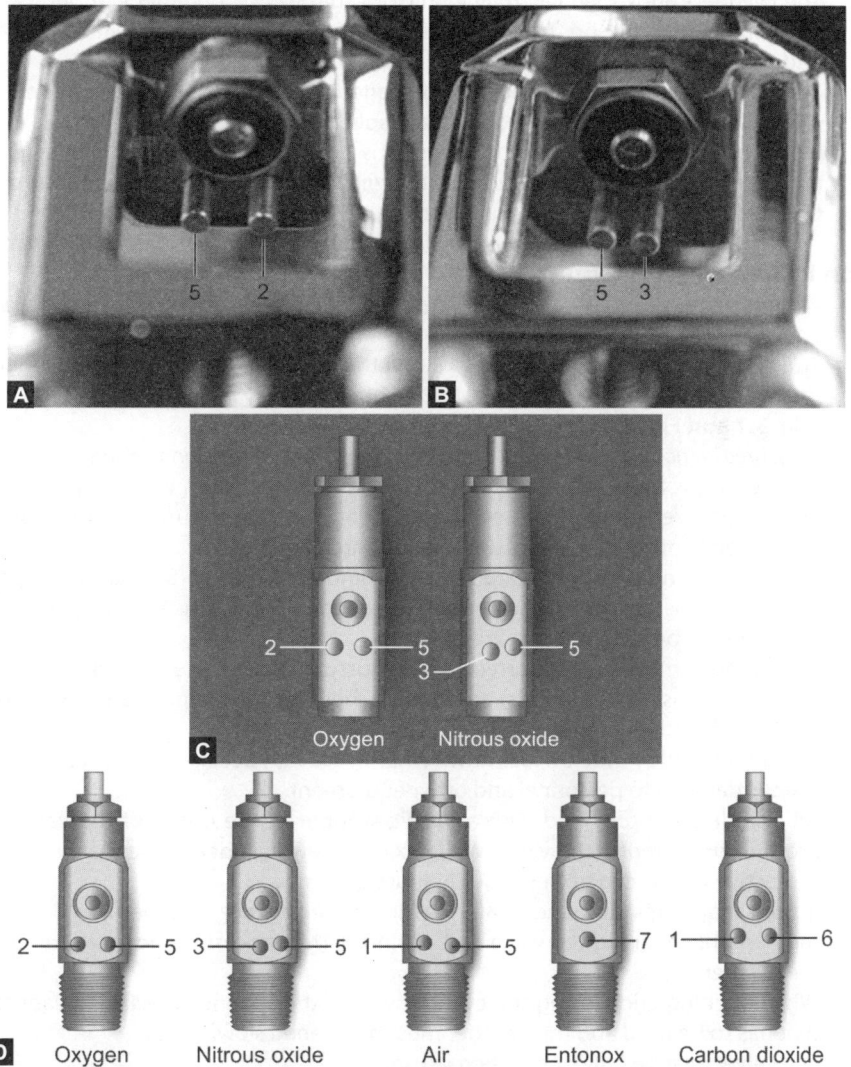

Figs 3.17A to D: (A) Yoke for Oxygen with mirror image pins for 2 and 5; (B) Yoke for nitrous oxide with mirror image pins for 3 and 5 (The striking difference in the position of pins may be noted); (C) Flush valve of Oxygen with holes 2 and 5; Flush valve of nitrous oxide with holes 3 and 5; (D) Configuration of pin index for various gases; (1) Oxygen 2 and 5; (2) Nitrous oxide 3 and 5; (3) Air 1 and 5; (4) Entonox 7; (5) Carbon dioxide 1 and 6

Pin Index

- O_2 - 2 and 5
- N_2O - 3 and 5
- Air   - 1 and 5
- CO_2 - 1 and 6
- Entonox - 7
- C_3H_6 - 3 and 6

Cautions and Rules to be Strictly Followed with Cylinders

- The cylinders are wiped carefully with cloth soaked in a detergent to clean any mud or any such dirt on the surface as soon as they reach the hospital premises and allowed to dry in shade.
- Then these cylinders are stored in the hospital in a clean well-ventilated room.
- All the cylinders must be stored vertically specially liquefied gases like N_2O.
- Before bringing it to the operating room, it is cleaned by dusting and wiping with a cloth soaked in any antiseptic. If not, it will increase the contamination in the operation theater.
- *All machines, including those on pipeline gases, should have full reserve cylinders attached, but turned off (Closed).*
- *Without a reserve full cylinder of oxygen (for any emergency) attached to the machine anesthesia should not be induced.*
- The cylinder should not be dragged along the floor. This will cause slow thinning out of the corners of the bottom of the cylinder and may result in danger bursting **(Fig. 3.1 and Fig. 3.3B)**.
- *Oil or grease should never be used on cylinders and pressure reducing valves,* as sudden release of gas from the cylinder and instant recompression into the pressure-reducing valve will generate enormous heat, which will burn the material in the presence of oxygen and cause a serious fire or explosion.
- A tag which indicates the status of the cylinder— 'Full'; 'In Service' or 'Empty' must always be present on the neck of the cylinder **(Fig. 3.18)**. An empty cylinder should never be left in the machine.
- The cylinder must be supported by the dorsum of foot and carefully fixed to the yoke by using two hands; one hand is holding the cylinder and the other securing the screw of the anesthetic machine.
- Insecurely fixed cylinders if falls down while in use may act like a missile and cause serious damage to personnel and other equipment.
- All cylinders are provided with a plastic stopper at the outlet of the valve to prevent dirt entering the valve. While fixing a new cylinder to the machine, the protective plastic cap from the outlet must be removed.
- If the stopper is not present, any dirt in the *flush valve* may be blown off by momentarily opening the valve and closing it. This process is known as *cracking the cylinder.*
- While opening and closing the cylinder valves, the spanner specially meant for that has to be used and the cylinder must be opened slowly.
- The valve must be fully open when in use.
- Too much force should not be used for closing or opening but must be optimum force of the wrist must be used.
- If there is any difficulty experienced in opening the spindle by the force of hand, a 'wooden hammer' or 'nylon headed soft hammer' may be used for opening by gentle repeated striking on the spanner **(Fig. 3.19)**.

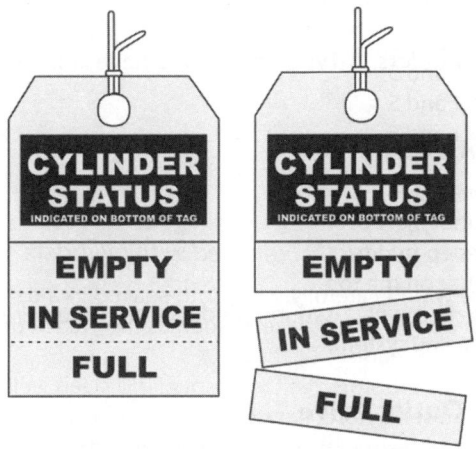

Fig. 3.18: The tag that indicates the status of the cylinder

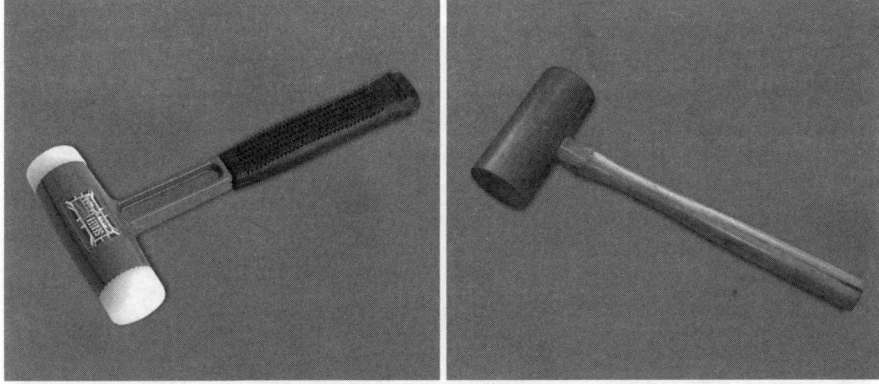

Fig. 3.19: Plastic hammer with nylon heads or wooden hammer. • If the force of hands is not sufficient to open the cylinder, no hard object must be used to strike the spanner; • These hammers with soft head must be used for gentle, repeated striking on the spanner handle for opening the valve

- No other hard objects should be used as it may permanently damage the spindle or the valve.
- It is important to note that in the older machines, yoke for oxygen cylinder is on the left side and nitrous oxide on the right side. In newer machines, this has been reversed that oxygen is on the right side.

Cracking the Cylinder

The protective plastic stopper may not present in the outlet of the flush valve. Hence, before fitting the cylinder to the yoke of the machine, just quickly open and close the valve so that a short burst of gases will blow away any dirt from the outlet. This is done pointing the outlet away from the user or any other person.

If this is not done, any dirt present in the outlet may get into the pressure reducing valve and other parts of the machine causing malfunctioning. This is referred to as cracking the cylinder.

Maximum amount of oxygen that can be stored inside a health care facility is 20,000 cu ft.

Other bigger cylinders, B-Type and above have only Bullnose type valves **(Fig. 3.20)**.

Bullnose Type of Valve

There are three types:
1. Straight with outlet on top
2. Straight with outlet on side
3. Angled with outlet on the top.

All these valves are mainly used in cylinders used for other purposes as in ward or in manifold of pipeline system.

Construction of Outlet Valve

It is made of brass metal, plated with chromium. The spindle is made of hard steel. The inner end of the spindle is cone shaped and it fits into a cone-shaped hollow in the cylinder outlet. Sometimes it may convex and fits on a flat opening of the cylinder. The leak of the gas around the spindle is prevented by a packing around it with a noncombustible material like asbestos rope or 'teflon' rope and it is tightened

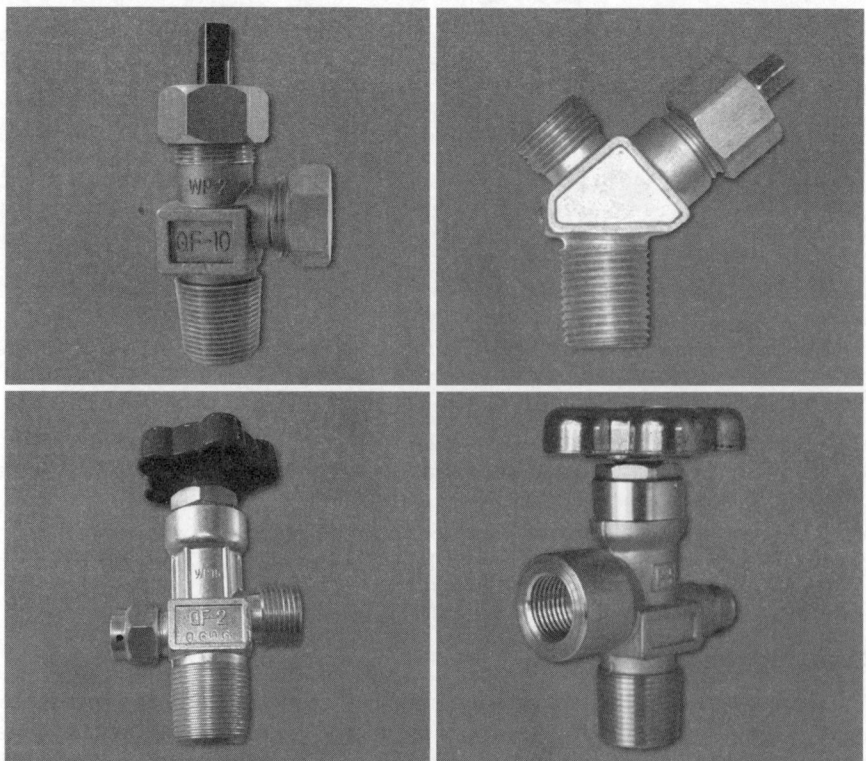

Fig. 3.20: Different varieties of 'Bullnose valves'. • Straight Bullnose, angled Bullnose and Bullnose with hand wheel; • The valves with hand wheels have safety valves attached on the back; • The vent hole of the pressure release valve could be seen

Medical Gas Cylinders

by a hexagonal gland nut. In medical cylinders, asbestos is eliminated because of the health hazard it may cause.

Oil or grease should never be used in any part of the valve. When the compressed gas under high pressure (from the cylinders) is released and recompressed instantly into a small closed space (high pressure chamber of pressure reducing valves), the heat of compression is not dissipated and enormous heat is generated in this process. This is called *'adiabatic compression'*. The heat generated in this process will ignite any combustible material like grease or oil if present in the vicinity and will cause fires or explosions.

Decanting or Filling of Cylinders

- A compressor pump is used for compressing gases into a cylinder to the required pressure.
- Liquid O_2 is evaporated and the gas is compressed into the cylinders by a pump until the pressure reaches 132 atm (1940 psi). Now the cylinder is said to be full. In recent years universally the filling pressure is standardized as 150 bar (atm)–2200 psi (approximately). After filling, the valve is covered with a metal cap to prevent injury or dust getting into the valve outlet (*See* **Fig. 3.2**).

Liquid O_2

Liquid oxygen is transported in vacuum insulated tanker. The tank is constructed with outer wall made of *steel* and inner wall made of *copper*. Activated charcoal is present between the walls, to absorb any trace of air making vacuum perfect.

1 Ton liquid oxygen = 26,540 cubic feet
1 Cubic foot = 28.3 L
Capacity of a tanker = 4–5 tons (approximate)

Since the critical temperature of O_2 is $-118°C$, it cannot be liquefied (compressed into a liquid) at room temperature of $20°C$. At $-118°C$ at a pressure of 50 atm, it is liquefied.

Oxygen Bottling Unit

- We can see liquid O_2 in open vessels, but there the temperature is very low.
- When liquid oxygen is transferred to a thermos flask open to atmosphere, it continues to boil furiously.
- But the latent heat of vaporization has to come from the liquid itself. So the temperature of the liquid falls rapidly.
- When the temperature falls below $-183°C$ (boiling point of liquid O_2) the liquid ceases to boil and at this point the vapor pressure at this temperature is no longer more than 1 atmosphere.

In a cylinder, liquid O_2 is not possible because;

- Pressure required will be 4000–5000 atm (60,000 psi)
- The storage at this pressure will be impractical (It will be like a bomb, may explode)
- The cylinder wall has to be extremely thick to stand this pressure.
- The packing gland nut for this pressure is difficult to construct.
- At this pressure O_2 causes spontaneous ignition of cylinder material.
- A risk of forming cracks in the cylinder is more.

Cylinders to stand 5000 atm have been made for experimental purpose. The cylinders in common use are thin walled.

Points to be remembered on oxygen and nitrous oxide cylinders
- The present day medical gas cylinders are made of *molybdenum steel alloy*, which has very high tensile strength, and stand very high pressure.
- Cylinders for both oxygen and nitrous oxide are manufactured in the same standards and subjected to the same type of tests for safety.

Oxygen Cylinders

- Oxygen is commercially prepared by fractional distillation of liquefied air. Before liquefaction, the carbon dioxide is removed.
- Afterwards, the oxygen and nitrogen are separated using the difference in their boiling points.
- The boiling point of oxygen is –182.5°C. The boiling point of nitrogen is –195°C.
- Therefore, the oxygen will escape first during evaporation.
- This gas is collected purified and compressed through a pump to a pressure of about 1800–2,000 psi and stored in the cylinders.
- Under normal conditions of temperature it cannot be liquefied so it is always in gaseous form in cylinders.
- The cylinders are *colored black body with white shoulder.*
- Oxygen cylinders are available in various sizes.
- There are only two sizes, which can be directly attached to the anesthetic machine.
  - 12 cu ft (AA Type)—This is no longer in use.
  - 20 cu ft (A-Type).
- These two types are supplied with *flush valves* that can be directly fixed to the yoke of the machine. The 12 cu ft (AA Type) is almost withdrawn as it is not economical.
- 40 cu ft (B-Type) are commonly used in wards for oxygen therapy.
- Bulk cylinders (D Type) are commonly used for feeding the manifold of the central pipeline supply of gases. These are fitted with *Bullnose valves.*
- When the cylinders are brought into the operating room, special and adequate precautions to maintain asepsis are to be taken as *these cylinders are transported and stored in different steps in very unclean atmosphere are responsible for contaminating the theater atmosphere.*
- Oxygen cylinder sizes and capacities
  - Height in inches: 18   31   34   49   57
  - Sizes: AA   A   B   C   D
  - Capacity (Liters): 340   680   1360   3400   6800
- The pressure of full cylinder is 150 kg/sq cm (2000 psi)
- A content of full cylinder, as the number of liters is noted on the valve. (e.g. 335 L)
- During the use if the pressure has fallen to 100 kg/sq cm, it indicates that 2/3rds of the contents remain inside. Approximately 200 L of gas.
- This is very useful information in the considerations of safety.

Nitrous Oxide Cylinders

- Nitrous oxide is a liquefiable gas.
- At a pressure of 750 psi, it is liquefied.
- The cylinders are colored *French Blue.*

- Though the pressure is low, same standard cylinder as for oxygen is used because if a cylinder is exposed to a high temperature as in hot sun, at 65°C, all the liquid is converted to vapor and a pressure of 2600 psi may be reached.
- AA" and "A" Type cylinders are in use with anesthetic machine. Most commonly used is "A" Type.
- For manifold of central pipeline "D" type bulk cylinders are used.
- There is difference in the position of yokes of oxygen and nitrous oxide between the older anesthetic machines and the newer ones manufactured after eighties.
- In older machines, the yokes for oxygen are on the left side of the machine and nitrous oxide on the right side.
- In newer machines, it is seen in the reverse, i.e. oxygen yokes are on the right side and nitrous oxide on the left side. (downstream position of oxygen)
- This change was made *as a safety measure to keep the flow meter of oxygen to be kept at the downstream, to reduce the chance of hypoxic mixtures being delivered to the patient* even if there is a small leak in the flow meter bank.
- Contents of the N_2O cylinder can be calculated by the weight of gas in the cylinder.
- From the total weight of cylinder deduct the tare weight–gives the weight of the gas.
- 455 L of nitrous oxide weighs 850 g. The content can be calculated.

Filling Ratio

In liquefiable gases like nitrous oxide, the liquid is not filled to the full volume of the cylinder.

The degree of filling of a nitrous oxide cylinder is expressed as *the mass of nitrous oxide* in a cylinder divided by *the mass of water* that the cylinder could hold. Normally, a cylinder of nitrous oxide is filled to a ratio of 0.67.

Filling ratio is defined as the weight of the gas in full cylinder/weight of water which the cylinder can hold.

This should not be confused with the volume of liquid nitrous oxide in a cylinder. A full cylinder of nitrous oxide at room temperature is filled to the point at which approximately 90% of the interior of the cylinder is occupied by the liquid, the remaining 10% being occupied by gaseous nitrous oxide.

Simply, filling ratio is the weight of the fluid in the cylinder divided by the weight of the water required to fill it.

Practical significance of the 'Filling ratio' has been discussed in detail in Chapter 1.

Critical Temperature

The temperature to which the gas must be cooled before it could be liquefied by pressure.

N_2O – 36.5°C
O_2 – –116°C

Critical Pressure

The minimum pressure which is required to liquefy the gas at it is critical temperature.

N_2O — 71 atmospheres (1000 psi)
O_2 — 50 atmospheres (750 psi)

Practical significance
- Critical temperature of N_2O is 36.5°C.
- At this temperature, 74 atm pressure is required to liquefy it.
- But at room temperature (20°C), 50 atm pressures is sufficient to liquefy it.
- There is a misconception that N_2O is always at 750 psi in cylinders (51 atms).
- The vapor pressure above the liquid like any other gas varies with the temperature.
  At –89°C, vapor pressure falls below 1 atm
  But above this at,

0° C	–	31 atm
10° C	–	40 atm
20° C	–	51 atm

- During *hot climate,* the working conditions will often be above the critical temp of N_2O (36.5°C) and the *contents of the cylinder will be wholly gaseous.*
- Although the cylinder contents change from liquid to gas, there is no sudden raise of pressure in the cylinder as the critical temperature is past.

35° C	—	72 atmosphere vapor pressure
37° C	—	76 atmospheres

- At tropical conditions, the cylinders may attain, high temperature as 65°C when pressure of a full cylinder is 175 atmosphere (2600 psi).
- On account of this, N_2O cylinders are also submitted to the same pressure test as O_2 cylinders.

When the N_2O cylinder in use in the machine is opened, the liquid is converted to gas rapidly to maintain a constant vapor pressure, and the consumption of heat is sufficiently rapid. The liquid N_2O and the cylinder temperature falls rapidly and the temperature of the air in the immediately neighborhood falls, so that water vapor condenses on the cylinders and snow may be formed on the wall of the cylinder. This corresponds to the level of the liquid gas in the cylinder. Water vapor in the gases as impurity may condense in the valve and choke the valve outlet. Nowadays, the purification is complete and it is perfectly dried. So such problems do not occur.

FURTHER READING

1. Baha Al Shaikh, Simon Stacey. Essentials of Anaesthetic Equipment, 1st edn. London, Churchill Livingstone, 1995.
2. Das S, Chattopadhyay S, Bose P. The anaesthesia gas supply system. Indian J Anaesth. 2013;57:489-99.
3. Howell RSC. Piped medical gas and vacuum systems. Anaesthesia. 1980;35;676-98.
4. Jerry A Dorsch, Susan E Dorsch. Understanding Anaesthesia Equipment, 4th edn. London. Lippincott Williams and Wilkins, 1999.
5. Jerry A Dorsch, Susan E Dorsch. Understanding Anaesthesia Equipment, 5th edn. London, Lippincott Williams and Wilkins, 2008.
6. John TB Moyle, Andrew Davey. Ward's Anaesthetic Equipment, 4th edn. London. WB Saunders Company Limited, 1998.
7. Lee's Synopsis of Anaesthesia. 11th edn, London. Butterworth- Heinemann Ltd., 1993.
8. Ward CS. Anaesthetic Equipment, 2nd edn. London: Balliere, S, 1985.

Medical Gas Pipeline System

chapter 4

Medical gas pipeline system (MGPS) is the provision of storing the medical gases oincluding oxygen, nitrous oxide and air in a central point, and supplying these medical gases through pipeline to the point of use through out the hospital.

As vacuum is included in this pipeline system along with the gases some name it as piped medical gas and vacuum (PMGV).

The vacuum is for suctioning as well as for scavenging waste gases.

This is governed by the law HTM 02-01 of UK (Department of Health. Health Technical Memorandum 02-01) and NFPA 99 (National Fire Protection Act Standards) of USA.

IS 12827 (1989): Nonflammable medical gas pipeline systems [MHD 11: Anesthetic, Resuscitation and Allied Equipment] is the law that governs this.

Medical gas pipeline system provides a safe, convenient and costs effective supply of medical gases. It eliminates many problems associated with the use of gas cylinders.

PIPELINE OF MEDICAL GASES

It includes three components:
1. A source of gas supply—cylinders
2. A pipeline extending from the source to the point of utility
3. A terminal unit at each point of use.

- In bigger hospitals, four pipelines would be running along the walls to operation theater, postoperative ward, intensive care unit (ICU) and other wards.
- These are pipelines carrying *oxygen, nitrous oxide, compressed air* and *vacuum* to various destinations.
- Usually pipelines to the operation theater supply the anesthetic gases—oxygen, nitrous oxide, compressed air and vacuum.
- Compressed air supplied by pipeline is used in modern anesthesia machines. It is used for driving pneumatic equipment such as drills and for operating ventilators as well.
- For other wards of the hospital, pipelines supply oxygen and vacuum necessary for applying suction.
- The central pipeline receives gas from large cylinders kept elsewhere in the hospital and that place is known as *Manifold room*.

Advantages of Central Pipeline Supply

Asepsis

- Cylinders transported from distant place of manufacture are likely to carry dirt and contamination.
- The large D-Type cylinders (also known as bulk cylinders or 50 L water capacity cylinders) are used in the manifold of central pipeline supply.

- They are not brought into the operating theater complex. Hence, this source of contamination is eliminated.

Simple
It is practically easier to use pipeline supply of gases in anesthetic machines by plugging probes and flexible hoses from the self-sealing valve of the outlet (Schrader self-sealing valve). Flexible hose carries the gas to the machine.

Economical
- Cost of gas in bulk cylinders are relatively less compared to the cost of gas in small cylinders used in anesthesia machines.
- Investment on cylinders is considerably reduced, as the number of bulk cylinders required is significantly less.

Efficient
Continuous uninterrupted supply is possible without much wastage of gases.

Reliable and Safe
Automatic changeover in manifold control panel maintains uninterrupted supply of gases and assures safety.

Saves Space
- Manifold room occupies relatively less space away from the main building.
- Storing small cylinders for anesthetic machine in large number is cumbersome and occupies more space.

Psychological Effects
- The sight of an oxygen cylinder causes a big psychological impact on the patient and relatives.
- Particularly an oxygen cylinder near the postoperative bed makes them feel anxious.
- In central pipeline system, the cylinders are far away from the sight of patient and relatives.

The station where bulk cylinders are kept for feeding the central pipeline is known as the Manifold Room.

MANIFOLD ROOM
- A convenient well-ventilated spacious room in the ground floor well away from the operation theater and wards for easy transportability of bulk cylinders.
- It is a fireproof room **(Fig. 4.1A)**, constructed with non-flammable material and must have easy accessibility for transporting vehicle to reach.

Gas Manifold and Control Panel
- When a number of cylinders are connected simultaneously into a single pipe through many side connections which has a single outlet, it is called a Manifold **(Figs 4.1A to C)**. It is a terminology of automobile industry.

Medical Gas Pipeline System 95

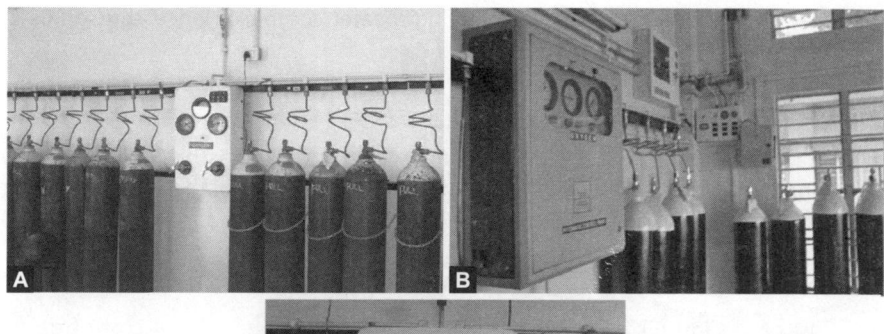

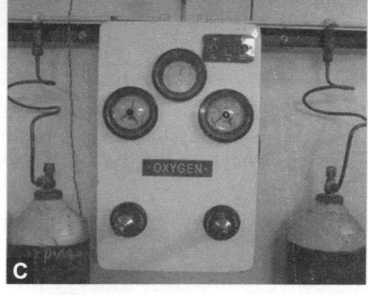

Figs 4.1A to C: Oxygen manifold in the manifold room: (A) Oxygen manifold with two banks and control panel; • The coiled copper tail pipes connect the cylinder to the manifold, manual control panel is seen; • (B) It is a well-ventilated room; • Manifold with electronic control panel; • Four spare cylinders are seen on the side; • There are three pressure gauges; • The two pressure gauges on the sides show the pressure of the cylinders in each bank while the one pressure gauge in the center shows the pipeline pressure; (C) Manual control panel (semi-automatic) with the three pressure gauges; • Three pressure gauges; two on the sides for manifolds with minimum contact gauge, the one on the center is for pipeline pressure; • There are three indicator lamps seen on the top; one in the center indicates that the pipeline is ON; • The other two warning lights are to indicate the exhausted bank of cylinders

- Usually, the manifold room houses the manifolds for oxygen and nitrous oxide.
- There are two 'manifold systems' with central control panel for oxygen and nitrous oxide.
- Ideally, the air compressor and tank for oil-free filtered air "medical air" and vacuum pump and vacuum tank are not housed in the same room, though some hospitals prefer to have it for convenience of operation.

Oxygen Pipeline

- Uninterrupted supply of oxygen through pipeline is derived from two manifolds that are provided on either side of an automatic device in the center known as Central control panel.
- *D-Type* cylinders (50 LWC or Bulk cylinders) with 'Bull nose' valves are connected to the manifold through especially designed coiled copper 'tail pipes' **(Figs 4.2A to C)**.
- The tail pipes have 'gas specific threads' and hexagonal nuts. It is not possible to connect a wrong gas in the manifold **(Figs 4.2A to C)**.
- To prevent 'transfilling'—flow of gases from one cylinder to another 'non-return valves' are used **(Figs 4.3A and B)**.

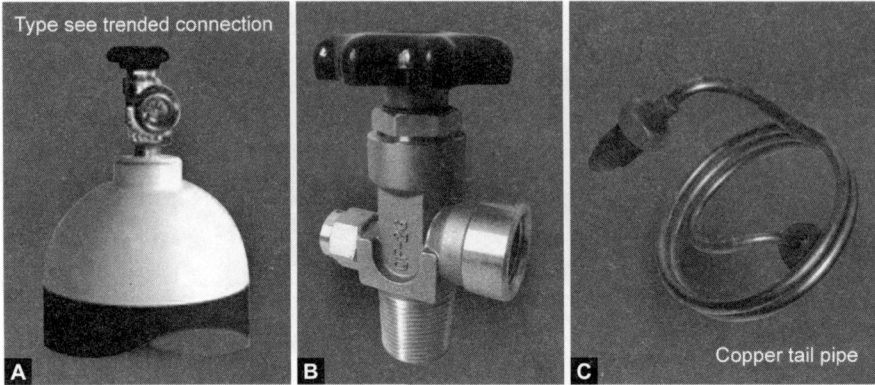

Figs 4.2A to C: Cylinder with Bullnose valve, bullnose valve and the tail pipe; • The cylinder has 'Bullnose' valve with hand wheel; • The bullnose valve has hand wheel and a pressure release valve; • Some Bullnose valves do not have hand wheel but special wrench is used to open

- The number of cylinders connected to each manifold depends upon the requirements of the hospital.
- Each side of manifold (known as 'bank of cylinders') must contain an average four day's supply and a minimum of two cylinders at least.
- One of the manifolds will be the *Running bank* of cylinders (Duty bank) from which the gas flows into the pipeline, while the other manifold will be the Reserve bank.
- A 'control panel' with double shut off valve and a central pressure reducer is used.
- When the *Running bank* is near exhaustion, the *Reserve bank* automatically takes over and maintains uninterrupted supply in the pipeline.
- Simultaneously, two warning lamps one situated on the control panel and another in the theater complex are activated to warn the anesthesiologist that the Running bank is getting exhausted.
- The double shut off valve makes the *Reserve bank to automatically* take over.
- A simple design of this unit with multiple cylinders on each side is shown in **Figure 4.1A**.
- The changeover done at the control panel may be fully automatic by electronic controls **(Fig. 4.1B)** or it can be partially automatic **(Fig. 4.1C)**.
- For automatic changeover during use, all the cylinders in both the manifolds will be kept open.
- Apart from the cylinders connected to the manifold, spare cylinders in the number equal to one bank must be stored in manifold room.
- While servicing of the manifold is being carried out, the outlet valve from the panel to the line may be closed.
- There will be provision for connecting a single bulk cylinder with pressure reducing valve in the pipeline for feeding the pipeline during this time.

Control Panel

It may be *Fully automatic electronic control panel* or *Semiautomatic mechanical control panel* **(Fig. 4.1)**.
Purpose
- Reducing the cylinder pressure to the pipeline pressure (60 psi or 4 bar—working pressure of the machines)
- Maintaining uninterrupted supply of gas in the pipeline.

Medical Gas Pipeline System

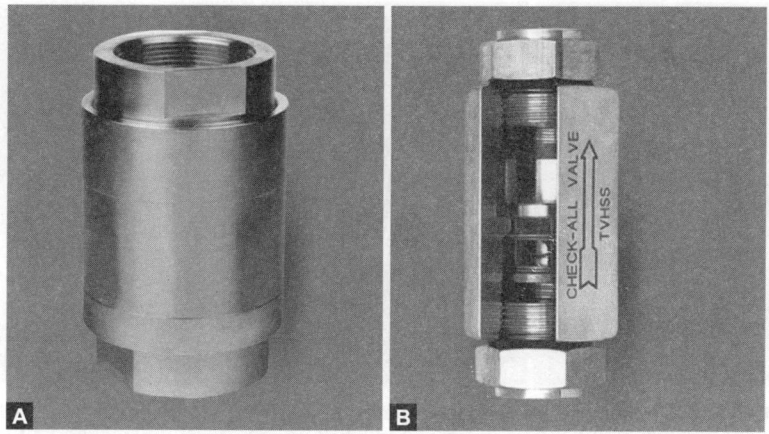

Figs 4.3A and B: Non-return valve. Non-return valve to be fixed in the manifold where tail pipe joins; • This valve prevents reverse flow of gases and transfilling of cylinders; • The mechanism is shown in the Figure B

The control panel consists of *six components:*
1. *Two pressure reducing valves* for reducing the output pressure of the two manifolds to a level just above the final outlet pressure.
2. *Two pressure gauges* to assess the pressure in each manifold **(Fig. 4.1C)**. This is a special gauge known as *'minimum contact gauge*. It is provided with *a central knob that can adjust set the pressure desired to activate the warning lamp*. Usually, it is set at a pressure little higher than the final out let pressure–say 5 or 6 bar. It will have electrical contacts which are connected to a low voltage control system to activate the warning lamp and alarm **(Figs 4.4A and B)**.
3. *A shuttle valve* to make the automatic changeover.
4. *A common outlet pathway with a central pressure reducing valve* that reduces the pressure of the common outlet as 4 bar (60 psi) **(*See* Fig. 4.1C)**.
5. *Two handles fixed to the pressure reducing valves* of the manifolds that can be turned to set the 'Running bank' and 'Reserve bank' as required.
6. *Two red warning lamps* for each manifold to indicate exhaustion and an amber lamp to indicate that the pipeline is on.

Modern control panels 'the pressure difference' between the running and reserve banks is used for automatic switch over of reserve bank when the running bank is exhausted **(Fig. 4.5)**.

Instead of 'Minimum contact gauges' sensitive 'Pressure switches' which work on low voltage DC current are used on the manifold outlets to activate warning lamps in present day manifolds **(Fig. 4.5)**.

For N_2O electrically operated, thermostatically controlled heating system maintaining at 47°C is used in the control panel to prevent freezing of gas within and choking the flow (In countries where ambient temperature falls very low to freezing levels).

Partial Automatic System

- When 'Running bank' is exhausted and the warning lamp is activated with alarm.
- Now, the technician will *manually* turn a lever of the pressure reducing valve (RV) of that side, so that the Reserve bank will now become the Running bank.

98 Anesthetic Equipment Made Easy

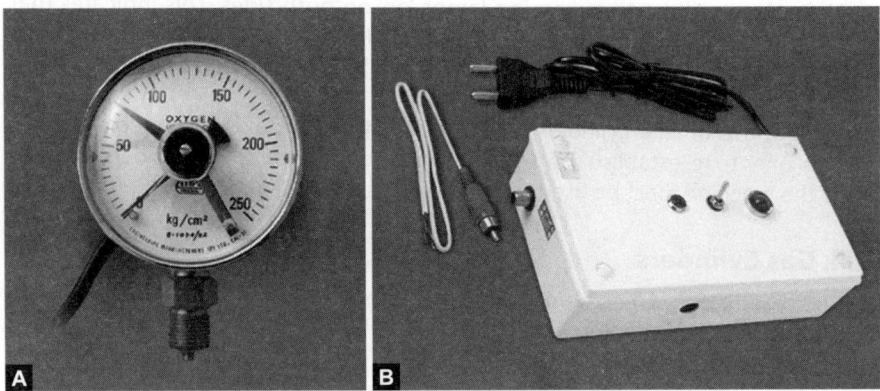

Figs 4.4A and B: Minimum contact gauge and its alarm device; • The central knob on the dial can be rotated to adjust the lowest pressure at which the electrical contact should be made to activate the audiovisual indication

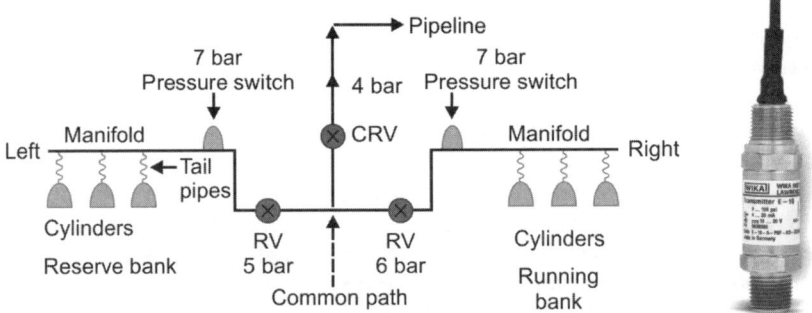

Fig. 4.5: Schematic representation of modern control panel and pressure switch
• The pressure reducing valve (RV) in the 'Reserve bank' is set as 5 bar • The pressure reducing valve (RV) in 'Running bank' is set as 6 bar (1 bar higher) • The central reducing valve (CRV) is set at 4 bar • On both sides the pressure switch is set at 7 bar to activate the warning lamp, • All the cylinders in both the banks (Reserve and Running) kept fully open. Because the Running bank outlet pressure is set higher (6 bar) than the outlet pressure of Reserve bank (5 bar), preferential flow occurs from the Running bank to the Central reducing valve (CRV) where it is reduced further to 4 bar and flows into the pipeline • When the pressure drops to 7 bar in the 'Running bank', the warning lamp is activated to indicate that the bank is nearing exhaustion • When the pressure drops below 5 bar automatically preferential flow from the Reserve bank will start and it will take over the supply

- Then he will replace the empty cylinders with full cylinders and open them and change the lever to 'Reserve'.
- Now the new cylinders connected will form the "Reserve bank".
- Once the reserve bank is full and is open, the warning lamp will go OFF.
- In case, the exhausted cylinders are not replaced with full cylinders, the warning lamp continues to be 'ON'.
- Now the 'Running bank' is empty and the supply to the pipeline is from the reserve bank.
- When the second bank also is nearing exhaustion, as it reaches the set pressure, it activates a second warning lamp.

Medical Gas Pipeline System

- Now, there will be two warning lamps 'on' on both sides. This indicates that central pipeline supply will fail soon, if the cylinders are not replaced.
- There are two sets of warning lamps (**Fig. 4.1C**) one set on the panel and the other set at the operation theater.
- Even at this time, if cylinders in the manifold room could not be replaced with new ones to re-establish the pipeline supply, the A-Type spare cylinders attached to the machine must be used as standby until the pipeline supply is restored.

Bulk Gas Cylinders

- The cylinders used for feeding the manifolds of central pipeline system are known as D-Type cylinders (Note that different countries have different names for this cylinder).
- In India, D-Type cylinders are of 50 L water capacity (LWC).
- In a cylinder with *1 L water* capacity *150 bar* pressure will compress 150 L of O_2 into it.
- The water capacity of D-Type cylinder is approximately 47 L and the exact volume is usually seen printed on the shoulder of the cylinder. However, for convenience, we take 50 L as the volume.
- Full pressure in oxygen cylinder is 150 bars (2,000 psi). Therefore, the full cylinder has $150 \times 50 = 7500$ L of gas.
- Hence, if there are four "D-Type cylinders in a bank, then the total gas available is $7,500 \times 4 = 30,000$ L (Approximately).
- These cylinders come with "Bullnose valves" which have screw threaded outlets to which the screw threads of "Copper tail pipe" is connected and tightened. These screw threads are 'gas specific' and cannot be connected other gas cylinders (**Figs 4.2A to C**).
- The outlets may be pointing upwards or on the sides and depending upon that the suitable type of tail pipes are used.
- At the manifold end, a 'non return valve' is incorporated to allow unidirectional flow and to prevent transfilling of cylinders (**Figs 4.3A and B**).
- There may be small variations in the tail pipes of different gas suppliers.

Safety Precautions in a Manifold Room

- The manifolds must be housed in a well-ventilated room constructed with fireproof material such as concrete.
- Ventilators must be provided at the top and bottom of the room.
- It must have adequate space for handling trolleys, bulky cylinders, for easy changing of cylinders on the manifold, keeping extra reserve cylinders, etc.
- No oil, grease, or any other flammable material should be brought into the room.
- There should be no "High Voltage" electricity cable in the vicinity.
- There should be no drains or gulleys where gas can collect.
- The compressors and reservoir for the central vacuum plant and the plant for medical compressed air should not be housed in the manifold room.
- Provision should be made for securing the cylinders to the wall (**Fig. 4.1A**).
- All the personnel should be made to understand that compressed gas, particularly; oxygen can be dangerous, if mishandled.
- Fire extinguishers of adequate size in adequate numbers must be available at strategic points.

INDICATORS AND ALARMS

- Since the manifolds are usually situated remote from the users and the staff who are responsible for changing the cylinders (a Senior Anesthesia Technician in the name of manifold room technician), indicators are installed to indicate and warn about the status of gas source in the manifold.
- Indicators will be available in manifold room and in operating theater suite so that the anesthesiologist as well as the person responsible for changing the cylinders is informed.
- The indicators or alarms are of two types: it may be "visual alarm" or "audible alarm". Commonly both are present in the same unit. If needed audible alarm may be silenced.
- The visual indicators are in the form of lights (green, red and amber).
- Normally, running is indicated by green light. Red light or flashing orange when a bank is nearing empty.
- When a cylinder bank nears exhaustion, as sensed by a predetermined pressure, the indicator is activated.
- It is activated by the minimum contact gauge. The system is shown in **Figures 4.4A and B**.
- When the cylinders are replenished, the alarm stops.
- The contact gauge has electrical contacts. It should be connected to the pipeline gas failure alarm, which has two signal lights, a buzzer and an "ON/OFF" switch **(Figs 4.4A and B)**.
- When the contact gauge is connected to the power supply and the ON/OFF switch of the alarm is switched "ON", green light will show indicating that the electrical supply serving the contact gauge and alarm are working correctly.
- The green light should show at all-times when the pipeline is in use.
- The other red light is a warning light which is automatically switched ON and the buzzer rings when the pressure in the running cylinder has fallen to a determined value.
- Put the switch to OFF position after which the reserve cylinders should be brought into operation (running) by turning the handle provided, promptly to ensure continuity of supply.
- After this, the empty cylinders are replaced with full cylinders in the exhausted bank and are opened fully. Now the warning lamp will go OFF. Switching the handle to "Reserve" will make the steps complete.

Pressure Sensors or Switches

- In modern manifolds, instead of the *Minimum contact gauge*, more sensitive and safe *Pressure sensor switches* working on low voltage are used on the manifolds of both right and left banks to activate the warning device **(Fig. 4.5)**.
- The desired pressure to activate the warning lamp can be set in the switch and connected to the warning lamps.
- When the pressure in the outlet of the bank falls below the set value (usually 7 bar), it activates a warning lamp on the panel as well as in the operating theater to indicate that the respective bank is nearing exhaustion (Empty).

Modern Control Panels

- Modern control panels are simplified.
- Double shut off valves are eliminated and automatic takeover is done by the drop in pressure of the manifold outlet.

Medical Gas Pipeline System

- Schematic representation shown in **Figure 4.5**.
  The pressures set in the system in the following way: (1 bar is approximately 1 kg):
  Pressure switches   - 7 bar
  Running bank reducing valve (RV) - 6 bar
  Reserve bank reducing valve (RV) - 5 bar
  Central reducing valve (CRV)   - 4 bar
- In the semi automatic control panel the reserve bank will start working as soon as the running manifolds outlet pressure becomes equal to the reserve banks outlet pressure (5 bar).
- As the running banks cylinder pressure has gone down the reserve bank takes over to feed the pipeline.
- It will not wait for the pressure to go down further as a very small differential pressure is sufficient for change over.
- The 'nonreturn valves prevent transfilling into the other side.
  The **Figure 4.5** shows the right manifold (Bank) and the left manifold having 3 cylinders connected by coiled tail pipes.
- The pressure switch is connected to manifold pipe on both sides before the pipe enters the pressure reducing valves (RV).
- The pressure switch is set at 7 bar. This means that when the pressure in the cylinders falls from 150 bar to a level below 7 bar (almost nearing empty), the switch will activate the warning lamp.
- The pressure of the cylinders in the bank (2000 psi or 150 kg/sq cm or 150 bar) is reduced by the pressure reducing valves RV.
- This outlet pressure in the pressure reducing valve is set a little lower than the pressure (7 bar) set in the set in the pressure switch.
- Taking right bank as 'Running bank' the outlet pressure in the reducing valve is set as 6 kg or 6 bar.
- The left bank is now the 'Reserve bank'. So, the outlet pressure in the reducing valve is set one kg lower, 5 kg or 5 bar.
- Both these outlets from the banks join at the centre and proceed as a single pipe (common path) towards the central valve (CRV).
- This central reducing valve (CRV) further reduces the pressure to 4 bar (60 psi) and allows to flow into the pipeline to the operating theater.
- When all the cylinders in both the banks are open, the outlet pressure of the running bank (Right) 6 bar, which is 1 bar higher than the outlet pressure of the reserve bank (Left) 5 bar. Hence, the flow from the left bank is opposed and there will be flow only from the right bank to the pipeline.
- This flow of gas will continue till the outlet pressure of the right bank drops a little lower than that of the left bank, say 4.5 bar.
- At this point, because the right bank outlet pressure is lower than the left bank outlet pressure, flow of gases start from the left bank and left bank automatically takes over.
- This allows uninterrupted supply of gases to the pipeline.
- Now, the empty cylinders in the right bank are replaced with new cylinders and the controls are set as "Reserve" on the right side and "Running" on the left side by turning the handles provided for that. This will reset the outlet pressure of right and left banks.

The most important things to be remembered at this point are:
- *The pressure switches are set at 7 kg and so the warning lamp will be activated sufficiently before the supply of the gas exhausts.* It means still there is gas present

in the cylinder (2 bar pressure) to feed the pipeline for some more time before the reserve bank takes over.
- So, when the running bank cylinders are nearing exhaustion, and sufficiently before the reserve bank cylinders takeover automatically, the warning lamp is activated, and indicates it in control panel of manifold room as well as in operation theater.
- At the earliest possible time, technician visits the manifold room, replaces the exhausted cylinders and fixes full cylinders to the manifold, and then turns the control in such a way that the newly fixed cylinders now become 'Reserve bank' and the other side is 'Running bank'.
- When this change is done the warning lamp goes 'OFF'.

PIPELINES AND ISOLATION VALVES

- The pipes are made of medical grade copper and the joints are made with gas welding.
- Copper to brass welding is generally not permitted on site as flux is used for brazing which can leave a residue, which will be difficult to clean and degrease on site.
- So copper-to-copper brazing only is permitted with a special CP104 brazing rod which has silver, copper and phosphorous alloy.
- The pipes of suitable size is used depending upon the volume of use and are color coded. Some countries use same color entire length where as in India 3" strip of color is painted at specific intervals.
- There are shut off valves which help to isolate specific areas of pipeline system for maintenance service purpose **(Fig. 4.6)**.

Terminal Outlets (Wall Outlet of Pipeline)

- From the main pipeline that runs near the roof, smaller pipes are drawn down perpendicular to the main line as drops in the required points of use in operating room, postanesthetic care unit (PACU), postoperative wards, ICU, etc.
- These pipes end in wall outlet units. All these outlets have self-sealing valve that prevent gas leak.

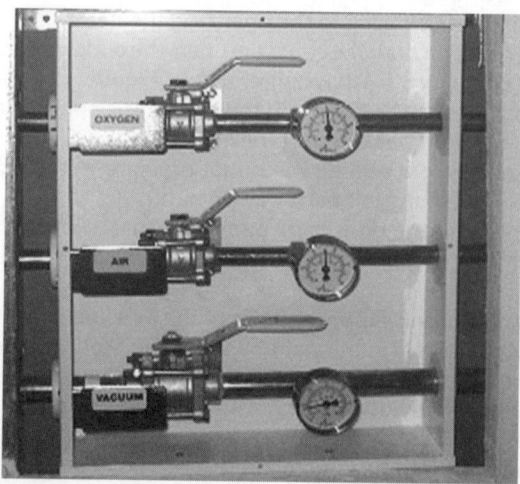

Fig. 4.6: Isolation valves (Regional shut off valve in a box) of the line. • These valves can be closed to isolate the region, so that there is no gas flows in the pipeline that region of supply; • Necessary service can be done in that region without interruption of supply to other regions

- Commonly "Schrader self-sealing valves" are in use **(Figs 4.7B and C)**.
- Usually, the terminal unit provided on the wall as a unit. All the outlets arranged in a row (oxygen, nitrous oxide, medical air and vacuum) **(Fig. 4.7A)**.
- Color-coded flexible hoses carry gases from the outlet point to the machine.
- There are color-coded hoses with gas specific; 'collar indexed' (diameter) probes at one end of the hose and pin indexed 'Yoke Block' **(Fig. 4.7F)** at the other end are used for connecting the machine to the wall outlet **(Figs 4.7D and E)**.
- The probes have a protruding "collar index" that is gas specific with different diameter for each gas **(Fig. 4.7D)**.
- It is impossible to connect a wrong probe (Collar indexed) into an outlet.
- Similarly, it is impossible to connect the 'Yoke block' (Pin-indexed) to the wrong yoke.
- The pin indexed 'Yoke block' **(Fig. 4.7F)** is kept fixed permanently in the yoke assembly and the probe is plugged into the wall outlet to make connection instantly.
- It is easy to insert or remove the probe using one hand. The Schrader valve socket assembly has a spring loaded outer ring which when depressed releases the mechanism that holds the probe and ejects it.

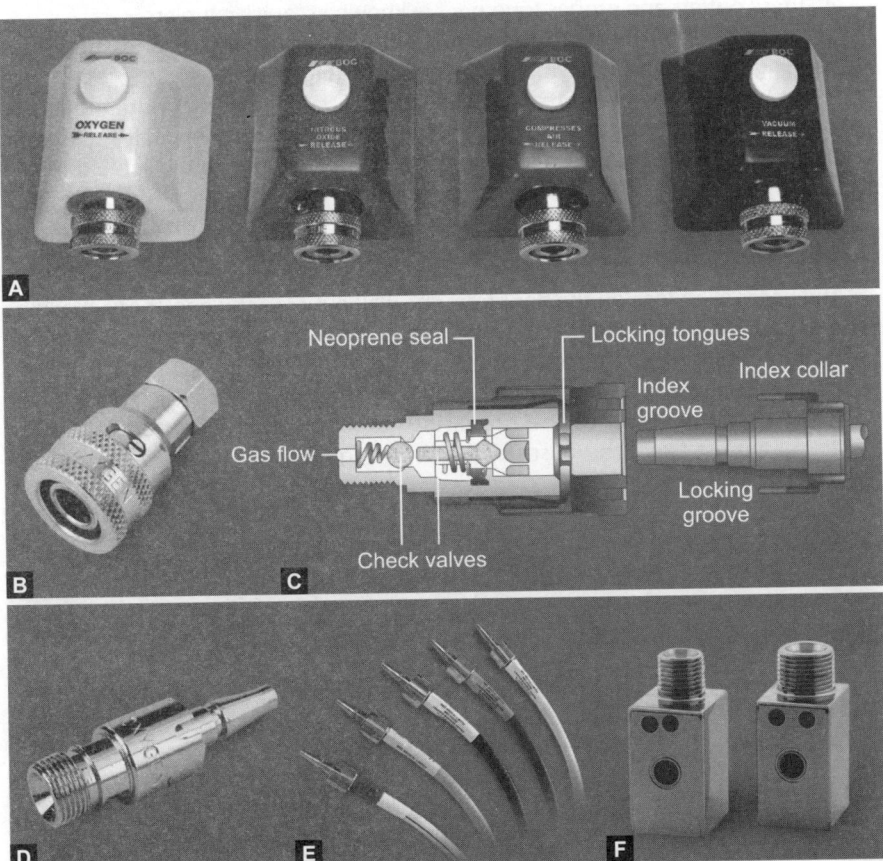

Figs 4.7A to F: Schrader type self-sealing valves, probes and hoses with probes. • Color-coded Schrader self-sealing outlet valve with color coded casing for oxygen, nitrous oxide, air and vacuum; • Schrader valve • The self-sealing mechanism of the Schrader valve • Diameter-coded probe 'Collar indexed' • Different 'Gas specific' - 'Collar indexed' probes fixed with color-coded hoses • Yoke Block with pin index

104 Anesthetic Equipment Made Easy

- In modern Anesthesia Workstations at the machine end of the hose non-interchangeable screw threads (NIST) are provided to prevent wrong gas connections **(Figs 4.8A and B)**.
- These are actually not noninterchangeable screw threads, but the unique connector probes are gas specific and non-interchangeable. The nuts have the same diameter and screw threads for all the gas services. Hence, the name NIST is a misnomer and misleading.
- For use in wards, for individual beds, usually oxygen and suction (vacuum) are provided as individual wall outlets.
- In Schrader self-sealing valves the probes can be plugged in from below.
- Some wall outlets have provision that the probe can be plugged in from the front **(Fig. 4.9)**.
- These valves (plugging from front) have double locking type with a 'parking, position. When the probe is plugged in with the first lock, it will stay on (parking), no gas flow will be there. When it is pushed to the second lock the valve opens and gas flow starts. Similarly to remove the probe both the locks have to be released.
- All these outlets and probes together are known as "quick couplers"
- Series of wall outlets in operating room may have one for anesthetic gas scavenging also. This has wider probe and tube **(Fig. 4.10)**.

It has to be remembered that except Schrader valves all other outlet units are not similar in dimensions. It varies with every manufacturer. Hence, it is essential to check whether the probe available in the machine belongs to the same unit and fits in.

Outlet Points from Ceiling

- The hoses lying lose on the floor from the wall outlet to the anesthesia machine may cause severe interference to the movement of personnel as well as sterile instrument trolleys, other equipment, etc.
- For preventing this, swinging overhead 'Hose Booms' were in use in earlier days.
- Now, as the position of the operating table and the anesthesia machine are all almost fixed, the gases delivery through flexible hoses is drawn from the ceiling.

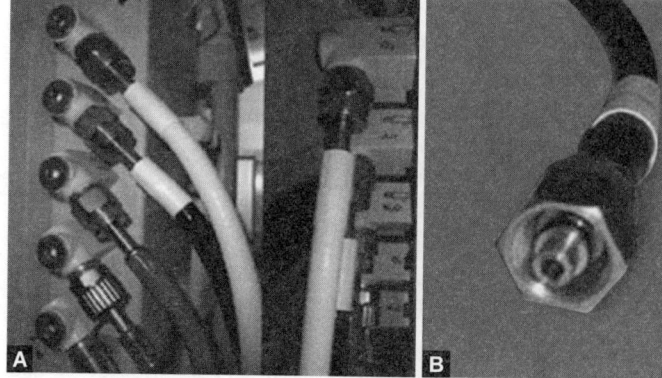

Figs 4.8A and B: Noninterchangeable screw-threaded hose connections

Medical Gas Pipeline System 105

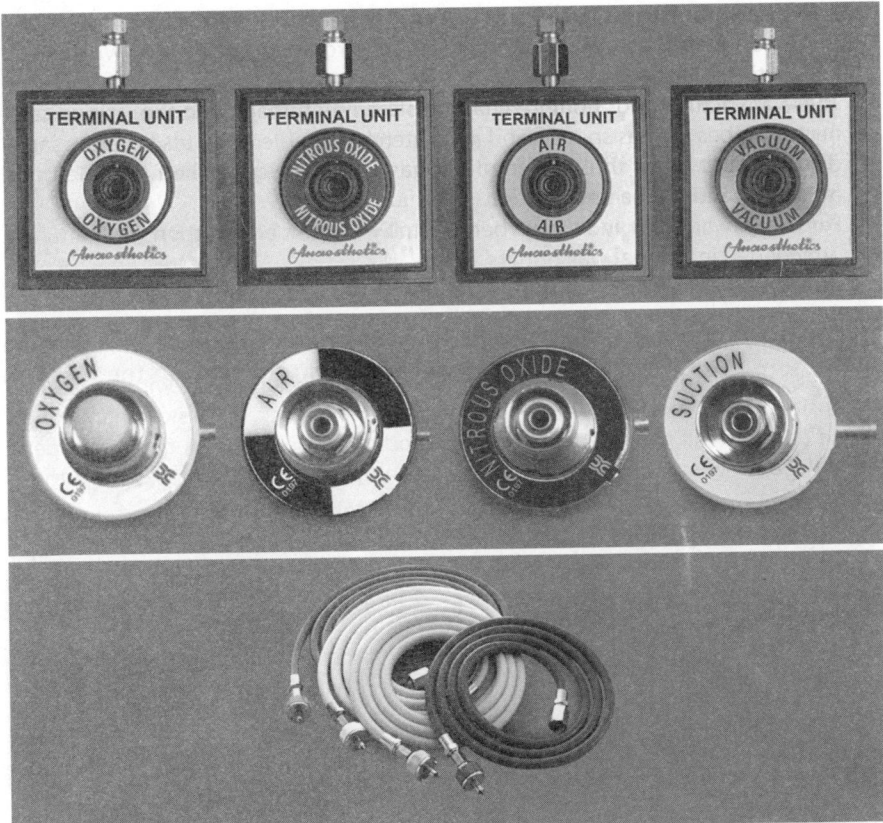

Fig. 4.9: Two types of wall outlet units for plugging in the probes from front. • The color-coded hoses with probes for wall outlets and NIST connectors at the machine end

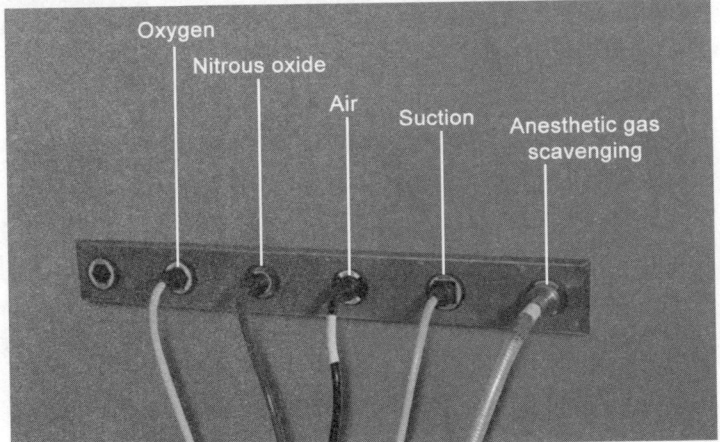

Fig. 4.10: Series of wall outlets with a provision for scavenging

Three Types Ceiling Outlets are Available

Pendants

- Pendants are rigid structures fixed to the ceiling of operating room at a suitable height.
- They are provided with the terminal outlets of the gases and also electrical sockets for use in the work stations and monitors.
- The rigid pendant may be fixed or retractable **(Figs 4.11A and B)**.

Ceiling Reel Type of Outlets

These are the gas outlets from the ceiling with long reel of hoses which can be pulled down to the required length for connecting the hose to the machine **(Figs 4.12A to C)**.

Swivel Pendants

- These pendants provide gas outlets, electrical outlets and platforms to hold monitors as well.

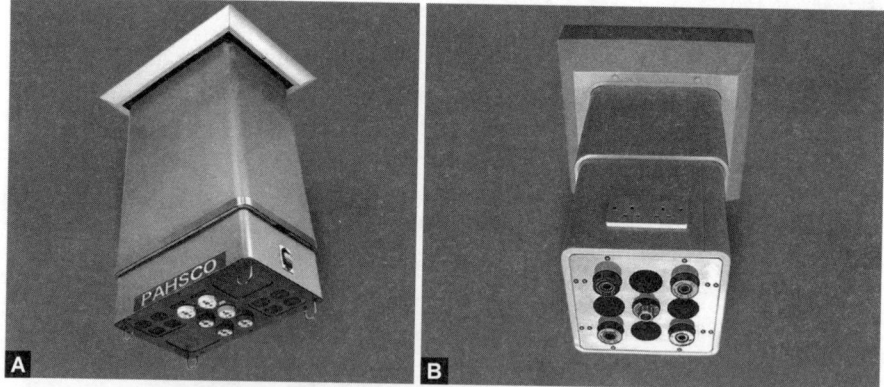

Figs 4.11A and B: Various types of ceiling-mounted pendants. • (A) Rigid ceiling column pendent; (B) Retractable ceiling column pendent

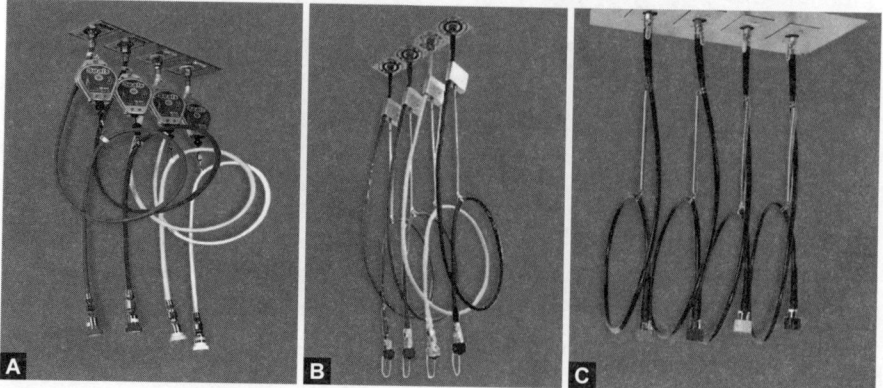

Figs 4.12A to C: Different types of ceiling reel outlets

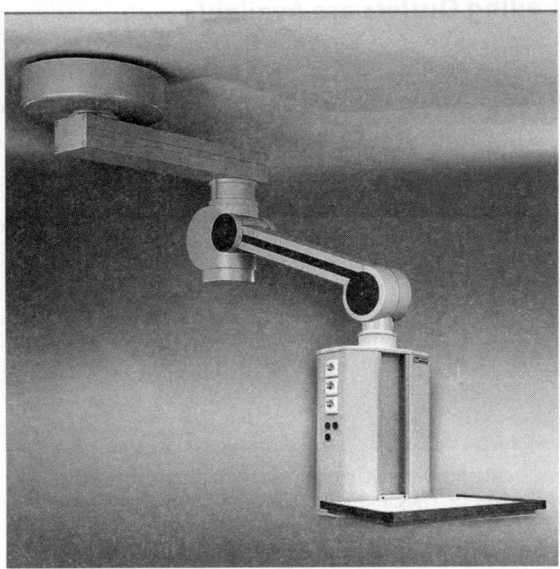

Fig. 4.13: Swivel pendant. • The pipeline and electrical line reach the pendant from the ceiling; • From the pendant outlets, the flexible hoses connect the machine; • Monitors are connected to the electrical outlets in the pendant; • Swivel pendant can have a wider movement

- Usually, it has three joints and three swivels so that it has a wider movement within the theater **(Fig. 4.13)**.

CENTRAL VACUUM (SUCTION)
- This unit consists of a motor (vacuum pump), which generates vacuum that is stored in a tank (reservoir)
- The capacity of the tank depends upon the usage requirement of the hospital in an average.
- Some of the units will have double pumps (motors) mounted on the tank **(Fig. 4.14)**. However, bigger units have the tank, pumps and the control panel mounted separately.
- One motor will be running (Duty) while the other will be at reserve (Standby).
- Usually, one pump is enough for the functioning of the system. The motors run alternating with each other for continuous use.
- There is an automatic control switch that maintains a constant negative pressure in the tank by switching ON or OFF the pump according to the necessity.
- Main vacuum pipes usually are two from two pumps (motors) will pass through two isolation valves and then a drainage trap **(Fig. 4.14)**.
- In *the drainage trap*, any aspirated liquid, condensed vapor, etc. may separate and can be removed.
- Then the pipes pass through bacterial filters to the vacuum reservoir (tank).
- The reservoir (tank) has at its bottom a drainage pipe with a manual drain valve, to evacuate any liquid that may collect.
- The drain provided in the tank is mainly for the purpose of draining water out of the tank after hydraulic pressure testing done on specific intervals.

108 Anesthetic Equipment Made Easy

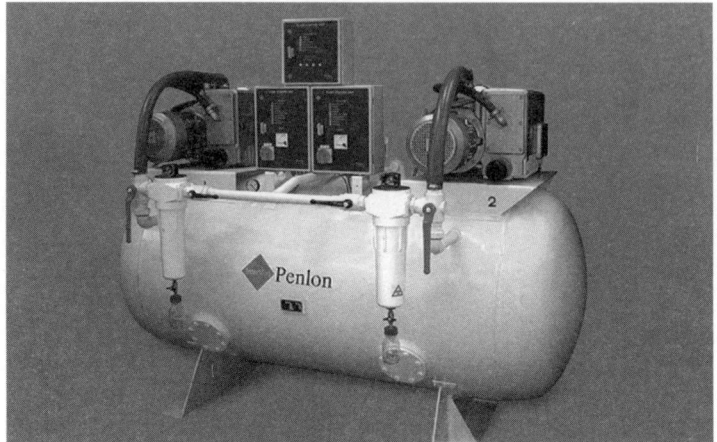

Fig. 4.14: Central vacuum unit with two pumps and two drainage traps. • There are two suction motors and isolation valves; • The drainage traps for removing any aspirated vapor or fluid are seen with collection bottles • The control panel has features to set the pressure at which the motor is to be activated and the duration for which each motor is to work

- Usually, the connection between the reservoir and the vacuum pumps is made through flexible hoses in order to reduce the vibration and the noise that may be transmitted through the pipeline.
- The outlet from the pumps after passing through a silencer is exhausted at a suitable point above the roof to prevent pollution of atmosphere, which the staffs breathe.
- The standard of vacuum that has to be maintained must be *at least 400 mm Hg* (negative) below atmospheric pressure.
- This pressure must be able to take a flow of *free air of at least 40 L/minute*.
- In the operation theater, there must be *one outlet for each operating table* and *one exclusively for anesthesiologist with a spare for recovery bed*.

Wall Outlet for Vacuum

- The outlet in the operating room is seen adjacent to oxygen and nitrous oxide outlets on the wall and is colored yellow or black **(See Figs 4.7 and 4.8)**. It will be provided in pendant also.
- By plugging in the probe with yellow-coded hose, it can be connected to the twin jar trolley mounted unit for surgical use.
- Wall mounting unit which can be plugged into the wall socket is also available which may be handy to the anesthesiologist.
- Both the types are provided with an ON/OFF switch, and a regulator to adjust the power of suction (negative pressure) **(Fig. 4.15)**.
- There is safety device in the form of a float inside the jar. When the jar is full with the aspirated fluid, the float lifts a valve that opens the jar to the atmosphere, thus preventing fluids being aspirated and entering into the pipeline.

COMPRESSED MEDICAL AIR

- Compressed air used for medical use is different from that used in industries.
- Industrial compressed air will contain water vapor and oil mist from the air compressor.

Medical Gas Pipeline System

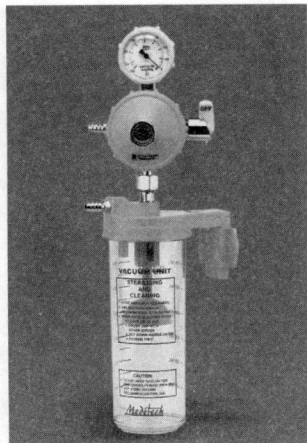

Fig. 4.15: Wall mounting suction unit with suction regulator. • The regulator has an ON/OFF switch, a knob to control the power of suction, and a pressure gauge. This can be directly plugged into the wall outlet; • The jar can be fixed to the lower end of the regulator by screwing in; • There is a float inside the jar, which lifts and opens the jar to the atmosphere when it is full, and thus prevents the fluid from entering into the pipeline

- Medical compressed air must have the highest degree of purity. Otherwise the oil mist will produce oil pneumonitis for patient ventilated with it. It may contaminate the surgical wound, if used for driving equipment.
- The pistons in medical air compressors are Teflon coated and have Teflon rings.
- Medical compressed air will be administered to the patients through either anesthetic machines, or ventilators in operation theater or ICU. A pressure of 60 psi is enough for this application.
- It may be used for operating some of the pneumatic surgical instruments. A pressure of 105 psi may be required for this.
- Because of this difference in pressure needed for the two different applications, generally two different terminal outlets are provided with different probes that misconnections are not possible.
- However, as the surgical instruments are infrequently operated with air, only outlets for 60 psi pressure are provided routinely.
- Pipeline medical air may be supplied from either a manifold of cylinders as it is for oxygen and nitrous oxide or by a compressor.
- In bigger hospitals, a compressor is economical, but at the outlet of compressor, it is dried and filtered to ensure purity.
- The compressors are oil-free compressors **(Fig. 4.16)**.

LIQUID OXYGEN

- It is transported in a specially insulated tanker and is delivered into a vacuum insulated container in the hospital known as vacuum-insulated evaporator (VIE).
- When cooled to very low temperatures, gases (oxygen and nitrogen) change to liquids.
- Oxygen has to be cooled to below −118°C to change to a liquid.
- When the *gas* changes its form to *liquid*, it occupies a much smaller volume.

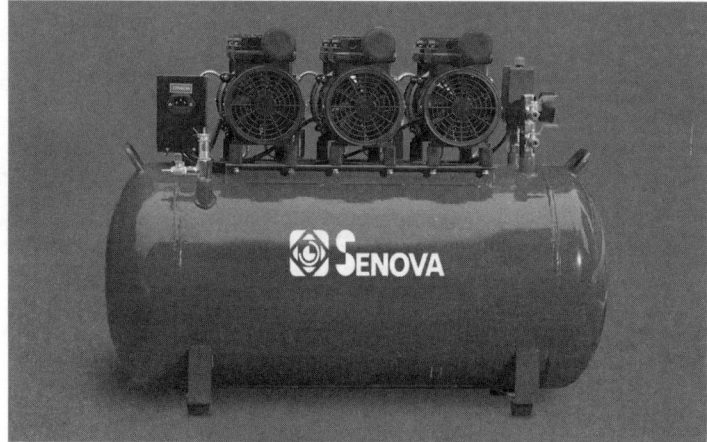

Fig. 4.16: Oil-free air compressors with tank for supplying medical air

- Therefore, when a small volume of liquid oxygen is warmed, it will make a very large volume of gaseous oxygen.
- In hospitals where the weekly requirement of oxygen exceeds 50,000 cubic feet, *liquid oxygen* is used.
- In the liquid form, a very large quantity of oxygen can be transported or stored in a low volume, although there are problems in keeping the liquid cold as explained below.
- Liquid oxygen is transported in *vacuum-insulated tankers*.
- The container has outer wall made of carbon steel and inner wall made of copper or stainless steel with vacuum in between.
- Activated charcoal is kept in the vacuum in between the walls to remove any residual air.
- Insulating material is filled in the space in between the walls to prevent heat transfer in spite of the presence of vacuum.
- One tanker holds 4 to 5 tons of liquid oxygen.
    - 1 ton = 26540 cubic feet of oxygen.
    - 1 cubic foot = 28.3 liters of oxygen.
    - 1 tanker holds approximately (26540 × 28 × 4 tons) 2972480 liters of oxygen.
- In hospitals, oxygen is stored as a liquid in a special container, vacuum-insulated evaporator (VIE).
- In vacuum-insulated evaporator, the liquid oxygen is allowed to evaporate and supplied through the pipeline at 60 psi pressure.
- No compressor or mechanical device is needed for that.
- A reserve of cylinders for four days requirement is kept as reserve in case the liquid oxygen is exhausted. This is to continue the supply until the liquid oxygen tanker reaches the hospital for refilling the tank after informing the company.

Vacuum-insulated Evaporator

- A vacuum-insulated evaporator (VIE) is a container designed to store liquid oxygen and to deliver it to the pipeline **(Fig. 4.17)**.

Medical Gas Pipeline System 111

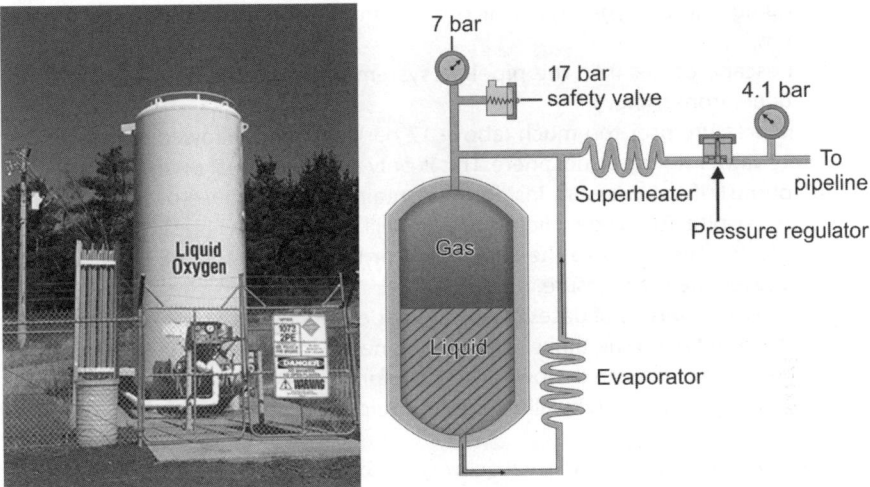

Fig. 4.17: Vacuum-insulated evaporator and the principle of VIE. • The gaseous oxygen is above the liquid oxygen; • The gas enters the pipeline system from the top; • If the demand is less, then pressure may build-up in the tank, which will be released by the safety valve; • If the demand is high and a large quantity of oxygen is needed, then liquid is drawn from the bottom, passes through the evaporator and the gas, then enters the pipeline

- The vacuum-insulated evaporator system is used in large hospitals which have a pipeline system, for which liquid oxygen is supplied from special vacuum insulated tanks transported on tanker lorries by road.
- The tank is designed to allow the liquid oxygen inside to remain very cold.
- It consists of two layers, where the *outer carbon steel shell* is separated by a vacuum from an *inner stainless steel shell, or copper* which contains the oxygen.
- In between the two walls, greatest degree of vacuum possible is maintained.
- The space is filled with a powder "Perlite" an inorganic insulating material, so that heat gain into the inner shell is minimized, even if the vacuum is lost.
- The oxygen temperature inside is about –183°C and the container is pressurised to 10.5 atmospheres (10.5 bar).
- The tanks are fitted with brass valves and copper interconnecting pipe work.
- There are three connections to the inner container namely, *the filling port, gas withdrawal line at top, and liquid withdrawal line* at the bottom (This will have a connection to supply line through evaporator).
- The fresh supply is filled through the filling port.
- Through the gas withdrawal line at the top of the container, gaseous oxygen above the liquid is passed through the superheater to raise the temperature to ambient (outside) levels.
- It then flows into the hospital pipeline system giving a continuous supply of piped oxygen to outlets on the wards and in theater.
- The "Superheater" is a length of copper tubing with diameter of 2.5 cm on which metallic fins are mounted to conduct atmospheric heat.
- This will raise the temperature of oxygen to the level of ambient temperature. Otherwise dangerously cold oxygen may reach the outlets in the theater.
- Because it is not possible to give perfect insulation to the tank, heat is always able to get into the container and provides the energy to evaporate the liquid oxygen,

- changing it into oxygen gas which is continuously drawn off into the pipeline system.
- This escape of gas into the pipeline system prevents the pressure inside the container from rising.
- If the pressure rises too much (above 17 bar), oxygen is allowed to escape via a safety valve into the atmosphere. This is only a very minimal quantity.
- In contrast, if the pressure inside the container falls because of heavy demand in the hospital for oxygen, liquid oxygen will be withdrawn, passed through the evaporator, then pass to the supply line or returned to the VIE in the gaseous form to restore the pressure.
- Considerable wastes of gases occur during delivery of fresh supply of liquid.
- The hose between the tanker and the VIE needs to be cooled below the critical temperature of oxygen (below $-118°$ C) before delivery could be effected.
- The cooling is achieved by allowing the liquid to escape through the hose to the atmosphere.
- It is estimated that 1/4th of total delivery has been wasted this way of pre-cooling.
- The amount of oxygen available in the container is estimated by weighing the container with an inbuilt device.

Precautions for Liquid Oxygen

- Liquid oxygen plant should not be housed inside a building. It should be at a distance of about 6 meters away from any combustible material.
- The floor must be of concrete or similar noncombustible material. Tar or asphalt should not be used as it will form explosive mixture with liquid oxygen.
- No smoking is permitted around this area.
- The plant should be surrounded by a fencing of non-combustible material with adequate access for the delivery tanker.
- There should be no overhead wires, drains or trenches within the prescribed area.

FURTHER READING

1. Al-Shaikh Baha, Stacey Simon. Essentials of Anaesthetic Equipment, 1st edn. London, Churchill Livingstone, 1995.
2. Das S, Chattopadhyay S, Bose P. The anaesthesia gas supply system. Indian J Anaesth. 2013;57:489-99.
3. Dorsch JA, Dorsch SE. Understanding Anaesthesia Equipment, 4th edn. London: Lippincott Williams and Wilkins, 1999.
4. Dorsch JA, Dorsch SE. Understanding Anaesthesia Equipment, 5th edn. London: Lippincott Williams and Wilkins, 2008.
5. Howell RSC. Piped medical gas and vacuum systems. Anaesthesia. 1980;35:676-98.
6. John TB Moyle, Andrew Davey. Ward's Anaesthetic Equipment, 4th edn. London. WB Saunders Company Limited, 1998.
7. Lee's Synopsis of Anaesthesia, 11th edn, London. Butterworth- Heinemann Ltd, 1993.
8. Ward CS. Anaesthetic Equipment, 2nd edn. London: Balliere, S, 1985.

Pressure Reducing Valves (Pressure Regulators)

chapter 5

The pressure of gases in the cylinders is very high (2000 psi for oxygen and 750 psi for nitrous oxide). Delivering such high pressure into the anesthesia machine is potentially dangerous.
- First, it may damage the delicate devices such as flow meters and vaporizers.
- Secondly, the fluctuations in the pressure may cause malfunctioning of the devices.
- More seriously such surge of pressure may accidentally be transmitted the breathing system and cause damage to the patient.

The first Boyle's machine (1917) had no pressure reducing valve. So, gross fluctuation in the output pressure was caused necessitating adjustment of the flow meter very frequently to keep the bobbin at the desired level.

PURPOSE

To provide safe, constant, reduced operating pressure (working pressure) inside the machine.

Benefits of Pressure Regulators
- The cylinder pressure is reduced to a desired value of *'the working pressure'* of the anesthesia machine.
- The outlet pressure is kept constant, even when the cylinder pressure diminishes as it runs down during use.
- The reduced pressure can be carried through the flexible hoses, to the flow meter, if needed. This is not possible without the reducing valve. The rubber tube may blow off with high pressure.
- If pressure reducing valve is not provided the patient's airway may accidentally be exposed to a high, dangerous pressure and it may cause barotrauma.
- Delicate instruments in the anesthetic machine such as flow meters, vaporizers, etc. may be damaged, if there is pressure surges or subjected to high pressure.

PRESSURE REDUCING VALVE (PRESSURE REGULATOR)
- The older anesthetic machines had the reduced working pressure as 14–16 psi.
- Now, in all anesthesia machines the working pressure is 50–60 psi (4 bar) as universal standard.
- Therefore, once the cylinder is opened, the high-pressure gas flows into the reducing valve and the pressure is reduced to a constant pressure of 60 psi to be delivered into the machine, as it is set (60 psi).
- The cylinder pressure will gradually fall as the gas is used.
- It may fall from 2,000 psi to any low level. The valve mechanism is such that even if, the pressure in the cylinder falls very low as 200 psi, the outlet pressure is constantly maintained as 60 psi.

- The modern pressure reducing valve is efficiently designed and when a pipeline with a pressure of 60 psi is connected to it, it behaves such as a bypass and allows the pressure to the outlet without alteration.
- The reduced pressure is necessary to prevent damage to the delicate components of the machine and to prevent damage to the patient's airway without causing "barotrauma" (pressure damage to the respiratory tract).
- As the pressure reducing valve not only reduces the pressure but also delivers a constant outlet pressure. Hence, the better name is *'Pressure regulator'*.

Basic Principle

Large pressure (force) acting over a *small area* counter balances *small pressure* (force) acting over a *large area* to provide a balance of forces across the flexible diaphragm.

$$P \times a = R \times A$$

(P = Large pressure, a = Small area, R = Small pressure, A = Large area)
- This principle is used in pressure reducing valves.
- 'High' pressure acting on a small diaphragm is balanced against a 'Low' pressure acting on a large diaphragm.

This can be explained by the following experiment. The pressure exerted by 10 inches high column of water on a diaphragm of 1 inch diameter balances the pressure exerted by 1 inch column of water acting on a diaphragm of 10 inch diameter **(Figs 5.1A and B)**.

Explanation

- There are two containers of water with freely moving pistons of different sizes at the bottom (H and L).
- These pistons are made to rest on either side of a balancing rod (B).
- The balancing rod is resting on a pivot and is free to move.
- On the left side, there is a high column of water (H) acting on a small piston (h) (diaphragm) which shows a high pressure on the gauge. This can be imagined as 10 inch column of water acting on 1 inch diaphragm.
- On the right side there is a low column of water (L) acting on a large piston (l) (diaphragm) showing a low pressure on the gauge. This can be imagined as 1 inch column acting on 10 inch diaphragm.

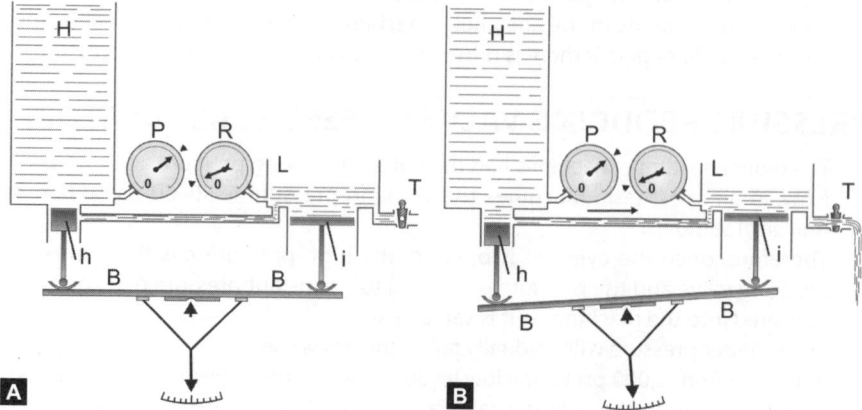

Figs 5.1A and B: Large pressure on small diaphragm balances small pressure on large diaphragm

- A communication through a small tube exists between the two containers. But it is blocked by the small piston when there is balance between the two pressures.
- A tap (T) is provided in the container on the right side which can be opened to let out water.
- As per the principle (P x a = R x A), the two pistons are in perfect balance **(Fig. 5.1 A)**.
- When the tap on the right side container is opened to let out a little of water, the height of the column drops and so the pressure acting on the diaphragm falls. As a consequence, the piston moves up a little.
- This will lower the piston on the left side so as to open the communicating channel allowing the water to flow to the right side which brings the balance between the two though at a lower level.
- Now the small piston moves up and closes the communicating channel.

The pressure reducing valves are made on this principle.
- In practice, a valve like this with the use of larger diaphragm produces a bulky regulator, so it is offset by some mechanisms where springs are used to balance the forces and the size is reduced.

Simple Pressure Reducing Valve

Simple design of a pressure reducing valve is explained in **Figure 5.2**. It has five components namely:
1. High pressure chamber (H)
2. Low pressure chamber (L)

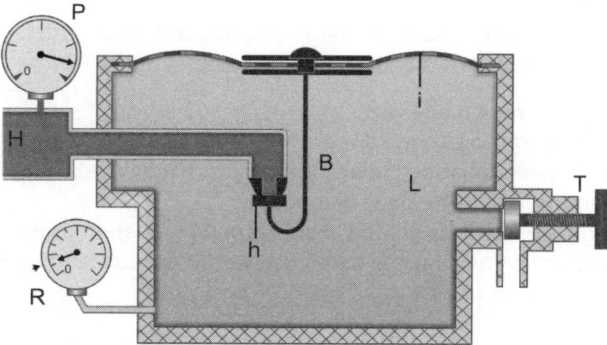

Fig. 5.2: Simple design of a pressure reducing valve. • High pressure chamber is the outlet from the cylinder entering the valve • High pressure chamber is opposed by the small diaphragm; • Low pressure chamber is the big chamber with a large diaphragm; • Two metal plates are fixed on both sides at the center of the large diaphragm and to this the 'J' shaped connecting rod is anchored. Incidentally it restricts the movement and flutter of the diaphragm; • The high pressure and low pressure are in equilibrium because the low pressure acting on the large diaphragm pulls the connecting rod and the small diaphragm closes the outlet of high pressure chamber; • There is a tap on the low pressure chamber which can be opened to let out the gas; • When the tap is opened to let out the gas, depending upon the amount of gas lost, the pressure drops in the low pressure chamber that lowers the large diaphragm; • This creates a small leak from the high pressure chamber that fills the lost gas to make up (balance) the drop in pressure; • If the tap is closed the balance is restored and the leak from high pressure chamber stops; • When the tap is opened to allow a fixed flow of gases continuously, then the leak continues in an attempt to restore the balance; • However, the pressure in the low pressure chamber will be restored once the tap is closed and the leak from the high pressure chamber to low pressure chamber will stop

3. Large diaphragm (l)
4. Small diaphragm (h)
5. Connecting device between the diaphragms (link) (B).

If a pressure reducing valve is constructed like this, it will be too 'bulky'. The movements of the diaphragm may cause flutter and will be 'noisy'.

Hence, the simple valve design must be improved in certain respects to rectify the defects and to supply the anesthesiologist with the practical reducing valve.

The Improved Type of Reducing Valves

- The outlet pressure should not get altered appreciably, while the cylinder pressure falls gradually during use.
- The reduced pressure must be adjustable at will, with certain limits *(Force balance)*. For example, in older machines, it is 14 psi and in newer machines, it is set as 60 psi but it is adjusted and set in the same reducing valve.

The *first* improvement made was:

The hydraulic force exerted by the reduced pressure is used principally to overcome some constant mechanical force.

- This mechanical force can be done with a *'weight'* or a *'helical spring'*.
- Helical spring is more convenient. This can be adjusted by a *'thump screw'*.
- This is known as main compression spring (S) and thump screw **(Fig. 5.3)**
- This makes the large diaphragm stable without fluttering.
- The 'Thump screw' helps in adjusting the output pressure. When the pressure on the helical spring is increased by tightening the screw, the output pressure increases and vice versa.

This improvement has made the large diaphragm stable. But still the 'J' shaped connecting rod is free to move and so the small diaphragm will flutter.

The *second* improvement made was:

A 'second short compression spring' acting in opposition to the "main compression spring" or "main regulating spring", is fixed just below the 'J' shaped connecting rod that prevents flutter of the small diaphragm.

- This spring counter balances the 'main compression spring' and the tension of this spring also can be adjusted with a screw that supports it **(Fig. 5. 3)**.

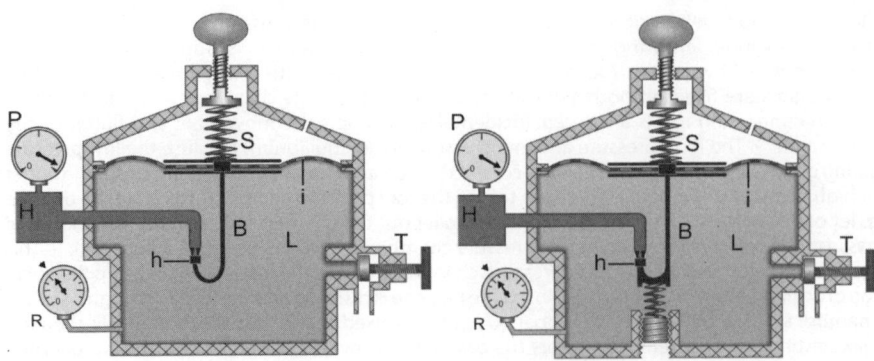

Fig. 5.3: The first and second improvements in the basic design

Pressure Reducing Valves (Pressure Regulators)

- The original metal diaphragm is replaced by a *rubber diaphragm* or *elastometal* or *canvas rubber diaphragm* (Nylon reinforced) that lasts longer.
- All these are meant to guard the degree of movements carefully so that finer movements and finer adjustments are possible.

The construction of any pressure reducing valve is based on these principles. But the new valve is slightly different in structure for making it compact, efficient and easily adjustable.

Therefore, the essential components of pressure reducing valve are **(Figs 5.3 and 5.4)**:
- High pressure chamber with small diaphragm High pressure inlet
- Low pressure chamber with large diaphragm
- Low pressure outlet
- Main compression spring and thump screw
- Second short compression spring (that prevents flutter of the diaphragm)

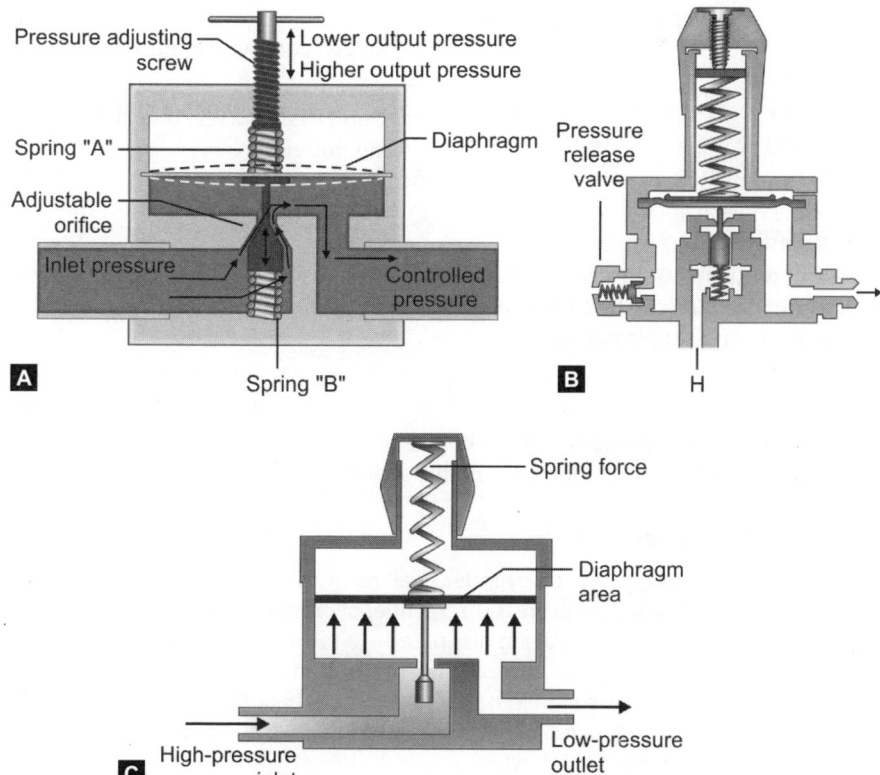

Figs 5.4A to C: The mechanism of modern pressure reducing valve. (A) The high pressure chamber, low pressure chamber, the large diaphragm, main compression spring with thump screw, and second short compression screw are seen; • The small diaphragm is represented by a conical valve sitting on the short spring linked to the large diaphragm; • This conical valve 'fits' well in a conical seating that permits regulated flow of gas (Poppet valve); (B) The section of a valve with the high pressure inlet at the bottom; (C) Has all the features except the short spring. But this figure illustrates how the valve works as a bypass when the cylinder pressure falls below the set outlet pressure (the pressure of low pressure chamber) of the valve

MODERN VALVES

Main Features
- Rubber covered canvas diaphragm.
- The diaphragm is clamped between two stout metal plates at the center to control the movements.
- The tension on the main compression spring is adjusted with the screw provided to fix the outlet pressure and a check nut is tightened to prevent changes.
- The outlet pressure (Low pressure chamber – R) is independent of input pressure (High pressure chamber–P).
- When the high pressure gets reduced slowly, when the cylinder is running down the output pressure remains constant till the P and R become equal.
- After this P and R get reduced simultaneously, now the reducing valve works as a by-pass.
- The R (Low pressure) can be fixed according to the requirement by using screw on the top of the main regulating spring, and then locking it with the help of the check nut provided **(Fig. 5.5)**.
- There are two pressure reducing valves for oxygen and two for nitrous oxide in a machine.
- The low pressure outlets from both the reducing valves join in a common tube leading to the back of the flow meters.
- This is known as 'Manifold' in the machine.

Advantages
- Input pressure can be varied (2000 psi or 60 psi)
- Output pressure can be fixed in a range from 6 psi to 60 psi
- Compact and simple mechanism.

Dangers
- Rupture of the diaphragm and loss of gasses instantly
- Adiabatic compression—Ignition of rubber diaphragm.

Adiabatic Compression
When a compressed gas from a cylinder is allowed to expand and recompressed instantly into a small space (high pressure chamber of pressure reducing valve) without the latent heat of compression being dissipated—enormous heat is generated in the space, which may ignite any combustible material present in that place and cause a fire accident. So no oil or grease should be used anywhere near the cylinder or pressure reducing valve. To prevent adiabatic compression, it is advised to open the spindle of the flush valve of cylinder very slowly.

Problems with Pressure Reducing Valves
- Usually foreign material such as dirt in the passage may cause excess or low output pressure by blocking the finer movement of the parts
- When a malfunctioning valve accidentally allows higher output pressure, it is likely to cause damage to the internal system of the machine such as flow meters, vaporizers, etc.

Pressure Reducing Valves (Pressure Regulators)

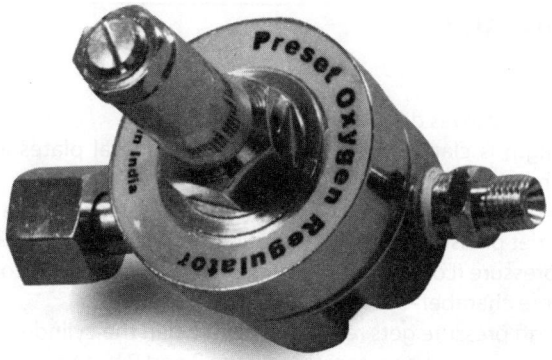

Fig. 5.5: The modern pressure reducing valve of an anesthetic machine. • The left side hexagonal nut connects to the yoke that leads to high pressure chamber; • The right side screw thread is the outlet from the low pressure chamber that connects to the manifold; • On the top is seen the screw for adjusting the tension of the main regulating spring to set the desired outlet pressure; • The hexagonal 'check nut' is to lock the setting after fixing (prevents accidental changes during use); • Some call this reducing valve as "Preset valve" which is a misnomer

- For preventing this problem, a safety device *known as* Safety valve or *Pressure release valve* or '*Pop off valve*' is used just beyond the outlet from the low pressure chamber to release the undue high pressure
- Normally, functioning pressure reducing valves may have minimal variations in the outlet pressure
- So, for giving allowance for these variations the release valve will be set at a little higher pressure than outlet pressure set for the valve
- When the outlet pressure of pressure reducing valve is 50–60 psi, the release valve will be set at 70 psi–about 20 psi more
- In traditional machines, it is situated in the 'manifold' which leads to the flow meter.
- This will release the excess pressure from any of the two pressure reducing valves into the atmosphere
- Some individual pressure reducing valves have the "Safety valve' incorporated in the low pressure chamber itself **(See Fig. 5.4B)**.

Mechanism of Safety Valve (Pressure Release Valve)

- This consists of a body where a gas outlet is closed with a rubber diaphragm mounted on a metal body (usually known as 'poppet') which is retained in that position by a compression spring that can be adjusted with a screw **(Fig. 5.6B)**.
- By adjusting the screw the pressure with which the diaphragm closes the outlet in the gas line can be modified.
- In other words, the pressure necessary to push the rubber diaphragm against the force of the spring to release the gas into atmosphere can be set and fixed. For example, it is fixed as 70 psi in the line leading to the flow meter bank in anesthesia machine.
- The whole mechanism, particularly the adjustment screw is covered by aluminum or brass-chromium housing which has vents to atmosphere **(Figs 5.6A and B)**.
- In some valves, the vent is in the body and adjustable screw is Allen screw that need not be covered and protected **(Fig. 5.6A)**.

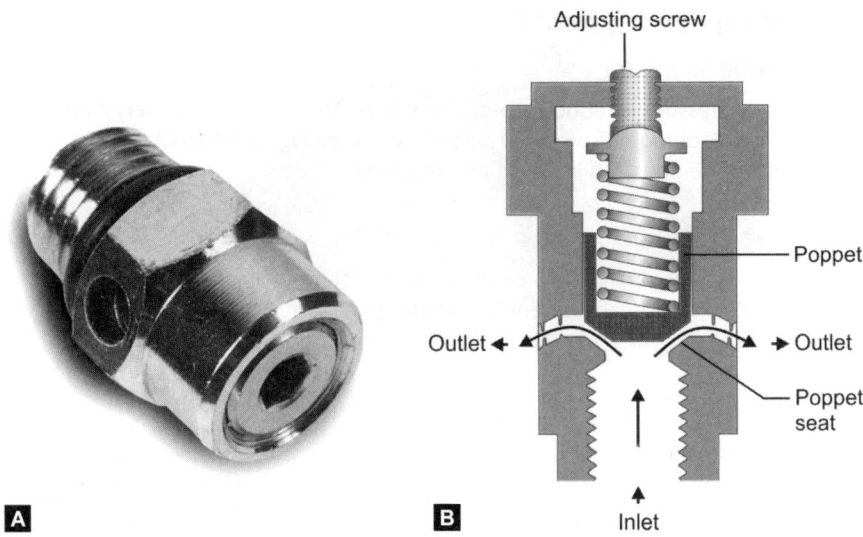

Figs 5.6A and B: Pressure release valve. • The valve has an adjustable screw at the top and a vent for the gas to atmosphere; • The required pressure can be set with screw on the top with an Allen key; • The section of the valve shows the rubber diaphragm at the outlet and the spring to retain it

Second Stage Regulator

- This is a safety mechanism present in modern anesthesia workstations (It is different from 'Two stage pressure reducing valve' which is discussed later)
- Modern anesthesia *Workstations* are provided with a second stage regulator for oxygen and some have it for nitrous oxide also
- It is located just upstream of the flow meters
- It receives the gas from the pipeline inlet or from the pressure reducing valves and further reduces to a low pressure
- The reduced pressure for nitrous oxide is 26 psi and for oxygen is 14 psi (old Boyle F machine had working pressure of 14 psi as standard)
- The purpose is to eliminate the fluctuations in the pressure supplied to the flow meters from the pipeline or from the pressure reducing valves.

TYPES OF PRESSURE REDUCING VALVES

Depending Upon the Outlet Pressure

Fixed Outlet Pressure Type

Though we can set the outlet pressure, we can not modify the pressure at usage.
Example: Pressure reducing valve in the Boyle's machine.

Variable Outlet Pressure Type

- The outlet pressure can be varied according to our need by using the thumbscrew with the handle.
Example: Pressure reducing valves used in the ward cylinders (therapy cylinders).

Depending Upon Type of Construction

Single Stage Regulator

Where high pressure is reduced to one low pressure which causes very high strain on the large diaphragm (from 2000 psi to 60 psi) (*See* **Figs 5.4A to C**).

Example: The one used in anesthesia machine

Two Stage Regulator (or) Multistage Regulator

- Here stepwise reduction in pressure using two or more diaphragms and chambers.
- From 2000 psi, it can be reduced at the first stage to 500 psi, and then from 500 psi to 60 psi or lower (**Fig. 5.7**).

Adam's Valve

This valve was in use in earlier Boyle' machines:
- Though the principle is the same, the construction and the mechanism of working are slightly different
- The large diaphragm is a rubber diaphragm
- A steel cone that occlude high pressure outlet is considered as small diaphragm.
- These two are linked by a toggle lever mechanism (**Fig. 5.8**)
- The movement of rubber diaphragm is transferred by means of a lever mechanism to a diminished movement of the high-pressure seating (smaller diaphragm) and that is known as '*Toggle lever*' or '*Lazy Tong*'
- For N_2O, a small plastic disk is embedded in a holder to occlude high pressure diaphragm
- The outlet pressure is pre-set. Minimal adjustment is possible but the inlet pressure cannot be varied much
- Hence, there must be two different valves—one for pipeline and the other for cylinder supply.

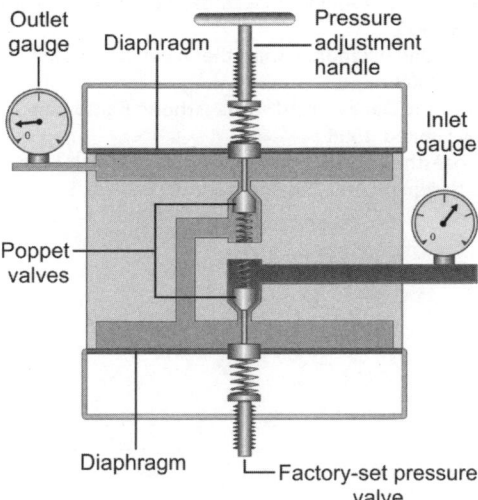

Fig. 5.7: Two-stage pressure reducing valve. (1) The first stage reducing valve seen inverted with the large diaphragm at the bottom; (2) The second stage reducing valve is seen on the upper half with the large diaphragm at the top.

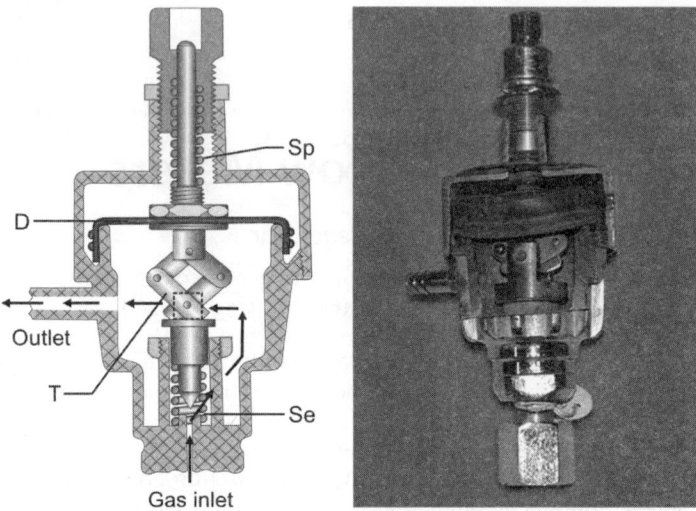

Fig. 5.8: Adam's pressure reducing valve. • The large rubber diaphragm anchored by stout metal plates in the centre; • The toggle lever links the two diaphragms; • The steel conical projection at the bottom of the small diaphragm moves down to seal the conical outlet of the high pressure chamber • The section of the valve shows the features

Disadvantages

- The diaphragm is a slack type and noisy
- The input variations cannot be very much.

FURTHER READING

1. Al-Shaikh Baha, Stacey Simon. Essentials of Anaesthetic Equipment, 1st edn. London, Churchill Livingstone, 1995.
2. Dorsch JA, Dorsch SE. Understanding Anaesthesia Equipment, 4th edn. London: Lippincott Williams and Wilkins, 1999.
3. Dorsch JA, Dorsch SE. Understanding Anaesthesia Equipment, 5th edn. London: Lippincott Williams and Wilkins, 2008.
4. John TB Moyle, Andrew Davey. Ward's Anaesthetic Equipment, 4th edn. London. WB Saunders Company Limited, 1998.
5. Lee's Synopsis of Anaesthesia. 11th edn. London. Butterworth-Heinemann Ltd. 1993.
6. Ward CS. Anaesthetic Equipment. 2nd edn. London: Balliere, S;1985.

chapter 6

Flow Meters

PRINCIPLES AND TYPES

Flow meters are instruments meant for measuring the flow rate of gases.

During anesthesia the fresh gas flow must match the respiratory requirements of the patient; otherwise irreparable damage may be caused to the patient.

Hence in anesthesia machines, the aim is to measure the flow rate of gases as L/minute before delivering to the patient. Flow meter is the device in the machine that can precisely measure the quantity of gas mixture delivered to the breathing system.

Physics

In physics, fluids means anything that flows; both liquids and gases. *Gases flow between two points of unequal pressures; that is from a higher pressure to a lower one.*

Flow of gases needs to have a path which is usually a *tube*. Occasionally, it may flow through an *orifice*.

Tube

Tube is a fluid pathway in which the length is many times greater than the diameter **(Fig. 6.1)**.

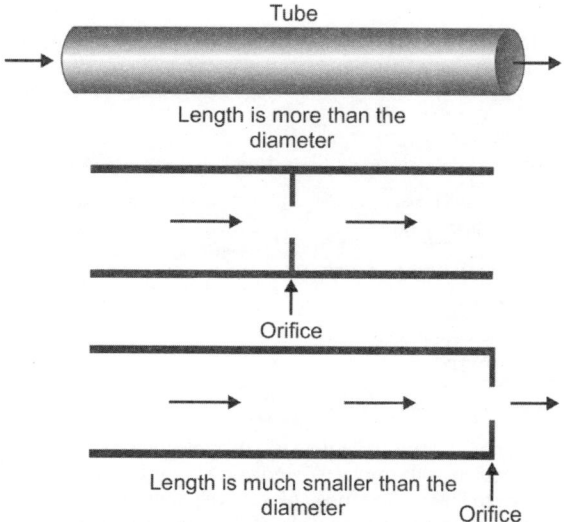

Fig. 6.1: Tube and orifice. • A tube with orifice in the middle, a tube with orifice at the end

Orifice

- Orifice is a fluid pathway where the diameter is greater than the length **(Fig. 6.1)**.
- The greater the diameter, the orifice is called as an ideal orifice.
  The flow of gases can be of two types—*Laminar flow* and *Turbulent flow*.

Laminar Flow

- When the flow of gas along the tube is smooth and regular, it is called 'Laminar flow'.
- Viscosity plays a main role in determining the flow.
- In laminar flow, the molecules move parallel to each other **(Fig. 6.2A)**.
- The molecules in the center move with high velocity.
- The wall of the tube offers greater resistance, so the molecules moving close to the wall have least velocity.
- Though molecules move smoothly, during the flow, there will be resistance offered by the molecules moving parallel.
- As a consequence, the molecules in the center will move faster and towards the periphery the velocity of molecules progressively decrease.
- This causes a convex moving head of the gas flow that is called as 'Parabolic curve' **(Figs 6.2A and B)**.
- Further, depending upon the diameter of the tube, when the gas flow reaches a critical velocity, the laminar flow becomes 'turbulent'.
- Resistance to flow is minimal in 'laminar flow'.

Turbulent Flow

- When the molecules of the gas move in an irregular and haphazard way, it is called 'Turbulent flow' **(Fig. 6.2B)**
- Resistance to the flow is higher in 'Turbulent flow'.

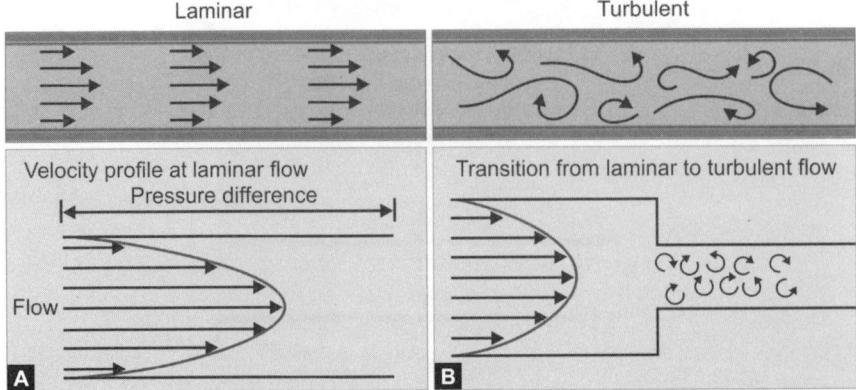

Figs 6.2A and B: Laminar and turbulent flow. • The molecules move parallel to each other- in laminar flow. During turbulence, the molecules move in a hap-hazard fashion, hit against the walls causing more resistance to flow; • The molecules move parallel to each other; • The molecules at the periphery have friction against the walls of the tube. So move slowly. The molecules in the center move faster; • This creates a convex moving head to the fluid that is called as "Parabolic Curve"; • When the tube is suddenly narrowed, flow becomes turbulent

Turbulent flow occurs
- In an orifice
- When the critical velocity of the flow is reached
- When there is a sudden narrowing of the tube
- In acute angles in the tube

The flow through an orifice depends upon:
- The diameter and thus on cross-section of the orifice.
- The difference of pressure on either side of the orifice.
    - The flow through an orifice is always partly turbulent and as the molecules are disturbed, there is inevitably considerable loss of energy, and therefore the pressure.
    - As soon as the flow becomes turbulent the *density* rather than *viscosity* plays great role in determining the volume of gas flow.
    - It indicates that lighter (less dense) gases have more rate of flow through an orifice.

Flow Meters in Anesthesia Machine

Before discussing the flow meters, it is essential to discuss the position and gas input to the flow meters.
- The gas beyond the pressure regulator is delivered in the manifold at 60 psi (4 bar) pressure. .
- The outlet from the two cylinders or one cylinder and the pipeline joined as a single pipe is known as manifold.
- This pressure is known as intermediate pressure system. This gas is transferred through metal pipes to the back of the pin valve of flow meter at the 'Flow meter block' on the back bar of the machine.
- The tube of each gas ends in 'gas specific' 'non-interchangeable' screw-threaded hexagonal nuts.
- The hexagonal nuts are gas specific, different in size as well as the screw threads that it is virtually impossible to connect the wrong gas to the pin valve. *This is a safety mechanism.*

Pin Valve (Needle Valve)

Though 'needle valve' is a part of the flow meter, it is discussed here as at this point, the 'intermediate pressure system' is changing to 'low pressure system'.
- The pin valve is a flow-metering application.
- A long tapered pin is fitting onto the similar shaped outlet occludes the flow of gases.
- The movement of the tip of the needle is controlled by screwing or unscrewing a very fine-threaded long screw.
- The fine thread of the screw gives a 'vernier effect'. That is when the flow control knob is turned anticlockwise one full circle; it will move the tip of the needle to a very small distance allowing very little gas to escape **(Fig. 6.3)**.
- The finer adjustment of the flow rate is possible by the needle valve.
- Incidentally the intermediate pressure of 60 psi is significantly reduced to 'Low pressure' of 12 psi so that patient's airway will not be subjected to surge of higher pressure.
- This is a safety mechanism.

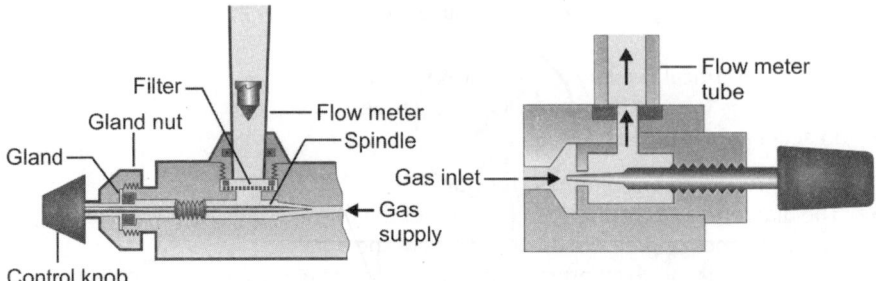

Fig. 6.3: Needle valve of flow meter

Classification of Flow Meters

The flow meters in anesthetic practice are basically two types (Based on the principle):
1. Fixed orifice with variable pressure difference (Not in use now)
2. Variable orifice with fixed pressure difference.

Fixed Orifice-variable Pressure Difference Type

This type consists of a tube with a constriction which is a true orifice interposed between the source of gas and point of delivery. There is a difference of pressure developed between the two sides of orifice as the gas flows thought it. This pressure difference is measured by a device usually a manometer or a pressure gauge placed at the upstream part of the tube proximal to the orifice. The pressure difference increases with flow rate. The unit of pressure difference is translated in terms of flow rate. The readings in the gauge are as flow rate and not pressure. Rate of flow is proportional to the square root of diameter of orifice **(Fig. 6.4)**.

Variable Orifice-fixed Pressure Difference Type

Though many variable orifice meters were in use earlier days, the only meter now in use anesthesia machines is the 'Rotameter'. A detailed discussion of rotameter is essential. The name 'Rotameter' is the trade name used by the manufacturer, Elliot Automation, but it has become synonymous with this type of flow meter.
- The principle was described by *Kuepper* in 1908. In 1910, it was used in industries.
- In 1910 in Germany, M Neu was the first to apply Rotameters for administration of nitrous oxide and oxygen but, his machine was not commercially successful since nitrous oxide was very expensive.
- In 1937, *Richard Salt* in Britain used, it in anesthesia with a little modification.
- Later on flow meters for cyclopropane and CO_2 were introduced.

In any anesthesia machine the flow meters for oxygen, nitrous oxide, and air are provided in a compact enclosure called 'Flow meter bank' usually fixed on the back bar of the machine.

The gases that leave the pressure reducing valve at 60 psi (intermediate pressure) are carried by narrow metal tubes reach the back of the corresponding flow meters in the flow meter block. These tubes are connected to the back of flow meter by screw threaded hexagonal connectors. These are agent specific having different size of hexagon and the size of threads. A tube carrying another gas cannot be connected to a flow meter by mistake.

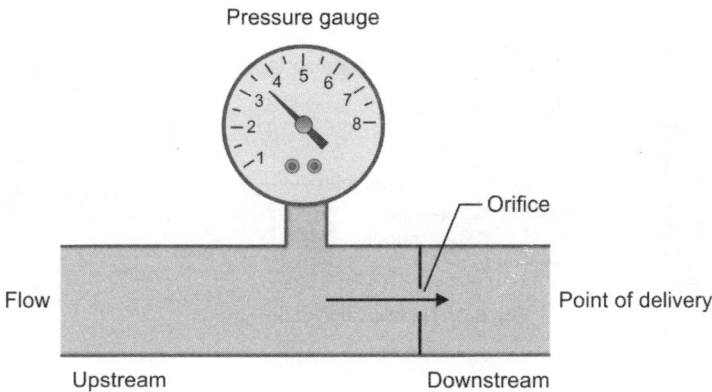

Fig. 6.4: 'Fixed orifice-variable pressure difference' type of flow meter. • During flow through the orifice, there is a higher pressure proximal to the orifice and lower pressure distally. So, there is a *'pressure difference'* between the two sides of the orifice; • When the flow increases, the pressure difference increase and vice versa; • The diameter of orifice is fixed (Fixed orifice) but the pressure difference is variable according to the flow; • Hence the name "Fixed orifice – variable pressure difference"; • The pressure gauge attached to the tube proximal to the orifice records the increase in pressure when the flow rate increases. The dial reads the flow rate

At the bottom of each flow meter, there is device called *Pin valve* or *Needle valve* which allows slow release of the gas into the flow meter tube. By rotating the knob of pin valve anticlockwise many times, the gas flows slowly into the bottom of the flow meter tube.

Flow Meters

- The "Flow meters" measure the flow of gases in L/minute.
- The amount of gas mixture necessary for each patient is calculated as L/minute.
- The flow meters are set to deliver the amount of gas mixture calculated for that particular patient as L/minute.
- The flow meters in present day machines are 'Rotameters'.

Rotameter

- It is a *"variable orifice, fixed pressure difference"* type.
- The float or bobbin is called a *Rotor* because it spins and rotates on its long axis.
- Usually, it consists of a long transparent tube with a tapered lumen and accommodates a spherical body called as *Float* or *Bobbin* (*Rotar* in Rotameter).
- Flow meter tube has a wider diameter on the top and smaller diameter at the bottom.
- The tube is arranged vertically with the widest portion uppermost like a funnel. The gas is admitted from the bottom of the tube.
- The tube is fixed on the outlet of the pin valve below with a 'O' ring for airtight fit.
- At the upper end, it is fixed to the common gas pathway with a 'O' ring for airtight fit.
- The wall may have *a constant taper* (uniform) or it may be *a variable taper* that suddenly widens at the top **(Fig. 6.5)**.
- The variable taper allows larger flow rates of gas at the wider portion.
- These tubes are calibrated and are not interchangeable.
- A bobbin or float made of aluminium or light plastic material kept in the tube that can freely move up and down within the lumen.

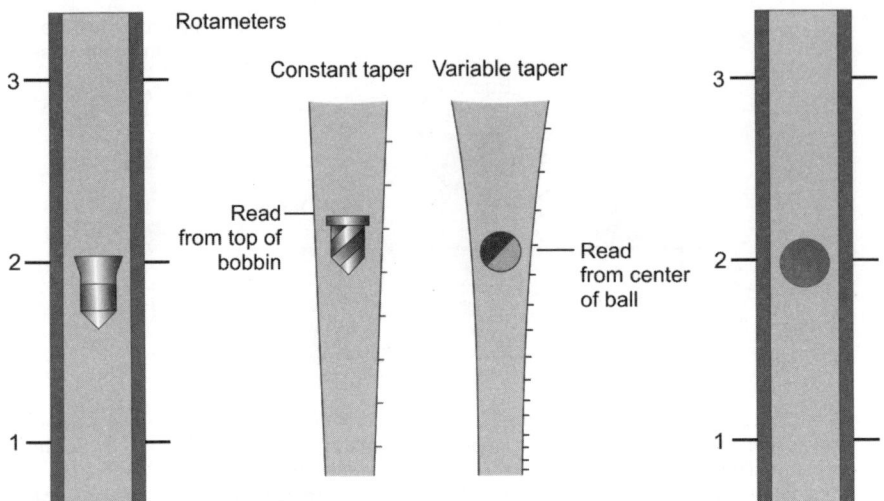

Fig. 6.5: Constant taper and variable taper of the flow meter tube;
- Reading the two types of bobbins spherical or cylindrical

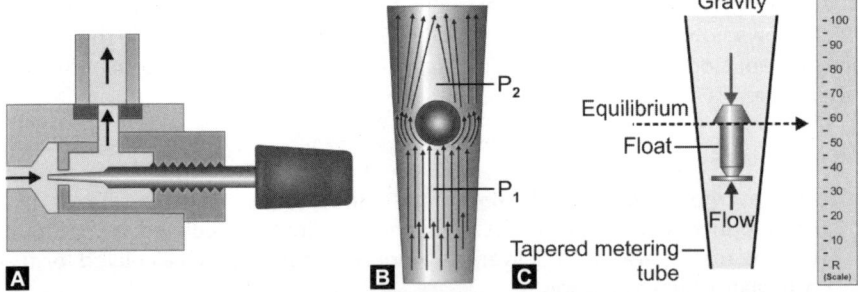

Figs 6.6A to C: 'Pin valve and flow of gas; Flow of gas around bobbin; Equilibrium of float • The P_1 at the bottom of the bobbin is higher than the P_2 at the top of bobbin, but the difference is always constant at whatever level the bobbin floats

- The bobbin usually rests on a short stout metal tube at the bottom or on a constriction present in the flow meter tube itself when the 'pin valve' is closed.
- When the control knob of pin valve is opened, gas enters into the tube lifting the bobbin and flows through the sides of the bobbin to reach the top of the tube **(Fig. 6.6A)**.
- As the gas enters, the float rises. The pressure at the bottom is higher than that at the top of the bobbin.
- When the flow increases the bobbin rises to wider portion of the tube and *the size of orifice* through which gas passes increases and the reverse occurs when the bobbin is lowered. This is *'variable orifice'* **(Fig. 6.7)**.
- In this process, there is an increased pressure at the bottom of the bobbin and a lower pressure at the top of bobbin. So, there *is a pressure difference* observed between the bottom and top of the bobbin **(Fig. 6.6B)**. The P_1 is greater than P_2.
- We can give an arbitrary value of *5 mm Hg* for the pressure difference developed between the bottom and top of the bobbin for the purpose of discussion.

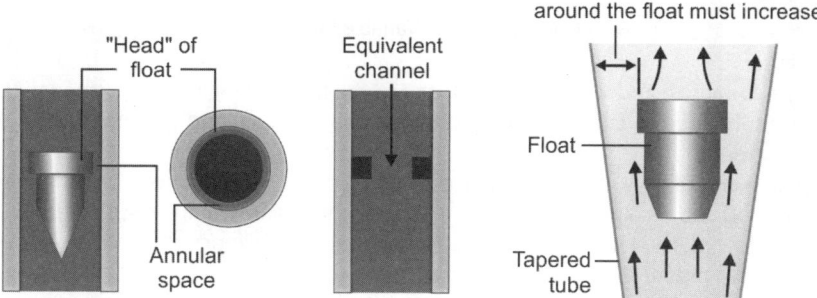

Fig. 6.7: The annular orifice around the bobbin that varies with is position

- The weight of the bobbin acted by the force gravity will pull the bobbin down.
- The gravitational force is overcome by the higher pressure at the bottom of the bobbin and the bobbin is lifted to float freely suspended on a *cushion of gas*.
- The *pressure difference* remains constant even when the flow is varied. In other words, the pressure difference between the top and bottom necessary to keep the float suspended is the same for a given float at any position in the tube.
- The float ceases to rise when the pressure on the underside of bobbin is sufficient to balance the effect of gravity upon the float.
- At each adjustment, the pressure on the underside of the float is readjusted to that value necessary for keeping it suspended.
- There will be equilibrium between the gravitational force and the pressure under the bobbin and it floats. That is why the bobbin is called as a "Float" **(Fig. 6.6C)**.
- The tube has graduations marked in liters and the position of the float shows the flow rate in liters/minute.
- When the flow rate increases and the bobbin rises, more pressure is needed to suspend it (P_1) and corresponding to that there will be a lower pressure at the top (P_2). But if we note the pressure difference it will be constant; 5 mm Hg (Fixed pressure difference).
- Depending upon the position of rotor, the flow rate may increase or decrease. But the *pressure difference between bottom and top of rotor is always constant (fixed)*.
- This pressure difference is constant irrespective of the position of the bobbin in the tube. In other words, irrespective the flow rate, there is a *fixed pressure difference* between P_1 and P_2.
- The space between the wall of the tube and the bobbin makes *a circular orifice* through which the gas flows. But the cross-sectional area of this orifice varies according to the position of the bobbin. Narrow orifice at the bottom and wider orifice at the top. That is why, it is called as *variable orifice* **(Fig. 6.7)**.
- The variations in the cross-sectional areas (diameters of the orifices) are determined and translated in terms of flow rate. This is read on the graduations on the flow meter tube.
- In larger orifice (at the top of the tube), the density of the gas determines the flow rate. Whereas, in smaller orifice (lower end of tube), the viscosity of the gas determines the flow rate as at this point, the orifice is more like a tube.
- The bobbin or float in a 'Rotameter' is specially constructed that gas flow around it makes it spin on its axis, and it rotates. Hence, it is named as "Rotor".

Variables

- The float need not be spherical. It may be cylindrical, conical, or in the form of disk.
- The form, size and weight of the float and the angle of inclination of the taper of the tube are the factors which determine the accuracy and performance of the flow meter.
- The scales of flow meters when used above or below atmospheric pressure need revision and recalibration as in mines, hyperbaric chamber and high altitude.
- The flow meter designed to be used when there is resistance to flow in the tube is called as pressure compensated flow meter.
- In practice, it is impossible to have an ideal orifice, so viscosity in addition to density play a role in altering the flow rates.

Practical Considerations

- At the lower part, viscosity plays a role in modifying the flow rate.
- At the upper part, density plays a role.
- The tube must be fixed perfectly vertical so that the bobbins do not touch the walls. If the bobbins come in contact with the walls, then it may cause friction and show relative low flow rate.
- Bobbins are made of aluminium or plastic material. Plastic may acquire static charges and may cause the bobbin to stick to the walls and may lead on to either low flow or high flow.
- Moisture or dirt may cause similar problems. No moisture or dirt must be allowed inside the flow meters.
- The possible error in these flow meters is + or –2%, so it is always essential to keep minimum inspired O_2% as 30% of the anesthetic mixture to prevent hypoxia.

Bobbins

The bobbins used in various types of flow meters may have various shapes **(Fig. 6.8)**.
- Disc with rod
- Bobbin-shaped
- Round (Globular)
- Oval (elliptical)
- Dumb-bell
- Conical
- Cylindrical with a head and tail (Rotor).

Bobbins may be of different shapes, but commonly 'cylindrical' or 'globular' bobbins are used **(See Fig. 6.4)**. In Rotameter, especially designed 'Rotor' is used.

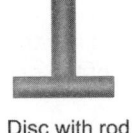
Disc with rod

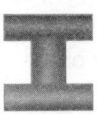
Bobbin

Round

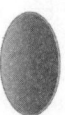
Oval

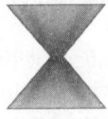
Dumb-bell

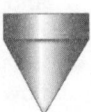
Conical

Fig. 6.8: Different bobbins used in flow meters

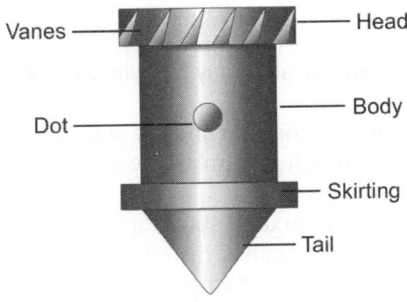

Fig. 6.9: Rotor

ROTOR (FLOAT)

- Rotor is the *bobbin* or *float* used in Rotameter.
- It is a float made of aluminium, light alloy or plastic.
- This usually has a specific design with *a head, body and a tail* (**Fig. 6.9**).
- The general shape is cylindrical with a tapering (conical) tail.
- The upper end has a slightly larger diameter than the body and is called as *head*.
- A number of *oblique grooves* are cut on the head.
- When the gas passes between the head and wall of the tube, the grooves act as the *blades of turbine* or *a set of vanes* the bobbin is set to spin in its long axis and rotate in its vertical axis.
- Its rotation is essential to prevent accumulation of static charges; otherwise, it may get stuck to the wall, especially if rotor is made up of plastic.
- The body is cylindrical.
- With the fast rotation and flow of gas around it the bobbin may have a wobbling effect.
- To prevent this effect and to stabilize it in its long axis a thin rim of a slightly larger diameter is present at the lower end of the body, called as *skirting* which is smaller than the head but bigger diameter than the body.
- The aerodynamically designed *conical tail* also helps preventing this problem. As the bobbin rotates while gas flows, it is named as *Rotor*.
- When there is no flow of gases, the bobbin will be at the bottom of the Rotameter tube, resting on a stout metal tube situated at the lower end of the tube, occluding the gas inlet. Sometimes, it may rest on a constriction in the tube at the lower end.
- To prevent the bobbin getting stuck at the top of the flow meter, a small helical spring juts into the tube from the top.
- To visibly ensure gas flow, a white dot is painted on the body that makes the rotation visible.
- To prevent the rotor getting stuck to the wall of the tube due to static charges, the inner surface of the tube is coated with "antistatic' material.

FLOW METER BANK

- As discussed earlier, the flow meters of all the gases are grouped in a protective enclosure assembly on the back bar of the machine known as *Flow meter Bank* or *Flow meter Block*.
- This accommodates all the pin valves, flow meter tubes and the common gas pathway at the top without any leak.

- On the back of the flow meter bank, the hexagonal connectors and screws for each flow meter are provided. The size of the nuts and screw threads are specific for each gas, and it is impossible to connect the wrong gas to the flow meter. This also is a safety feature.
- This assembly is usually situated at the left end of the back bar for convenience and the common gas pathway continues to the right end.
- A *fluorescent plate* placed in the back of the assembly illuminates the flow meters so that the position of the rotors is visible even in dark environment. This is a safety feature.
- In the older machines, the oxygen flow meter is on the left side and nitrous oxide on the right side (Upstream). In newer machines, as a safety feature, it is reversed. Oxygen is on the right side and nitrous oxide on the left side (Downstream) **(Figs 6.10A to C)**.
- This is to keep the *oxygen flow meter in the downstream* of the flow meter bank. Even if, there is a leak in the nitrous oxide flow meter, oxygen will flow into the common gas path. This is a safety feature to prevent hypoxic mixture in the case of any leak in nitrous oxide flow meter.
- For this reason, the oxygen cylinders are also shifted from left side to right side in the newer machines.
- The gases from the flow meters mix in the common gas path at the top of the flow meter bank and proceeds towards the common gas outlet of the machine.
- The control knobs of modern oxygen flow meters are specially designed. Larger ones which protrude out of the other control knobs. It is 'fluted' which means there are less number of deep grooves on it that can be easily identified by touch even in darkness **(Fig. 6.11)**. It is a safety feature.

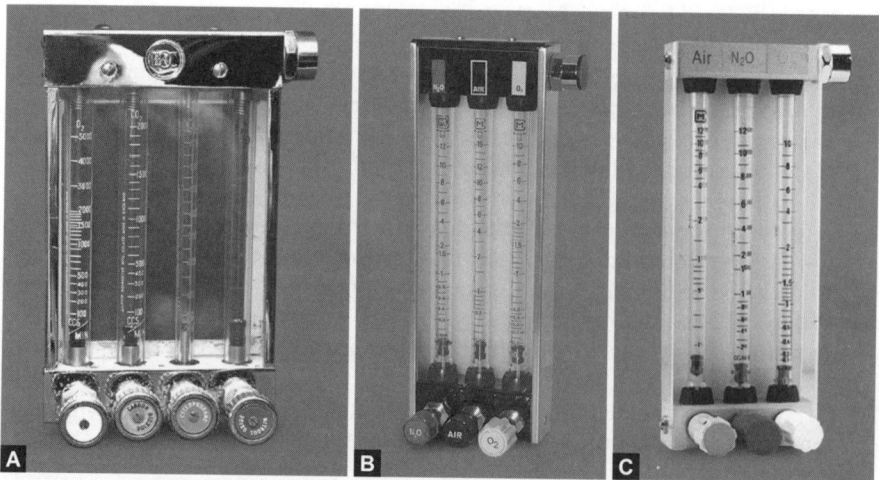

Figs 6.10A to C: Flow meter bank. (A) The flow meter bank of Boyle F machine with oxygen at the left end and nitrous oxide at the right end; • In between the carbon dioxide and cyclopropane flow meters are positioned; • All the control knobs are of same size and shape; (B) The oxygen flow meter is on the right end, nitrous oxide flow meter on the left end and for Air is in the middle; • Especially designed control knob for oxygen is used; (C) Flow meters are in the order; Air, nitrous oxide and oxygen from left to right

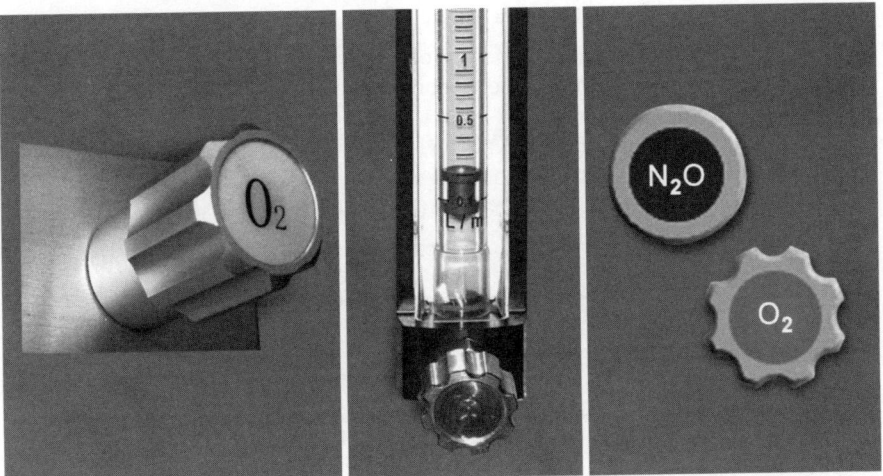

Fig. 6.11: The 'Fluted' control knob for oxygen and round knob for nitrous oxide

The two types of flow meters based on the principle may be dry flow meters or wet flow meters. In early days, some flow meters were constructed with jar containing water for measuring the gas flow and were known as wet type flow meters.

Though theses flow meters discussed here have no relevance to modern anesthesia, it is important to know the developments in history.

Fixed Orifice with Variable Pressure Difference:
- Pressure gauge meter   - Dry type
- Water depression meter   - Wet type
- Foregger meters   - Wet type

Variable Orifice with Fixed Pressure Difference
Coxeter Bobbin   -   Dry type
Heidbrinks meter (1868)   -   Dry type
Connell meter (1930)   -   Dry type
Rotameter (1908) by Kuepper -   Dry type
Water sight feed meter   -   Wet type

Fixed Orifice Dry Type

Pressure Gauge Type of Meter

A pressure gauge which reads in flow rate and not in pressure is attached at the upstream portion (proximal) of the orifice. This has the *Disadvantages that smaller flow rates cannot be accurately measured. These are not used in anesthetic machines* **(Fig. 6.12)**.

Fixed Orifice Wet Type (Also Known as Hydraulic Flow Meters)

Hydraulic flow meters, wet flow meters, aqua meters all refer to the same wet flow meter supplied by Foregger.

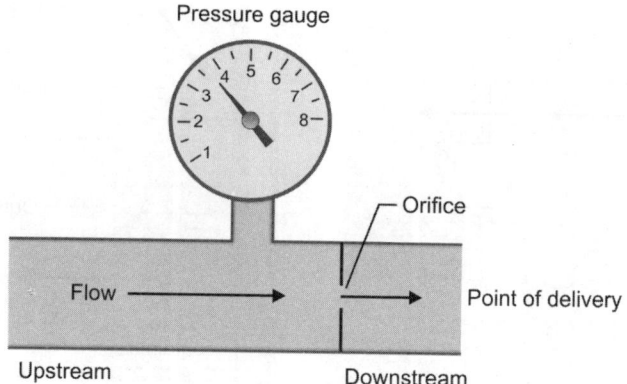

Fig. 6.12: Fixed orifice dry type flow meter (Pressure gauge type).
• The pressure gauge reads in units of volume

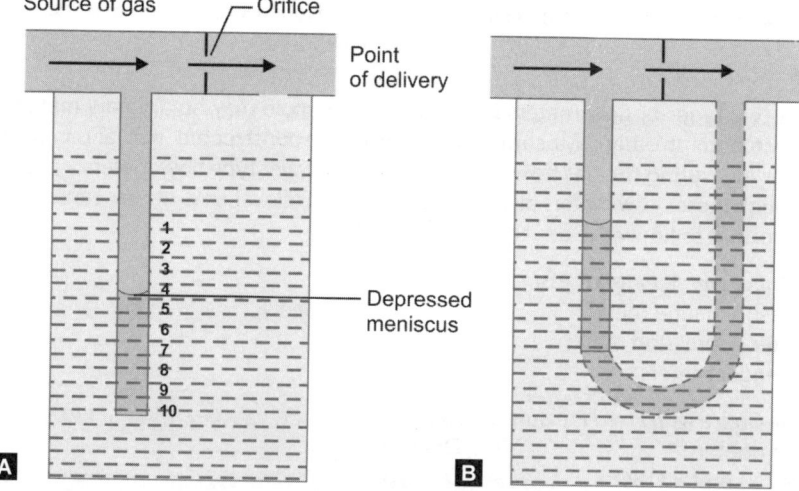

Figs 6.13A and B: (A) Inside flow meter (Water depression meter); (B) The principle; • (A) The depression of water meniscus in the vertical tube indicated the pressure and it is translated in volume per minute. The reading is etched on the tube or read on a scale; • (B) Explains how the tube is working similar to a 'U' tube manometer

Inside Flow Meters (Water Manometer)
- A slender glass tube fixed at right angles to the delivery tube proximal to the orifice.
- This glass tube is open at bottom and is immersed in a sealed jar of water.
- The depression of the meniscus results in proportion to the flow rate. Actually, it is a modified U tube manometer.
- The calibrations are marked on the tube or on a scale fixed behind the tube.
- If flow rate is higher than the maximum reading, then the excess gas will bubble through and reach the outlet **(Figs 6.13A and B)**.

Foregger Flow Meter (Outside Tube Flow Meter)
It works on the same principle but the construction is a little different **(Figs 6.14A and B)**.

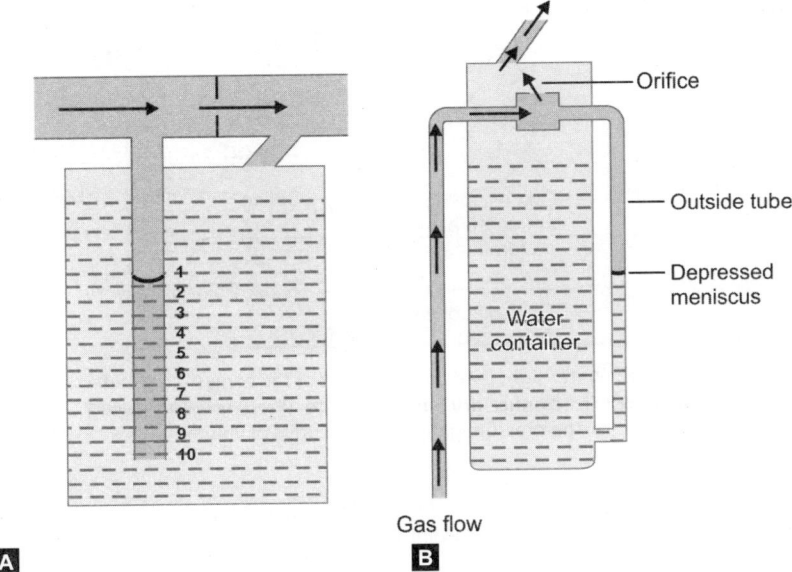

Figs 6.14A and B: Foregger flow meter (Wet type); (A) The simple principle of the meter; (B) The actual construction of the meter where the tube with the water meniscus is outside the container; • The flow rate is either etched on the tube or read against a scale

VARIABLE ORIFICE TYPE

Wet Type

Hydraulic Sight Feed Meter (Water sight Feed Meter) (Wet)
- With this one exception all the other types of wet flow meters are of fixed orifice principle.
- This is introduced by Foregger and called as "Sight Feed Meter". It was one of the earliest flow meters used for anesthesia.
- It consists of a slender metal tube with *perforations* at regular intervals along the length.
- The upper end directly communicates with the source of the gas.
- It is vertically immersed in water.
- Flow of gas depresses the meniscus to the first perforation in the tube and gas bubbles from it to the delivery tube.
- As the flow rate increases the meniscus is depressed further and activates further perforations **(Figs 6.15A and B)**.
- The cross-sectional area of the orifice increases as each successive perforation is activated. So variable orifice.
- The pressure difference remains constant.
- The number perforations which are bubbling is an index for flow rate.
- Several tubes may be assembled in one container when more than one gas is used.
- *Disadvantage:* Finer graduations are obviously impossible. It is of very little value in present day practice.

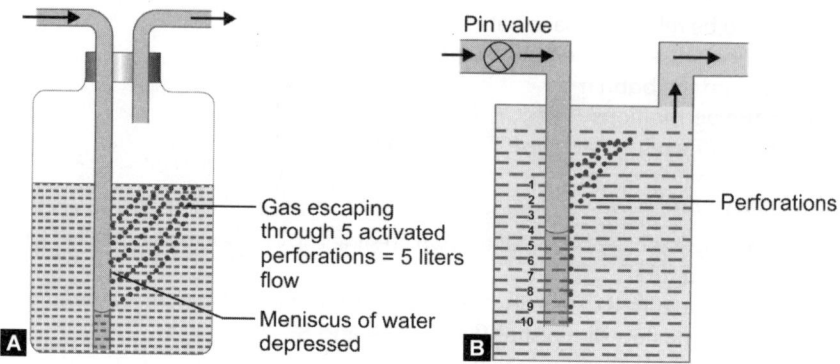

Figs 6.15A and B: Water sight feed meter; • One of the earliest flow meters used in ansethesia; • The only one 'variable orifice type in wet flow meters

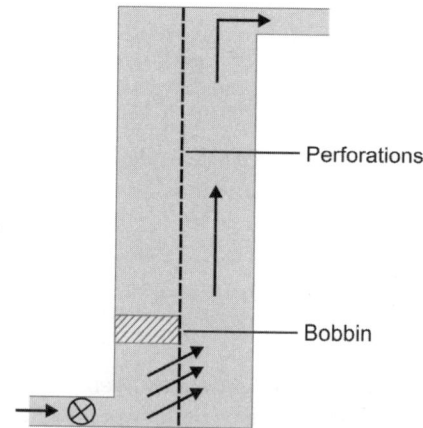

Fig. 6.16: Coxeter bobbin flow meter

Dry Type

Coxeter Bobbin Meter

- This operates basically in the very same principle as sight feed flow meter.
- A vertically placed transparent tube of uniform bore with series of perforations at regular intervals throughout its length.
- A cylindrical float or bobbin is snugly accommodated in the lumen to prevent gas passing around it **(Fig. 6.16)**.
- But it must slide up and down in the tube without resistance. The gas is admitted at the lower end and the upper end is sealed.
- As the flow rate increases the bobbin rises and the gas escapes through the perforations.
- The pressure difference is constant (Fixed pressure difference).
- The cross-sectional areas of the orifice vary with the number of the activated perforations.
- Each flow meter has tube calibrated separately for the gas to be used.

This is likely to be relatively inaccurate because of:
- Impedance caused by the bobbin and wall of tube.
- Leak around the bobbin
- Dirt in the perforations
- Rate of flow increases stepwise. Difficult to clean

Heidbrinks Meter

- The float consists of a horizontal disk which slides up and down a vertically placed metal tapered tube.
- A metal rod attached to the disc moves up when flow of gas increase and moves down when the flow diminishes **(Figs 6.17A and B)**.
- Behind the rod a scale calibrated in flow rates is fixed and the tip of the rod shows the flow rate.
- Density and viscosity both play a role in measuring the flow rate, because the thickness of disk produces turbulent passage at the narrow portion and so the viscosity in low flow rate.
- When the disk is in wider portion, the cross-sectional area through which the gas passes is greater and the influence of the thickness of disc is minimal, and so, density in high flow rate.

Connell Meter

- A tapered glass tube is used and is mounted on an inclined plane.
- The bobbins are a pair of stainless steel balls **(Fig. 6.18)**.

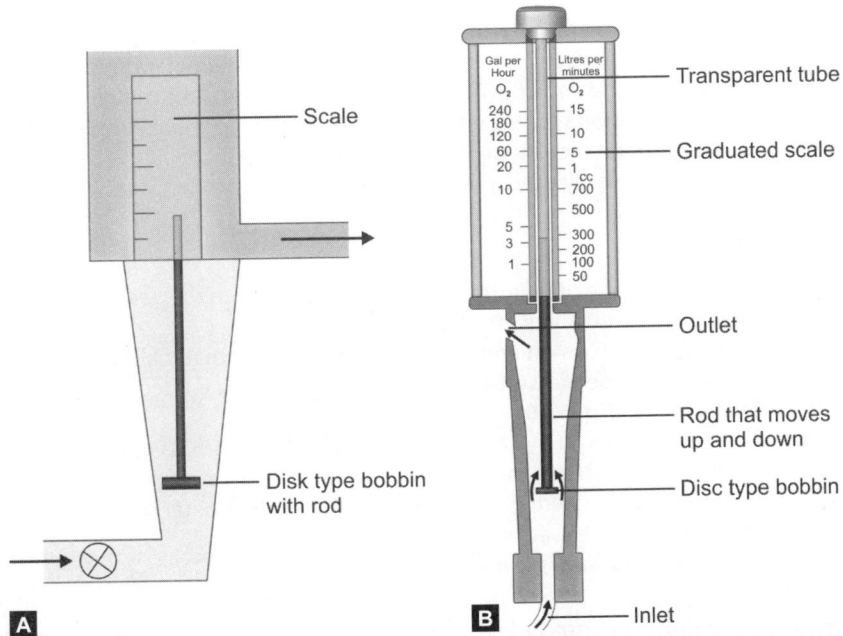

Figs 6.17A and B: Heidbrink flow meter. • The metal tube is of varying diameter with a thin disc type bobbin; • A rod attached at right angle to the disc moves up and down against a transparent graduated tube that shows flow rate

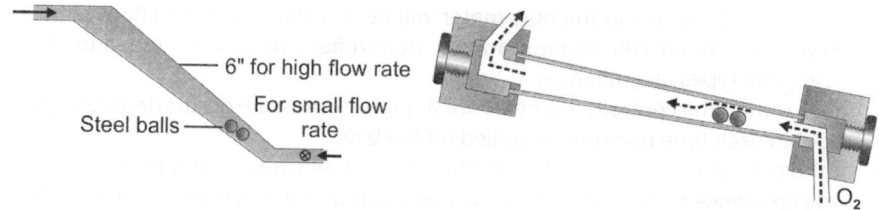

Fig. 6.18: Connell meter

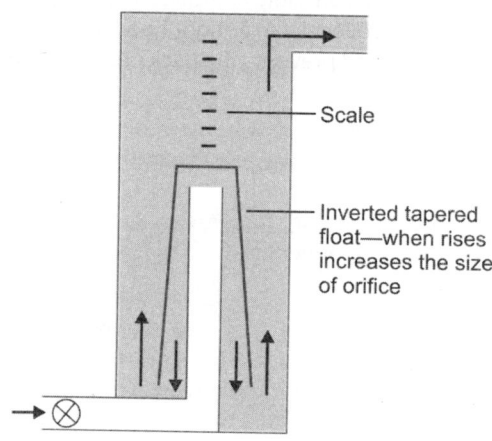

Fig. 6.19: McKesson meter

- The gas passes in front of them instead of around them.
- The bore of the tube is not increasing uniformly as in the Rotameter, but compound, so that both small and large flows can be measured in the same meter which is 6" long. The lower portion spreads out uniformly but upper portion flares out wildly in a short distance for measuring high flow rates.
- These are not commonly used in anesthetic machines.

McKesson Meter

- This has a vertical tube of uniform diameter through which the gas enters.
- This tube covered with an inverted glass like float.
- The float has tapered lumen and is made of light weight material. When the gas enters the vertical tube pressure builds up in the float, and it is lifted up depending upon the flow rate **(Fig. 6.19)**.
- The whole unit is covered by an air tight hood like cover with an outlet.
- The construction is such that the main tube has uniform diameter and the float has variable diameters (tapered) gradations are etched on the outer hood.
- Flow rate is read with reference to the top of the float.
- This flow meter is not suitable for low flow rates.

Back Pressure Compensated Flow Meter

- Any restriction placed at the outlet of the flow meter causes a pressure to be built up behind the constriction. So the fixed pressure difference of the flow meter is lost.

- The flow rate shown in the flow meter will be less than the actual flow. In other words, the meter will under read, e.g. humidifiers, nebulizers, jets and other restrictive types of appliances
- Even during the controlled ventilation, slight back pressure occurs depressing the bobbin each time pressure is applied on the bag.
- If the pin valve (flow control) is situated at the downstream from the flow meter. Any resistance to outflow will not be transmitted to the bobbin, so false reading is unlikely.
- This type of flow meters is known as 'Back pressure compensated' **(Fig. 6.20)**.
- There are other means of back pressure compensation. Allowing the gas from the outlet of the flow meter to collect in an airtight hood around the flow meter tube and having an exit in the hood prevents the back pressure **(Fig. 6.21)**.

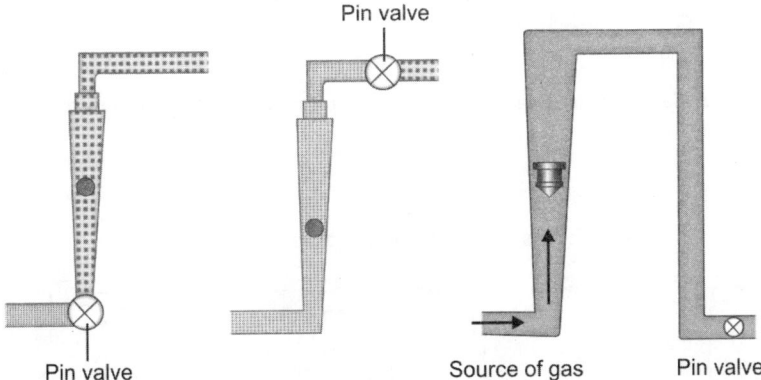

Fig. 6.20: Back pressure compensated flow meter. • The pin valve (flow control) is situated at the upstream (bottom) of flow meter. Any resistance to the flow will be transmitted to the tube cause depression of bobbin results in false reading; • The pin valve (flow control) is situated at the downstream from the flow meter. Any resistance to outflow will not be transmitted to the bobbin, so false reading is unlikely

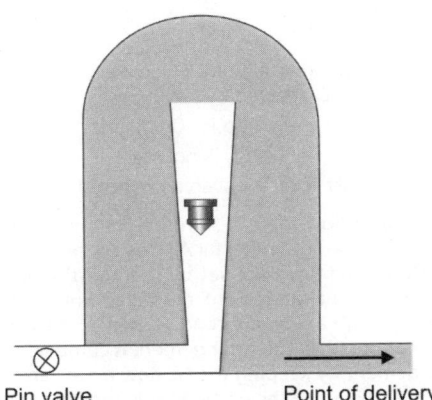

Fig. 6.21: Back pressure compensation using a hood. • The gas collects within the hood before delivery does not cause back pressure

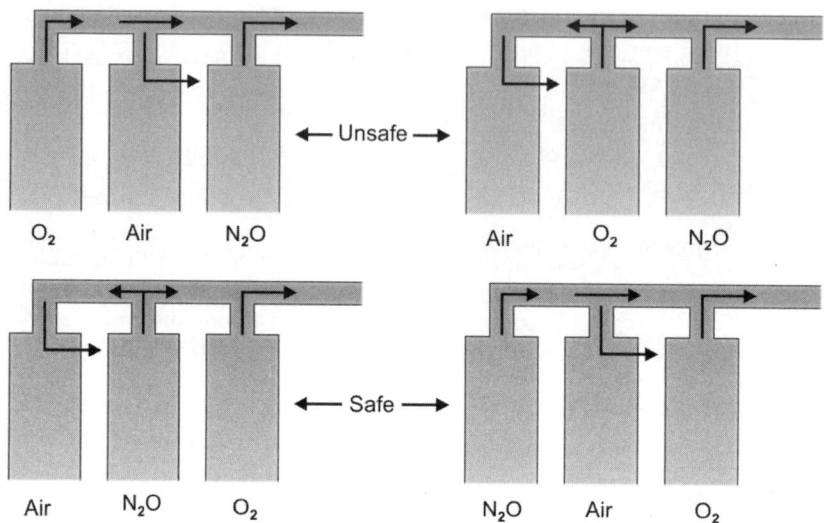

Fig. 6.22: Safety of positioning oxygen flow meter downstream of the flow meter bank

Problems related to position of flow meters and leaks

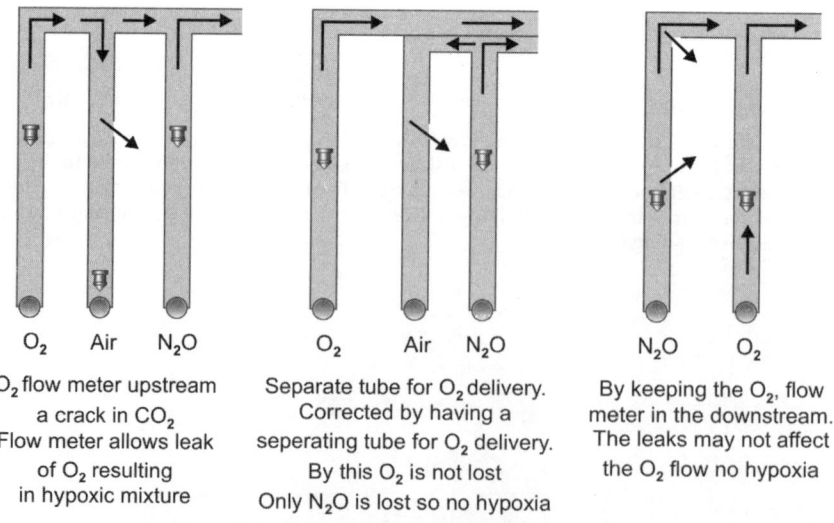

O_2 flow meter upstream a crack in CO_2 Flow meter allows leak of O_2 resulting in hypoxic mixture

Separate tube for O_2 delivery. Corrected by having a seperating tube for O_2 delivery. By this O_2 is not lost Only N_2O is lost so no hypoxia

By keeping the O_2, flow meter in the downstream. The leaks may not affect the O_2 flow no hypoxia

Fig. 6.23: Safe arrangement of flow meters. • In the first arrangement O_2 flow meter is in upstream. When there is a leak in the flow meter for Air may cause loss of oxygen into atmosphere though the flow meter shows the flow rate set by the anesthesiologist leading to hypoxic mixture delivered; • In the second arrangement, the outlet from O_2 flow meter is delivered to the common gas pathway through a separate conduit. Hence, any leak in the flow meter of Air or N_2O hypoxic mixture is not possible. This arrangement is cumbersome and so not commonly used; • In the third arrangement by keeping the O_2 flow meter, any leak in the flow meter of N_2O or Air will not affect the delivery of the oxygen set in the flow meter. Hence, the chance of forming hypoxic mixture is less

Problems Related to the Position of Oxygen Flow Meter

- If oxygen flow meter is positioned on the left end of the flow meter bank, in case of any leaks in the downstream flow meters, varying volume of oxygen may be lost into the atmosphere.
- The remaining volume of oxygen that mixes with the other gases, and reach the common gas outlet may constitute a hypoxic mixture which is potentially dangerous.
- In modern machines as a measure of safety, oxygen flow meter is always positioned on the right end of the flow meter bank (downstream).
- This arrangement of flow meters is likely to prevent the delivery of hypoxic mixture—in case of leaks **(Figs 6.22 and 6.23)**.

FURTHER READING

1. Al-Shaikh Baha, Stacey Simon. Essentials of Anaesthetic Equipment, 1st edn. London, Churchill Livingstone, 1995.
2. Dorsch JA, Dorsch SE. Understanding Anaesthesia Equipment, 4th edn. London: Lippincott Williams and Wilkins, 1999.
3. Dorsch JA, Dorsch SE. Understanding Anaesthesia Equipment, 5th edn. London: Lippincott Williams and Wilkins, 2008.
4. John TB Moyle, Andrew Davey. Ward's Anaesthetic Equipment, 4th edn. London. WB Saunders Company Limited, 1998.
5. Lee's Synopsis of Anaesthesia, 11th edn, London. Butterworth- Heinemann Ltd. 1993.
6. Ward CS. Anaesthetic Equipment, 2nd edn. London: Balliere, S;1985.

chapter 7

Vaporizers

INTRODUCTION

All inhalational anesthetic agents at standard room temperature and pressure are in liquid state.
- Most of them are relatively volatile liquids and known as volatile anesthetic liquids
- An inhalational agent has to be transformed to a state that can be inhaled, i.e. Vapor
- The process of transforming the liquid agent into vapor form is 'Vaporization'

In modern anesthesia, newer volatile anesthetic agents which are highly potent are being used. This means highly calibrated vaporizers are required for delivery of precise concentration of the anesthetic agent into the anesthetic breathing system for reasons of safety and economy.

HISTORY

The first inhalational volatile liquid agent known to this world is Ether introduced in 1846 and the next was Chloroform in 1847

1846 *WTG Morton* used a simple glass inhaler with sponge inside and a non-return valve.

1847 *John Snow* designed an inhaler in which concentrations could be controlled.

1941 *Sir Robert Macintosh* (appointed as Professor in Oxford University) along with Ebstein and Mendelson designed the Oxford vaporizer which had a temperature compensating device.

1952 *Macintosh* and *Epstein* introduced the EMO vaporizer (Epstein Macintosh Oxford) incorporating water jacket and temperature compensating device (thermostat) for vaporizing ether in atmospheric air. This was in use till recent days for vaporizing ether in atmospheric air as carrier gas.

Purpose

To vaporize the volatile anesthetic liquid into a vapor and deliver, it in the desired concentration into the anesthetic breathing system along with the carrier gases which may be oxygen or oxygen and nitrous oxide or air.

Process of Evaporation

- Vaporization of a liquid occurs only on the surface.
- When the molecules collide, then they transfer energy to each other. Sometimes during the transfer, molecules near the surface end up with enough energy to escape.
- The energy of individual molecules is all about evaporation.

Means to Enhance Vaporization

- Increasing the surface area of the volatile liquid agent so as to make the liquid-gas interface larger will increase evaporation by enhancing the number of molecules escaping out of the liquid.
- Keeping the temperature of the liquid near its boiling point as far as possible.
- Providing heat energy to compensate the heat loss by utilization of 'latent heat of vaporization'. This will increase the kinetic energy of the molecules, thus increase the number of molecules capable of escaping from the liquid sate.
- Diverting variable quantity of gases onto the volatile liquid depending upon the need to have a constant vapor concentration.

All these efforts will enhance vaporization and maintain a relatively constant vapor concentration.

Methods to Increase the Liquid-gas Interface

Drops make the liquid into smaller units with individual globular surface-liquid gas interface.
- Increasing the surface area of the volatile liquid in a wider container in vaporizer. (sump) this will increase the number of molecules escaping from the surface **(Fig. 7.1A)**.
- Vapor pressure does not get altered for a given temperature, but the vaporization increases **(Fig. 7.1B)**.
- Using a 'wick' dipped in the liquid agent. By capillary action the liquid ascends up on to the lint cloth thereby increases the surface area available for evaporation.

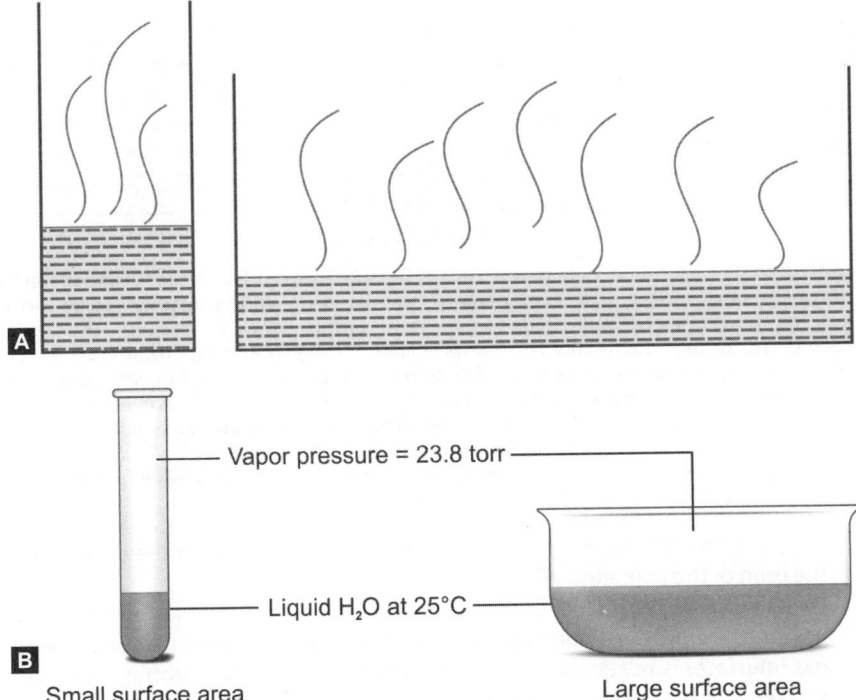

Figs 7.1A and B

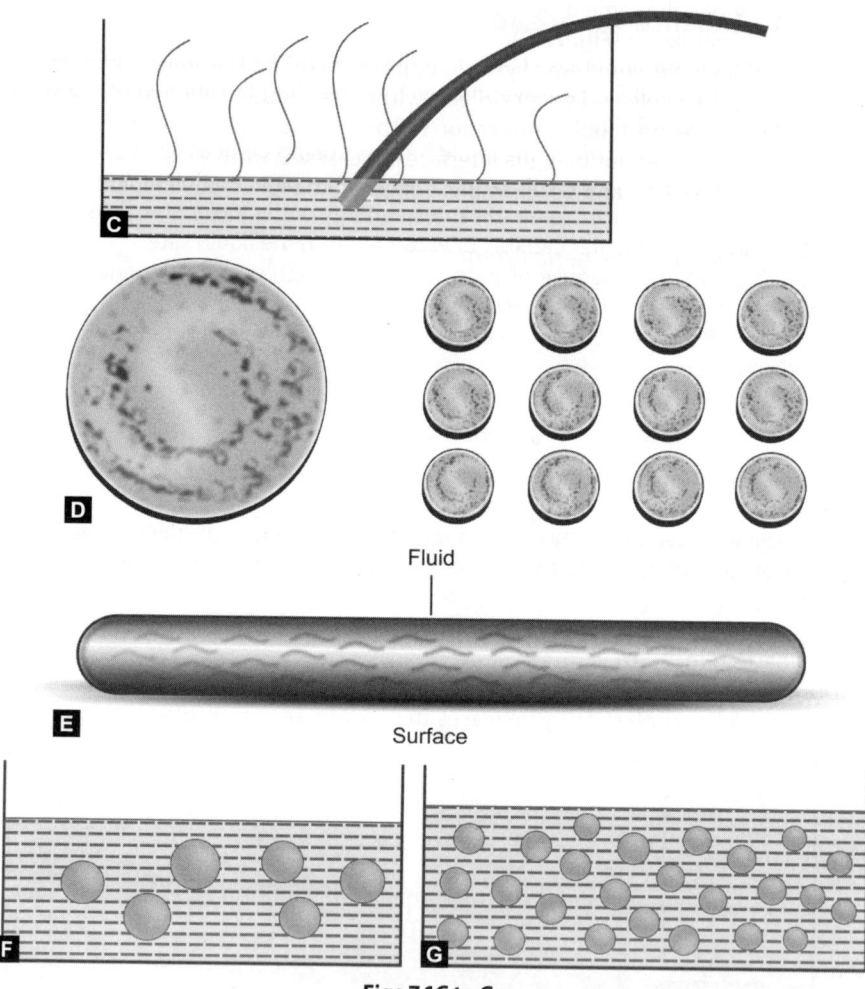

Figs 7.1C to G

Figs 7.1A to G: Methods to increase the Liquid–Gas interface (Surface area): (A and B) Narrow Container—small surface area—very minimal evaporation; • Wide container—large surface area—very good evaporation; (C) Wide container with a wick; • Wick is a lint cloth—the capillary action draws up the liquid—very large surface area; • Exaggerated vaporization by the vast surface area caused by the lint cloth; (D) Big drop—small surface; Same drop split into smaller droplets—larger area; • Big single drop provides small surface area—liquid gas interface-minimal vaporization; • Same drop split into many droplets make the surface area very large—very good vaporization; (E) Same large drop spread into a thick film-large area; • This also increases the surface–greater vaporization; (F) Large bubbles—small surface; (G) Smaller bubbles—large surface • Bubbles are opposite of drops. The interface is within the liquid

Simple example is dipping one end of a lint cloth and leaving the other end on the brim of the container **(Fig. 7.1C)**.

- Drops make the liquid into smaller units with individual globular surface – liquid gas interface. When a liquid is present as a big single drop the surface area (liquid-gas interface) is relatively smaller, whereas, if the same big drop is broken into smaller droplets, there is an enormous increase in the surface area compared to the single drop **(Fig. 7.1D)**.

- Similarly when the same drop is spread on to a surface as a film, again the surface area becomes larger **(Fig. 7.1E)**.
- Gas bubbles in the liquid are physically opposite of drops. The liquid –gas interface is within the bubble and vapor collects within the bubble. When there are larger bubble is inside the liquid, vaporization will be minimal, whereas if the bubbles are broken into smaller bubbles, the interface increases enormously and vaporization increases **(Figs 7.1F and G)**. Example: Copper Kettle for Ether vaporization.

Volatility of Liquid Anesthetic Agents

If the boiling point is low, the liquid is more volatile
- Ethyl chloride   -   12.5°C
- Ether   -   36.5°C
- Trilene   -   87.5°C
- Chloroform   -   61.0°C
- Halothane   -   50.2°C
- Enflurane   -   56.5°C
- Isoflurane   -   48.8°C
- Sevoflurane   -   58.9°C
- Desflurane   -   28.9°C

Definitions Related to Vapor and Vaporization

Vaporizer

It is a device used to evaporate a volatile-liquid anesthetic agent into its vapor so that it can be delivered in the desired concentrations into the anesthetic breathing system and to the patient.

Vapor

It is a liquid in its gaseous form (At normal room temperature and pressure it is a liquid).

Vapor Pressure

The molecules of vapor are always in a state of violent motion. The bombarding force which they exert on a unit area of the wall the container is called as vapor pressure.
 Pressure = Force × Area

Explanation

A liquid has its molecules closely bound together by the cohesive forces—force of mutual attraction between molecules.

Still they continue to be in motion. These molecules bombard the wall of the container. When the surface of the liquid is exposed to a gaseous atmosphere, there forms a liquid-gas interface. The molecules which are in movement may reach the surface of the liquid where they are likely to enter the gaseous compartment. In this process, they do a little work and lose kinetic energy. These molecules that enter into the gaseous compartment above the liquid are called as vapor.

In this process of entering the gaseous compartment, as they do work and lose kinetic energy, the temperature of the liquid falls. The molecules in the gaseous compartment have less mutual attraction and so they move violently to exert pressure on the wall of the container.

Saturated Vapor Pressure

The volatile agent at its boiling point will have a saturated vapor pressure that is equal to the atmospheric pressure (760 mm Hg).

Boiling Point

It is the temperature at which the saturated vapor pressure of a liquid equals to that of the atmospheric pressure. For example, Ether 36.5° C; Water 100° C.

Explanation

When the mouth of a container which contains a certain amount of liquid and gas is closed, there will be continuous escape of molecules into the gaseous compartment which will exert vapor pressure. When the gaseous compartment is fully saturated with molecules from the liquid no further molecule could escape into the gaseous compartment. When no further molecules could be accommodated, the pressure exerted is known as *saturated vapor pressure* for that temperature. Even at this stage, a number of molecules may escape out from the surface of the liquid and because equal number of molecules will re-enter the liquid compartment, it maintains equilibrium. This is called as *saturation*. This varies according to the temperature at which the liquid is exposed. At its boiling point it equals atmospheric pressure.

Latent Heat of Vaporization

The amount heat energy in calories required for converting one gram of the liquid into its vapor form without altering the temperature of the liquid.

Specific Heat

It is the number of calories required to increase the temperature of one gram of a substance by 1° C.

Thermal Capacity

It is defined as a product of specific heat and mass, represents the amount of heat stored in the vaporizer body.

If a substance or material has high specific heat or heat storage capacity, it can supply heat for a longer time to the anesthetic agent for vaporization.

Copper has specific heat 0.092 cal/g and water has specific heat 1 cal/g. So, copper and water are used as reservoirs of heat in vaporizers.

Thermal Conductivity

It is a measure of the speed with which heat flows through a substance. The higher the value, the better the substance conducts heat.

The thermal conductivity is measured in watts per meter per Kelvin (W/m/K). Copper 385, brass 109, aluminum 205, steel 50.2.

The body of a vaporizer should be made of good conducting material to conduct heat energy from the environment to the agent and also material of good specific heat. It should be bulky enough to store a good amount of heat.

Practical Application

In the construction of any vaporizer, whether crude or calibrated, there are a few considerations for the efficient functioning. When the surface area of the liquid is

more, more vaporization occurs. So in the construction basic principles followed are only two:
- Surface area of the liquid-gas interface has to be increased.
- The temperature of the volatile liquid anesthetic has to be near its boiling point.

When the liquid vaporizes the latent heat of vaporization is derived from the liquid, the container of the liquid and the surrounding structures and even from surrounding air. When the temperature falls very low, the water vapor from the atmospheric air condenses on the surface of the container.

This can be well observed in Boyle Bottle vaporizer in the anesthetic machine, particularly, when ether is used. With prolonged use, the temperature of the liquid and the bottle drops to very low level about 5°C or lower and water vapor of atmosphere condenses on the bottle. Sometime ice crystals form at the bottom of the bottle. At this low temperature, there will be negligible or no vaporization of ether with the boiling point of 36.5°C.

For preventing this problem, modern vaporizers are built with material having high specific heat and high thermal conductivity like copper. The body is made very heavy with this metal as that forms a good heat sink providing the heat for vaporization. More over the body of the vaporizer easily conducts the external temperature to the liquid.

Classification of Vaporizers

(Based on the flow of gases)
- *Draw over* vaporizers
- *Flow over* vaporizers—also known as *Plenum vaporizers*.

Draw Over Vaporizers

- The carrier gas is drawn over the surface of the liquid by a negative pressure created at the point of delivery.
- This is usually the negative pressure developed by the inspiratory force of the patient. For example, Schimmelbusch mask, Cyprane inhaler.
- It can be a negative pressure created by a bellows as in EMO ether inhaler.

Examples

Schimmelbusch Mask

- This is one of the earliest and simplest vaporizers.
- A wire framed, gauze covered mask for open drop ether administration.
- It is a oval metal frame with a hood and a device for clamping layers of gauze.
- About 8 to 12 layers of gauze is spread over the hood, stretched and clamped in position. The edges are trimmed. This completes the mask **(Figs 7.2A and B)**.
- A rectangular gamgee pad with a longitudinal slit to expose only mouth and nose is placed on the face to protect eyes and to fill the contour of face. The mask is kept on this pad to cover the mouth and nose.
- The liquid ether is allowed to fall in drops from a dropper bottle and spreads on the layers of the gauze covering the mask by capillary action **(Figs 7.2A and B)**.
- This process enormously increases the surface area of the liquid and so the liquid-gas interface.
- Patient's inspiratory negative force draws the air—the carrier gas—through the gauze layers which vaporizes the ether.

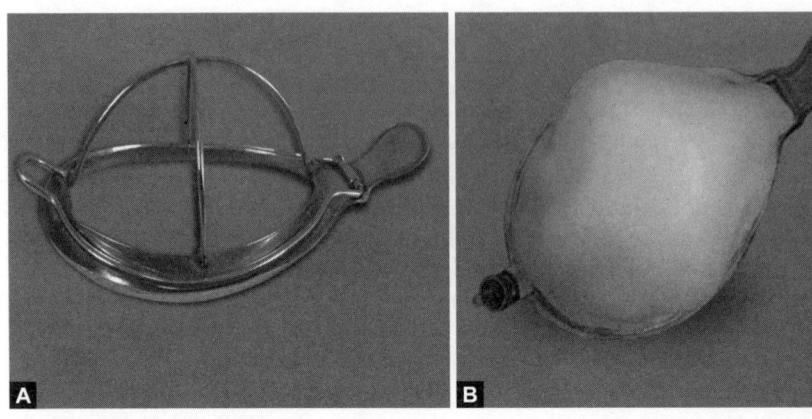

Figs 7.2A and B: Schimmelbusch mask. Frame A and Frame covered with gauze B. • Available in different sizes for adults and children; • Useful for administration of diethyl ether, ethyl chloride and chloroform

Advantages

- Simplicity
- Portability
- Flammability of ether is less when compared in use with oxygen.

Disadvantages

- Pollution of atmosphere
- Injury to the eye
- Wastage of volatile agent
- Increased resistance to respiration with prolonged use
- 8-10 layers of surgical gauze have to be used to optimize vaporization.

Cyprane Inhaler

- Draw over, wick in jar vaporizer for Trilene in air **(Figs 7.3A and B)**.
- This vaporizer was the first introduced by Bill Edmondson after setting up his company "Cyprane" in Yorkshire in 1947.
- Weight is less than 1/2 of a pound.
- Vaporizing chamber holds 15 mL of trilene.
- Boiling point of Trilene is 86.5°C, very less volatile but very potent.
- In this vaporizer, Trilene (Trichloroethylene) is vaporized in air and is used for self administration of obstetrics analgesia by patients.
- The patient holds the vaporizer and inhales at the onset of uterine contraction patient inhales from it so that analgesia is effective in full contraction.
- It gives adjustable output between 0.22% and 0.54% of Trilene in air. Adjustment is done with a key provided and locked.
- Patient's inspiratory negative pressure draws the carrier gas—atmospheric air—through the wick in jar type vaporizing chamber.

EMO Vaporizer

- The EMO inhaler (Designed by Dr HG. Epstein, Physicist in Oxford Department and Professor Macintosh at Oxford) introduced in 1952 **(Fig. 7.4)**.

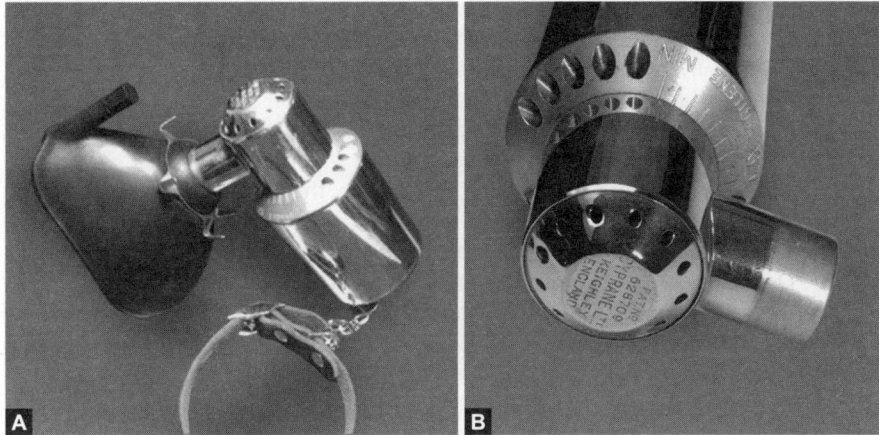

Figs 7.3A and B: Cyprane inhaler. • The patient fastens the hand strap and keeps the mask on the face to inhale Trilene in air; • When the patient becomes drowsy, the handstrap keeps the inhaler from falling out; • There is a key to set the percentage concentration and lock. There are five holes provided as air inlet

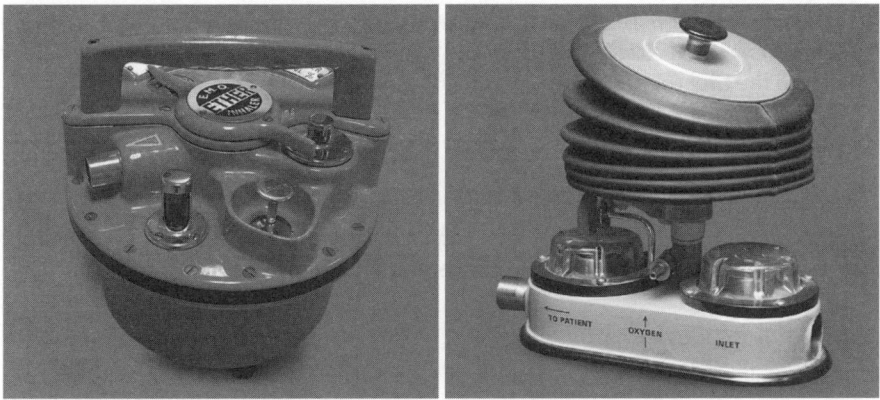

Fig. 7.4: EMO vaporizer and the Oxford inflating bellow

- It was one of the most popular draw over vaporizer widely used all over the world for using ether. In some places, it is in use even now in field situations.
- It has an annular ether vaporizing chamber lined with wicks.
- Surrounding this is a water compartment which can be filled to a capacity of 1200 mL.
- To maintain constant temperature of the liquid, a water bath is provided which serves as a heat sink.
- This, in conjunction with an automatic thermocompensating valve prevents any rapid fall in temperature even when higher concentrations are delivered. (Temperature compensation).
- The temperature compensation is done by a metal bellows filled with Freon gas or ether itself. It regulates the bypass of gases depending upon the temperature.
- It is designed for 'draw over' use in which flow is created by suction (patient's inspiratory effort) at the outlet rather than applying pressure in the inlet, and the air passages are relatively large, offering *a low resistance* to breathing.

- Concertina bellows with non-return disc valves to ensure that the direction of gas flow is correct, and hence that there is no rebreathing of expired air.
- It was originally intended for use with a simple spring loaded expiratory valve, but a non-rebreathing valve is preferred.
- The magnet is provided to immobilize the distal disc. The magnet must be fitted, whenever a non-rebreathing valve is used.
- When the control lever is placed in OFF position, the ether chamber is sealed off to prevent spillage during transport.
- The percentage setting is from 2% to 20% of ether in air.
- The Oxford inflating bellows is used for IPPV with EMO inhaler **(Fig. 7.4)**.
- Here the air is drawn through the vaporizing chamber by the negative pressure created by Oxford bellows.
- This Oxford bellows can be used for artificial ventilation in resuscitation.

Flow-over Vaporizer (Plenum Vaporizer)

- Plenum is a terminology used in air-conditioning which means pressurized chamber where air is pumped in, cooled and let out.
- Flow-over chamber (Plenum) forms the basic principle of construction of a modern vaporizer **(Fig. 7.5)**.
- The carrier gas is blown into the vaporizing chamber containing the liquid anesthetic and it collects the vapor and gets out through the exit which may deliver it into the breathing system.

Simple Plenum

Methods to Improve the Rate of Vaporization

Simple plenum vaporizer will have many disadvantages such as inconsistent vaporization with progressive fall in concentration as time passes.

Flow-splitting Device

- In simple plenum vaporizer, there is no control for the gas flow. All the fresh gas flows through the vaporizing chamber and carries the vapor. This results in higher concentration of vapor in the beginning and as time passes, when the temperature of the liquid drops, the concentration falls.

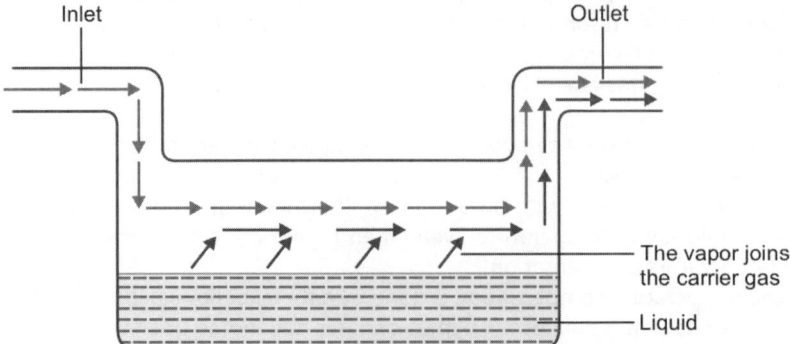

Fig. 7.5: Simple plenum chamber (Vaporizing chamber). • As the gas flows above the liquid, the vapor is also carried along with it to the outlet

- As a first step, the fresh gas flow into the vaporizing chamber is controlled by a flow-splitting device.
- This mechanism splits variable percentage of the carrier gas mixture that is flowing through the machine that could be blown into the vaporizing chamber by adjusting a lever.
- That allows only part of the fresh gases to flow into the plenum and the remaining portion flows through the bypass to join the outlet of the vaporizer.
- When the concentration falls in the course of time, the flow-splitting lever is adjusted to allow more flow into the plenum to carry more vapor **(Fig. 7.6)**.
- Depending upon the necessity more or less percentage of gases could be allowed to pass through the vaporizing chamber (plenum) to collect the vapor and join back to the mainstream of gases.
- The splitting can be varied from 0 to 100%. For example, Boyle's bottle vaporizer **(Figs 7.7 and 7.8)**.

Cowl

- Cowl is present in Boyle's bottle vaporizer.
- Fresh gas flow after passing through the 'Splitting device' enter the bottle (vaporizing chamber) through a J-shaped tube.
- A cowl is an inverted hood such as tubular structure that covers the outlet of the J tube so that the gas flow is directed towards the surface of the liquid in the container and impinges more forcefully on the liquid.
- This cowl can be moved up and down by means of a plunger. Moving down causes more impinging on the surface and more vaporization.
- When it is fully lowered the gas is allowed to bubble through the liquid carrying more gases. For example, Boyle's bottle vaporizer **(Figs 7.7 and 7.8)**.

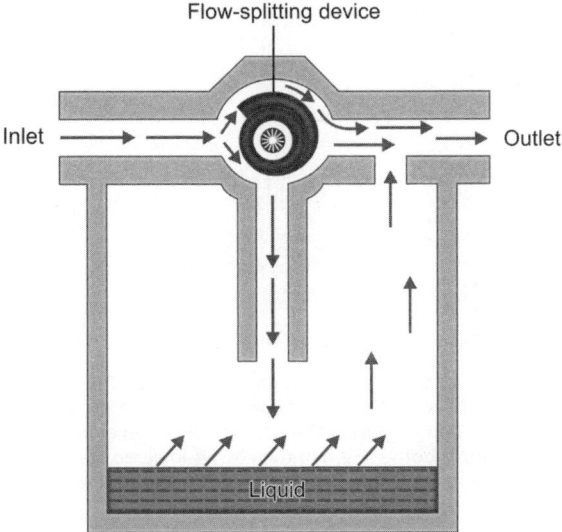

Fig. 7.6: Flow-splitting device. • The main flow of gases is split to various proportions and delivered into the vaporizing chamber; • Clockwise rotation of the 'cam' will increase the proportion of the gas entering into the chamber; • Full anticlockwise rotation will close the gas entering into the chamber

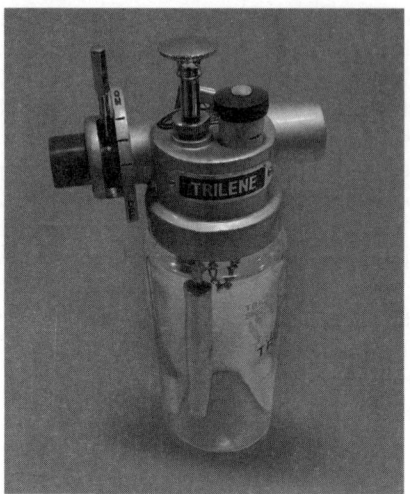

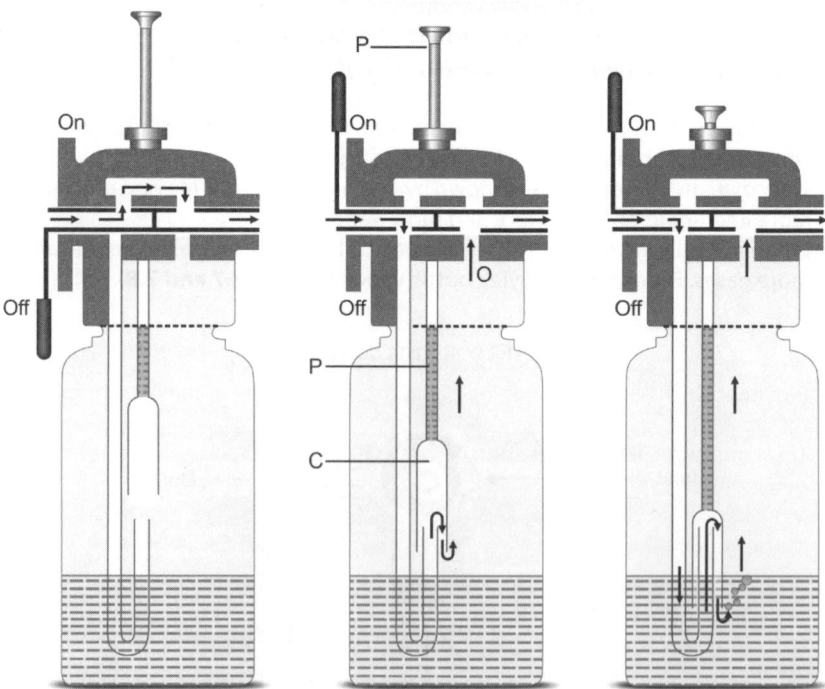

Fig. 7.7: Flow splitting device of Boyle bottle vaporizer. • When the lever is in OFF position, all the gases pass through the bypass • When the lever is in ON position, all the gases pass through the vaporizing bottle • Depending upon the position of the lever varying proportions of gas passes through the vaporizer bottle • When the cowl is lowered, gases impinge more on the liquid, and when the cowl is fully lowered, gases bubble through the liquid • P – Plunger; C – Cowl

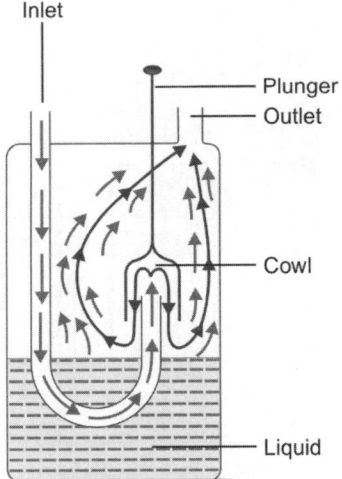

Fig. 7.8: 'Cowl' for directing the gas to the surface of liquid

Increasing the Surface Area of the Liquid

Baffles

In a plenum vaporizer in between the inlet and outlet, a series of baffles are provided from the roof and bottom of the container so that the gas is made to impinge repeatedly on the surface of the liquid carrying more vapor. For example, Ether vaporizer (vaporizer inside circuit) in Mark II circle absorber **(Fig. 7.9)**.

Baffles with Wicks on it

- Wicks by the capillary action absorb the liquid into it.
- Providing wicks on the baffles increases the surface area of the liquid exposed to the gas.
- This considerably increases the rate of vaporization when compared to the presence of baffles alone **(Fig. 7.10)**.
- Most of the modern vaporizers except TEC 6 and Aladin Cassette have wicks in the vaporizing chamber. These are known as "Wick in jar" type of plenum vaporizers.

Wicks

- The wicks may be made of linen, cotton, synthetic material or even fine metal mesh.
- The wicks are usually supported by a metal helical structure in the plenum.
- Multiple wicks are made to dip in the 'sump' (the liquid at the bottom of the plenum) so that by capillary action the liquid anesthetic agent is drawn up and spread all over the wick thereby increasing the surface area (liquid-gas interface) enormously **(Fig. 7.11)**.
- The carrier gas 'Flows over' this large surface are of the liquid to vaporize the liquid.

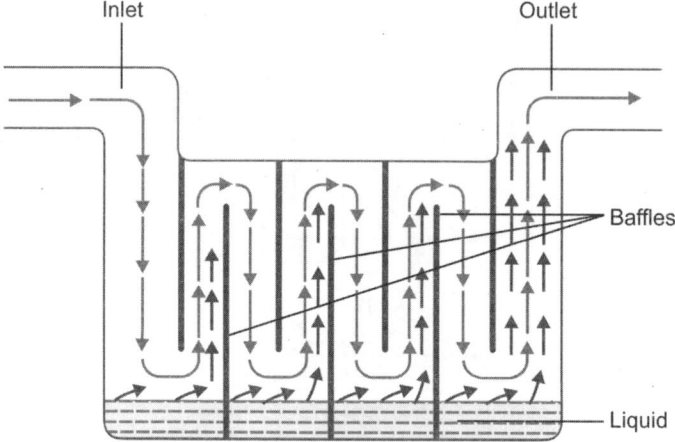

Fig. 7.9: Baffles in plenum

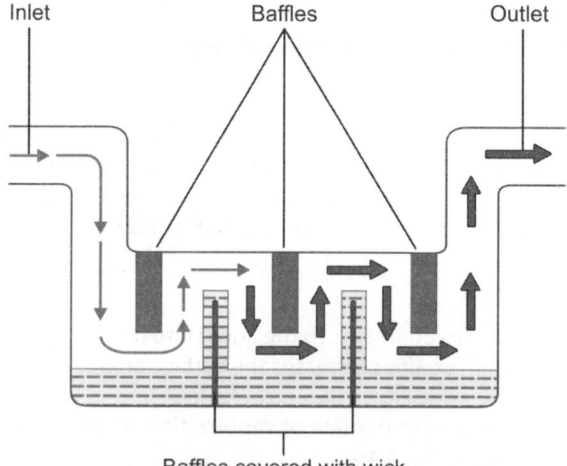

Baffles covered with wick

Fig. 7.10: Baffles with wicks on it in the plenum

Bubble through Device

- Gases are delivered through a tube which is immersed in the liquid anesthetic and opens into a wider outlet covered with 'sintered porex' or any other microporous material.
- This makes the gases escape through the liquid in the form of minute bubbles **(Fig. 7.12)**.
- These bubbles enormously increase the liquid-gas interface enhancing the vaporization. For example, Copper Kettle vaporizer for ether.

Atomizer Vaporizer (Venturi or Injector Device)

- It works on Venturi principle where a stream of gas picks up the liquid from the container through a capillary tube, makes it into a spray which is blown against a

Vaporizers

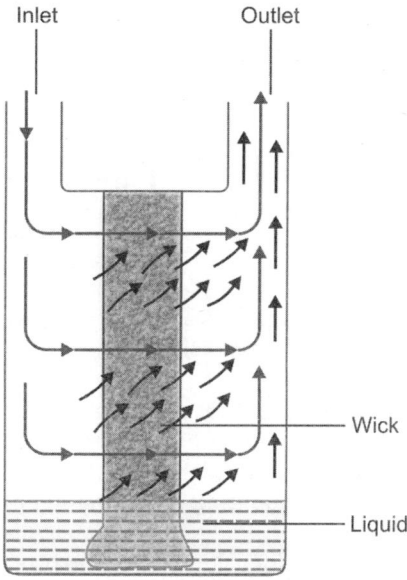

Fig. 7.11: Wick in Jar. • The wick dipping into the liquid in the sump takes up the liquid by capillary action and increases the surface area; • The carrier gas passing through the vaporizing chamber is exposed to the large area takes up more vapor

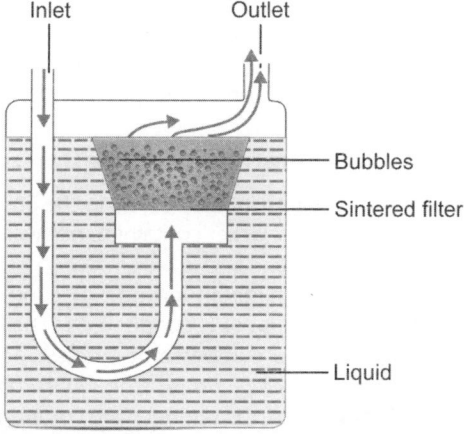

Fig. 7.12: Bubble through vaporizer

 solid ball where it is broken into minute particle thereby increasing the liquid-gas interface and improve vaporization **(Fig. 7.13A)**.
- It is the reverse of 'Bubble through' where the gas is broken into minute bubbles.
- Though not exactly this way, but the Venturi principle (Injector) is used a little differently in Siemens vaporizer **(Fig. 7.13B)**.
- A calibrated throttle valve is opened or closed by the anesthetist. This is activated by the concentration control dial.
- When the throttle valve is closed more, the resistance to the FGF is increased (P_1).
- This higher the pressure of the FGF is transmitted into the sump (container) of the vaporizer.

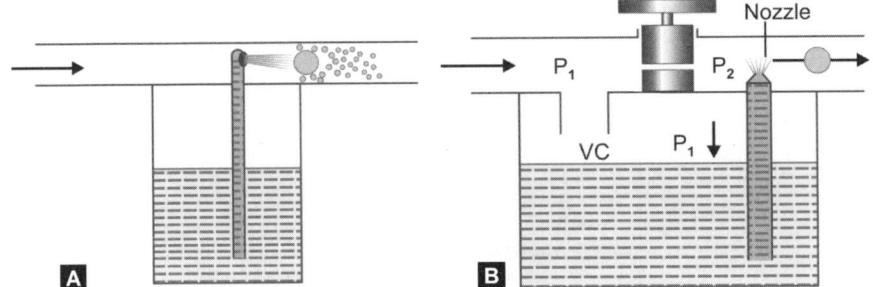

Figs 7.13A and B: Injector type vaporizer
Courtesy: IJA

- Liquid forced by the pressures ascends up to the injector nozzle and is atomized into fine fume (microparticles) and vaporized by the fresh gas flow at low pressure (P_2) but high velocity. (Venturi principle).
- Thus, since the liquid is not vaporizing within the sump, thermal compensation is not necessary.
- These vaporizers are available for halothane, enflurane and isoflurane.

Dropper Type (Not in use now)

A liquid anesthetic from a container is allowed to drop on a metal mesh which is kept on the passage of carrier gases. The mesh makes the liquid to spread by capillary action increasing the surface area and vaporization. The vapor gets added to the gas. Depending upon the requirement, to vary the concentration the number of drops may be increased or decreased using a stopper **(Fig. 7.14)**.

Methods to Keep the Temperature Near the Boiling Point

In earlier days, heat required for vaporization was fed to the liquid by:
- Surrounding the container with a jacket containing hot water.
- Warming the agent using a flame.
- Making the container (sump) with metals having high conductivity like copper so that the heat from the ambience is easily conducted to the liquid.

Supplying heat to the liquid is a cumbersome process. *To maintain a constant percentage output of vapor when the temperature of the liquid drops some compensatory mechanism must be used*. That is known as temperature compensating device.

Temperature Compensation

Later, the containers of vaporizers were made with *metals of high conductivity* and with very thick walls to have a better *heat sink*. This is the reason for the vaporizers being very heavy. Apart from this, *temperature-compensating devices* were included.
- A thermostatic valve which allows additional flow of gases into the vaporizing chamber when the temperature of the liquid falls and vice versa.
- In this mechanism, the thermostatic valve automatically adjusts the flow-splitting device and allows varying amount of gases into the chamber depending upon the temperature of the liquid and maintains the set percentage of vapor at all times. In the course of use, when the temperature of the liquid drops, this *temperature compensating valve* allows suitable quantity of additional flow of gases into

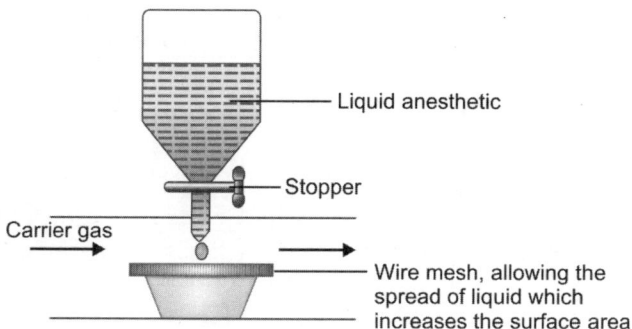

Fig. 7.14: Dropper type vaporizer

the vaporizing chamber to collect additional vapor so that the percentage is maintained constant.

At this point, it is important to remember that *Thermostatic device* and *Temperature-compensating device* are not the same.

If an *electrical-heating element* is used in the vaporizer which *thermostatically* controls the desired temperature, no other compensations are needed. This is not achieved all vaporizers except TEC6 vaporizer.

In all other vaporizers, *when the temperature of the liquid drops* during use, the rate of vaporization is *compensated* by allowing more gas to pass through the vaporizing chamber.

Bimetallic Strip Valve

Usually, the temperature-compensating device is a valve made of *bimetallic strip* with two different metals having different temperature coefficient of expansion (usually 'zinc-copper' or 'zinc-brass'). When the temperature of the liquid drops, the bimetallic strip bends backwards to open the valve to allow more gas and vice versa **(Fig. 7.15A)**.

Metal Bellows

Metal bellows filled with *Freon* gas is another device for temperature compensation. This bellows will expand or contract depending upon the temperature of the liquid which either opens or closes the inlet for additional gas to the vaporizing chamber. In EMO vaporizer the bellows is filled with ether vapor **(Fig. 7.15B)**.

Factors Modifying the Rate of Vaporization

- Volatility of the liquid
- Temperature of the liquid
- Temperature of the gas flowing over the liquid
- Area of liquid-gas interface
- Shape and volume of the space above the liquid

Ether vaporizer bottle in Boyle's machine is larger to have large surface for evaporation. Though ether has high volatility, it is less potent and need higher concentration for anesthesia.

Trilene vaporizer is smaller. Though trilene is less volatile, it is a potent agent and less concentration is needed for anesthesia.

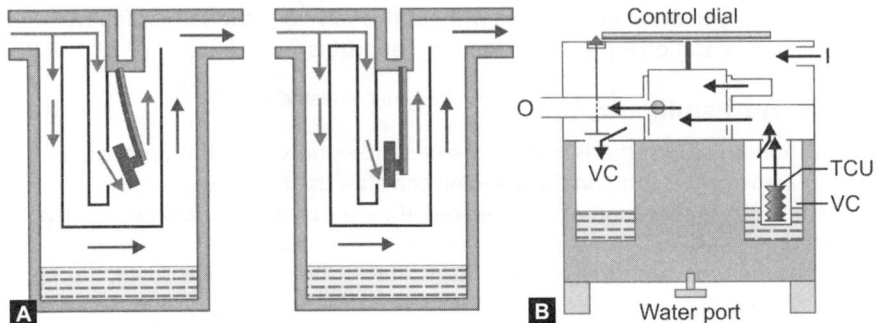

Figs 7.15A and B: Bimetallic strip and metal bellows for temperature compensation. • (A1) Temperature of the liquid is high. So more gas is allowed in the bypass; • (A2) Temperature of the liquid is low. So less gas is allowed in the bypass and more gas enters into the vaporizing chamber; • (B) Temperature compensation by metal bellows *filled* with *Ether* vapor or Freon gas
Courtesy: IJA

VAPORIZERS

Criteria for an Ideal Vaporizer: It must be:
- Fully calibrated
- Flow compensated
- Temperature compensated
- Back pressure compensated
- Stable - Anti-spill provision.

Fully Calibrated Vaporizer

- The concentration set on the dial is delivered to the common gas outlet.
- It must be independent of the possible variables with adequate compensation.

Flow Compensation

Irrespective of the variations in the flow rate of carrier gases used, the set concentration of the vapor is delivered.

Temperature Compensation

Irrespective of the variations in the temperature of the liquid anesthetic in the sump and variations in ambient temperature, the set concentration of vapor is delivered.

Backpressure Compensation

- When the patient is ventilated (IPPV), each time the positive pressure applied to the airway is transmitted to the vaporizer by back pressure.
- This will cause a variable back flow into the vaporizer and increased pressure in the vaporizing chamber (Pumping effect). This phenomena will pick up more concentration of vapor each time positive pressure is applied on the airway. There must be a mechanism to prevent this pumping effect.
- The modern machines do have a valve to prevent the back pressure into the machine.

- This is likely to occur in machines without this valve or if the valve is faulty.
- This compensation is present in modern vaporizers.

Stable (Anti-spill)

- All modern workstations have sect-a-tec provision where the vaporizer of the required agent is fixed on the machine and after use it can be changed.
- In the process of changing the vaporizers, there is a chance of the vaporizer getting tilted.
- Even when the vaporizer is accidentally tilted or tipped upside down, the liquid anesthetic from the sump should not spill into the breathing system.
- If this is not provided, liquid anesthetic may accidentally flow into the breathing system and may cause dangerous rise in concentration of anesthetic.
- Modern vaporizers (TEC5 and later models) are provided with this safety feature.

BOYLE'S BOTTLE VAPORIZER

- It is a crude vaporizer (plenum vaporizer without flow or temperature compensation) with a flow-splitting device. There are two such vaporizer bottles, one for ether and another for trilene **(Fig. 7.16)**.
- It is a crude, non-calibrated, flow over type, plenum vaporizer.
- This vaporizer is used for ether, trilene and chloroform in Boyle's anesthesia machine.
- There is a 'flow-splitting' device, which allows varying proportions of the gas mixture to be delivered into the vaporizer bottle by adjusting a lever on the top **(See Figs 7.7 and 7.15)**.
- The gas inlet to the bottle is through a J-shaped copper tube. A metal cowl is kept inverted on the outlet.
- The cowl can be moved up and down on the outlet by a plunger attached to it **(See Fig. 7.8)**.
- The cowl can be lowered into the liquid ether so that the gas bubbles the liquid carrying more vapor **(See Fig. 7.7)**.

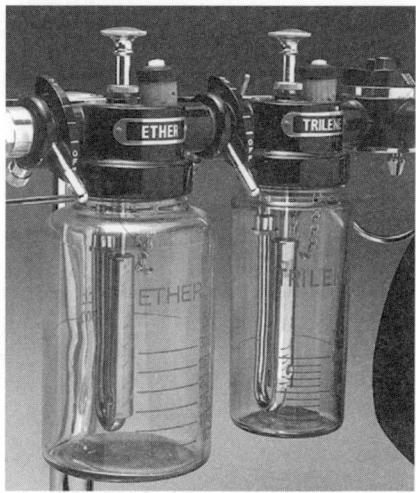

Fig. 7.16: Boyle Bottle vaporizer

- Apart from using the flow-splitting device using the plunger the concentration of ether delivered to the patient can be increased or decreased. When the cowl is lowered on the 'J' tube's outlet, more gas impinges on the liquid to take more vapor.
- In the ether vaporizer bottle, the tubes are made of copper as copper itself is a stabilizer of ether from chemical degradation. The tube in trilene bottle is made of copper with thick chromium plating, as trilene reacts with copper.
- Ether vaporizer bottle in Boyle's machine is larger to have large surface for evaporation. Though ether has high volatility (BP 36.5°C), it is less potent and need higher concentration for anesthesia.
- Trilene vaporizer is smaller. Though trilene is less volatile (BP 87°C), it is a potent agent and less concentration is needed for anesthesia.
- Ether bottle is kept in the upstream in order and trilene bottle comes next. If trilene with higher boiling point is kept in the first bottle, by mistake, if the gas mixture containing trilene enters the second bottle containing ether, the trilene vapor condenses and gets dissolved in ether causing contamination.

COPPER KETTLE VAPORIZER

- In 1952, Dr Lucien E Morris designed the Copper Kettle, which produced known volumes of saturated vapor, then diluted to calculated concentrations necessary for anesthesia. Originally it was designed for chloroform.
- Morris' design incorporated a separately metered flow of carrier gas through the vaporizer to produce known volumes of saturated vapor for introduction into the fresh gas flow delivery.
- It is a bubble through vaporizer. Oxygen is allowed to bubble through a sintered bronze bubbler **(Fig. 7.17)**.
- The container is made of copper which is a good heat sink.
- It is usually fixed to the metal top of the anesthesia machine for better heat conductivity.

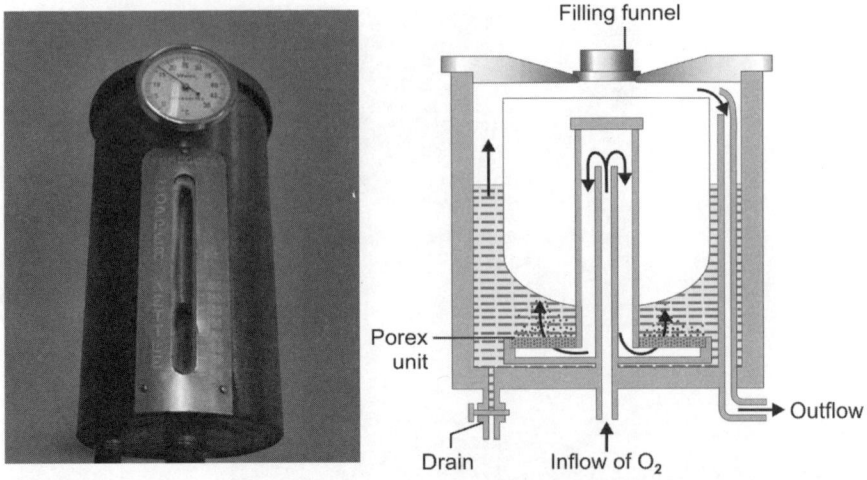

Fig. 7.17: Copper Kettle Ether vaporizer. • The Copper Kettle with level indicator and temperature gauge; • The internal structure is seen in the second picture

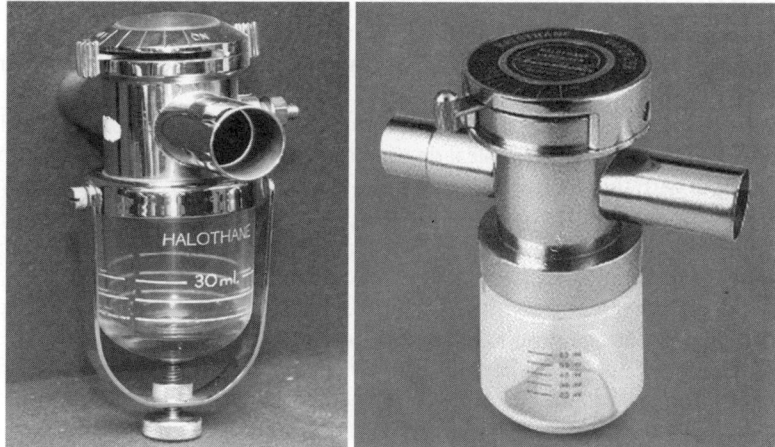

Fig. 7.18: Goldman halothane vaporizer. • The 'stirrup' holds the container in one and the other is screw type

GOLDMAN VAPORIZER

- Dr Victor Goldman (1903-1994) an English physician who specialized in dental anesthesia introduced the first model of his small halothane vaporizer for dental use in 1956.
- His second model 'Mark II' introduced in 1962 is in use now. It is small enough and could not deliver a dangerously high concentration of anesthetic.
- Simple and inexpensive vaporizer for halothane **(Fig. 7.18)**.
- It is not a temperature compensated vaporizer.
- Offers minimal resistance to flow and output is influenced by gas flow rate (not flow compensated).
- Though it is not a calibrated vaporizer, its advantage is that higher concentrations cannot be delivered. (0.5 to 2% only).
- At the flow rate of 8 L/ minute the maximum concentration achieved is 2.5%.

TEMPERATURE COMPENSATED VAPORIZERS

These are plenum type, variable by pass, concentration calibrated, direct reading dial-controlled vaporizer. TEC means 'temperature compensated'. Originally, it was introduced for halothane and was known as 'Fluotec' vaporizer.

First Fluotec was designed by Cyprane Company, for halothane. Later all the TEC vaporizers were manufactured by Ohmeda. These are temperature compensated calibrated vaporizer delivering a constant concentration fixed by the user.

Characteristics

- Plenum
- Wick-in-Jar
- Flow compensation (not fully compensated)
- Temperature compensation.

This original Fluotec was calibrated for fresh gas flow down to two liters per minute. With lower flow tares, the concentration delivered fell off quickly and so it was not suitable for completely closed breathing system technique of anesthesia, where very low flow rates are used.

Fluotec Mark 2 was developed for eliminating this limitation in 1959.

Fluotec Mark 2

It is a calibrated agent specific vaporizer for halothane introduced in 1959. But the calibration had certain limitations in low flows.

Limitation

- Temperature compensation is complete.
- Flow compensation is incomplete.
- The percentage of halothane delivered will be higher than that set on the dial, when the flow rate of fresh gas is less than 2 L/minute.
- When the flow rate is less than 500 mL/minute, there will be no vaporization.
- Between 500 mL and 2 L/minute, the concentration delivered is higher than that in the dial setting.
- A chart on a plastic card attached to the vaporizer shows the actual value at the particular flow rate so that suitable adjustments may be made in the dial setting.
- The dial setting is from 0 to 4%.
- The concentration control knob (dial) adjusts the valve of splitting ratio between the vaporizing chamber and the bypass.
- The gas passing through the chamber flows through a series of wicks to ensure that it is fully saturated.
- The gas flow through the vaporizing chamber is controlled by the bimetallic strip valve (Made of strips of two different metals having different temperature coefficient so that expansion or contractions are unequal).
- As evaporation proceeds and temperature of the liquid falls, the valve opens allowing more vapor to flow.
- This keeps the output concentration constant by temperature compensation.
- There is *no back pressure compensation*. So pumping effect and pressurizing effect are possible.
- Funnel filling system. Not keyed. No interlock.

Characteristics

Agent specific (Halothane), flow over, variable bypass, wick in jar, flow compensated, temperature compensated. *No* back pressure compensation.

- Dial (control knob) is present on the front near the top **(Fig. 7.19A)**.
- Dial setting range is from 0.5 to 4%.
- The filling port is funnel-shaped with screw-threaded stopper situated near the bottom of the vaporizer. The danger of inadvertently filling the wrong agent is possible.
- The drain cock is situated at the bottom of the sump.
- Charging volume required for a new vaporizer is 600 mL (Too high).
- Range of flow rate for effective vaporization is from 2 to 15 L/minute.
- Bimetallic strip for temperature compensation is situated within the vaporizing chamber. Corrosion of this valve by thymol (preservative present in halothane) may cause sticking of the valve.

- If the flow rate is less than 500 mL, no vaporization occurs. 500 mL to 2 L delivers higher concentration.
- Made of copper with thick chromium plating (high density heat sink).

Fluotec Mark 3

Some of the problems of Mark 2 are rectified.

Characteristics

Flow compensated, temperature compensated, Back pressure compensated, *Not* spill proof.
- Dial is situated on the top of the vaporizer **(Fig. 7.19B)**.
- Filling port and drain are combined as one piece (In earlier models, agent specific-filling device was not available. In later models agent specific keyed-filling device was introduced by Cyprane in 1980).
- Charging volume of a new vaporizer is 150 mL (approximately).
- In the vaporizing chamber, there are two concentric wick skirts. These tubular wicks are supported by a nickel-plated copper helix in between.
- This assembly forms a long spiral channel through which carrier gas flows before entering the chamber preventing back pressure problems.
- Bimetallic temperature sensitive valve is situated outside the vaporization chamber in the bypass.
- Works efficiently with flow rates from 250 mL to 15 L/minute.
- The percentage generated ranges from 0 to 5%.
- There is no anti-spill mechanism available.
- 'Select-a-tec' provision is available but optional (The vaporizers for more than one agent can be mounted on the back bar of the machine by hooking on. There is an *interlock mechanism* available, that prevents switching ON more than one vaporizer at a time. Ideally one vaporizer is mounted on the back bar and in case of necessity, it can be removed and another for other agent may be mounted in the same place).
- Anti-spill mechanism is not available.
- Back-pressure compensation is available (no pumping effect).

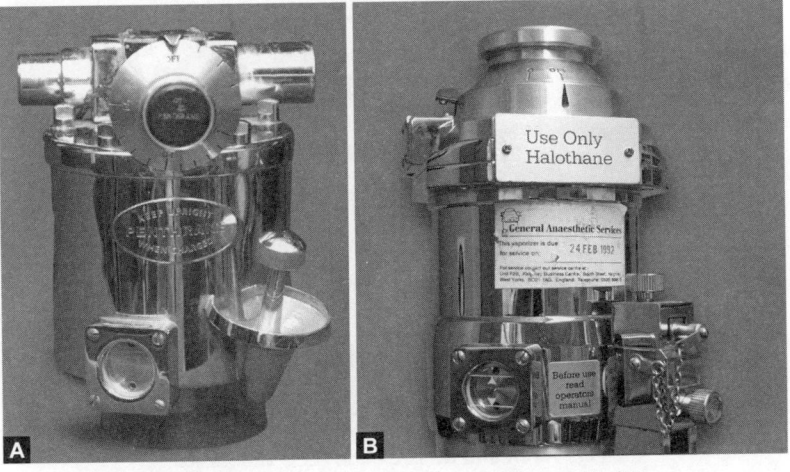

Figs 7.19A and B: Fluotec Mark 2 and Fluotec Mark 3

TEC 4

Characteristics (All the Compensations are Present)

Flow compensated, temperature compensated, back pressure compensated, with *Anti-spill* mechanism and provision for *Select-a-tec*. Introduced in 1983.

Anti-spill is a safety mechanism which prevents spilling of the liquid anesthetic flowing into the bypass channel and into the breathing system even when accidentally the vaporizer is tipped upside down.

- Dial is situated on the top of the vaporizer.
- Filling and draining port in a single piece with *agent specific keyed-filling device* **(Fig. 7.20A)**.
- *Select-a-tec vaporizer interlock mechanism* is present (Many vaporizers can be fixed on the back bar but only one can be operated at a time because of an interlocking device).
- Charging volume of a new vaporizer is 135 mL.
- Available for different agents. *Dial settings*: Halothane: *0 to 5%*; Enflurane: *0 to 7%*; Isoflurane: *0 to 5%*.

TEC 5

All compensations are available along with Select-a-tec feature.
- Similar in appearance to TEC 4 **(Fig. 7.20B)**.
- Improved wicks (hollow cloth tube kept opened by a steel wire spiral helix that prevents collapse of the cloth).
- Two additional features are added. One is *improved keyed-filling device* (Geometrically keyed—wrong agent cannot be filled) and the other is the control knob that can be adjusted with single hand.
- Color coding is present for safety (Bottle, vaporizer and key)
- *Halothane: Red; Enflurane: Orange; Isoflurane: Purple*

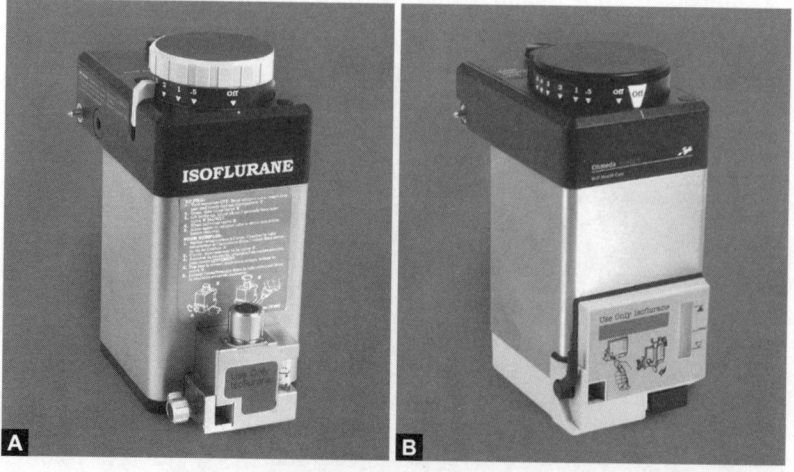

Figs 7.20A and B: TEC 4 and TEC 5 vaporizers

TEC 6

Designed for the newer agent—Desflurane (1993)
- This appears similar to other TEC vaporizers, but is *totally different in principles, functioning and construction* **(Figs 7.21A to C)**.
- Specifically designed for Desflurane (Boiling point: 23.9°C)
- Can be fixed on a *select-a-tec* back bar.
- It has a electrically heated sump with a capacity of 450 mL.
- Heated to a constant temperature of 39° C (Saturated vapor pressure is 1550 mm Hg at this temperature).
- It is a fully computerized device.
- Vapor pressure at 20°C is 664 mm Hg.
- Back up battery (9 Volts)—takes up in the event of power failure.
- Fresh gas flow does not flow into any chamber (No Plenum)
- Computer-controlled percentage mixing is shown in **Figure 7.21C**.

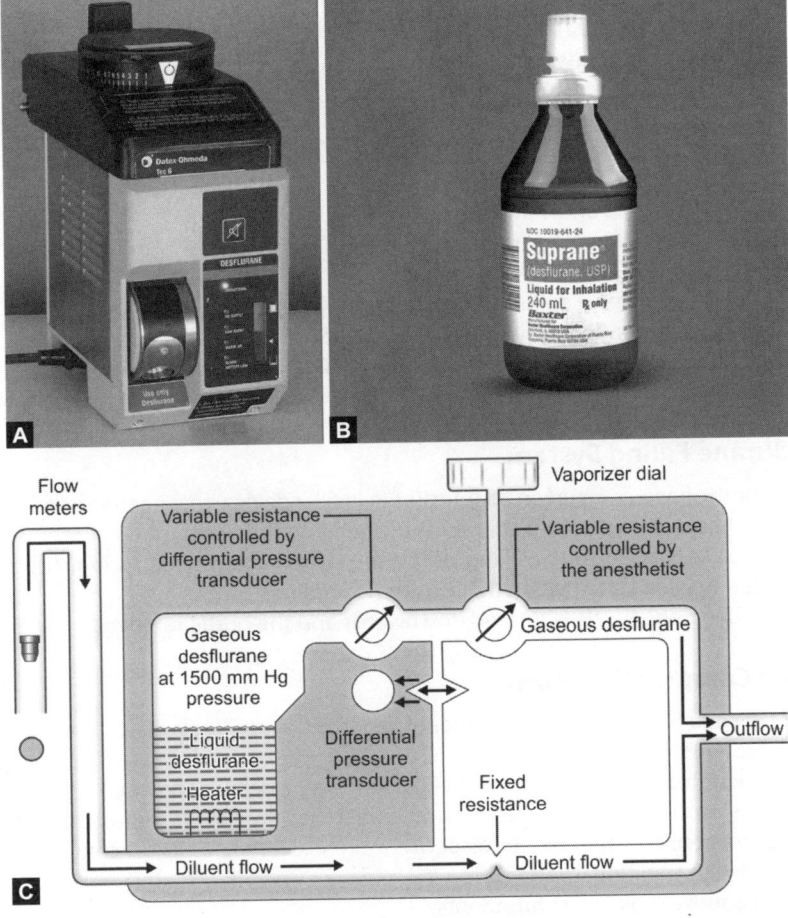

Figs 7.21A to C: TEC 6 and desflurane bottle with built in filler device.
- The internal structure computerized percentage mixing of TEC 6 is shown

- Vaporizer will not start functioning until the temperature reaches 39°C which takes about 5–10 minute (Depending upon the ambient temperature). This is known as *'Warm-up time'*.
- The *Amber* LED is on when connected to the main power. The *Green* LED is illuminated to indicate that the vaporizer has reached 39°C. The *Red* LED with an audible alarm indicates that there is no vapor delivered.
- Percentage concentration—0 to 18% (1% increments till 10%; 2% increments from 10 to 18%)
- Rotary-filling device is present. Drain also can be done through the same port by rotating it downwards.
- Even when the device is switched on, it can be filled.
- Not to be used in the presence of MRI. Physical damage to the scan or distorted images because high magnetic field will be absorbed by the metals. Damage to the vaporizer may occur due to the high magnetic field affecting the computer.

TEC 7

- Introduced by GE Datex Ohmeda for Halothane, Enflurane, Isoflurane and Sevoflurane **(Fig. 7.22)**.
- It is provided with 'Easy—fil' system for minimizing the agent leak during filling.
- For sevoflurane, it is available with 'Quick-fil'
- Provides consistent output throughout with the flow rate from 200 mL to 15 L/minute.
- Equipped with a large diameter control dial, with fine graduations of 0.2% between 0 and 1% and 0.5% from 1% to 8%.
- The dial for sevoflurane is marked in steps of 0.2% up to 1% and in steps of 1% between 1% and 8%.
- The Tec 7 Vaporizer accommodates 225 mL of anesthetic agent.
- Select-a-tec mounting provision is available **(*See* Fig. 7.24)**.
- Non-spill system limits movement of liquid agent, even if the vaporizer is tilted or inverted.

Desflurane Filling System

- The bottle has a 'crimped on adapter' (built in filler device) that has a spring-loaded valve that opens when the adapter is pushed into the filling port.
- The bottle is fitted to the filling port and pushed against the spring. Then it is rotated upwards and held in that position for filling.
- After filling, the bottle is rotated downwards and the bottle removed.

Aladin Cassette Vaporizer

Datex-Ohmeda has replaced conventional vaporizers with *Aladin* vaporizer cassettes in their S/5 *Anesthesia Delivery Unit*.

The cassettes are more lightweight (2–3 kg), are virtually service-free and have no restrictions for tilting. Integrated electronic fresh gas flow measurement of varying gas mixtures enables the unit to dispense more accurately a dialed concentration, compared with traditional vaporizers.
- This vaporizer has two components.
    1. An *electronic control system* which is installed in the machine.
    2. A *portable cassette* which is a liquid sump without control mechanism.

Vaporizers **167**

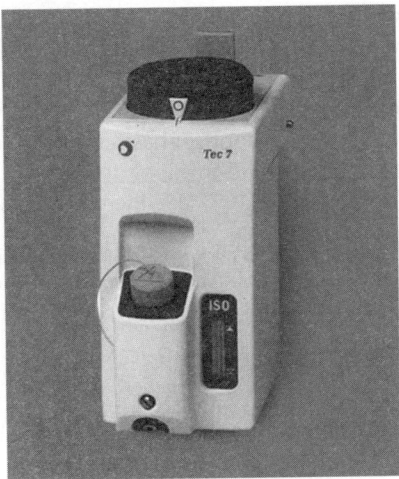

Fig. 7.22: TEC 7 Vaporizer

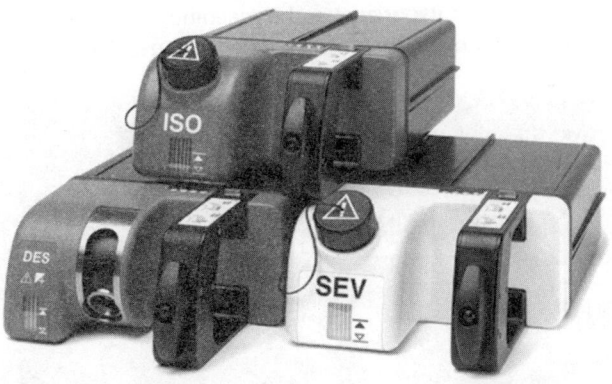

Fig. 7.23: Aladin cassette vaporizer

- A single electronic control system (CPU) installed in the anesthesia workstation can be used for all anesthetic agents including Desflurane.
- The flow at the outlet of the vaporizing chamber is controlled by the CPU.
- The vaporizer looks very different externally, but functionally similar to the conventional vaporizers that it has a vaporizing chamber and a bypass.
- This is designed for halothane, enflurane, isoflurane, sevoflurane and desflurane **(Fig. 7.23)**.
- Electropneumatic proportional flow valves controlled by microprocessors regulate the anesthetic vapor concentration.
- The agent is in a portable cassette that is inserted into a slot in the anesthesia machine.
- The cassette holds up to 250 mL when full.
- The cassette is color coded and magnetically coded.
- A magnetic sensor identifies the cassette.

- The control dial is on the machine next to the slot where the cassette is placed.
- The cassettes for halothane, enflurane and isoflurane have keyed fillers or the Easy-fil system.
- Sevoflurane cassettes may be equipped with either keyed filler or the Quik-fil system.

SELECT-A-TEC SYSTEM

- This system provides convenience for mounting the vaporizer of the required agent on the back bar of the machine according to the necessity **(Fig. 7.24)**.
- The mounting system has channel for the fresh gas from the flow meter towards the common gas outlet.
- The vaporizer is mounted on two vertical stout knobs with 'O' rings at the base for airtight fit.
- One is for inlet and the other is for outlet and has self-sealing valves in it.
- When the vaporizer is mounted and turned 'ON', two plungers push the valve of the mounting knob down to open the channel for gas to pass through the vaporizer.
- If no vaporizer is mounted or the vaporizer is in 'OFF' position, the gas passes directly through the channel of the mounting system.
- Less space is needed for vaporizers in the machine. Vaporizers can be mounted or removed very easily even during the conduct of anesthesia.

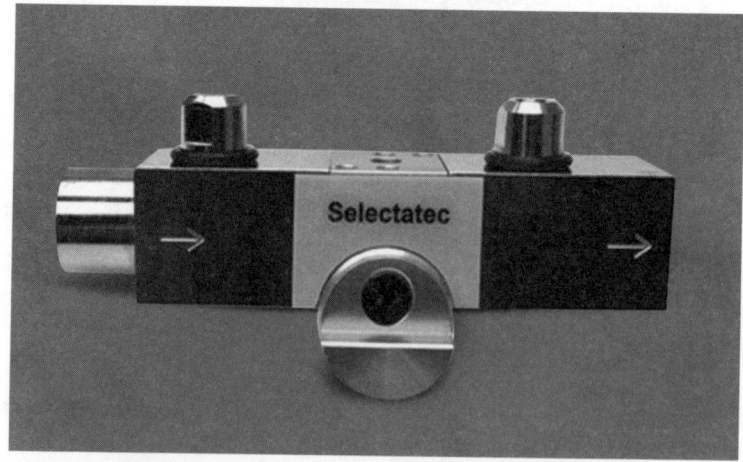

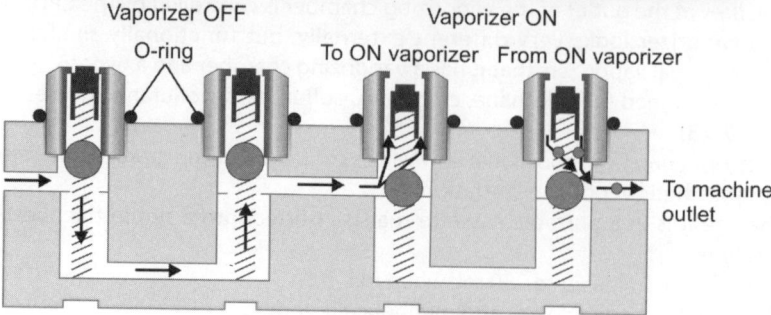

Fig. 7.24: Select-a-tec mounting and the mechanism

- Interlock system permits only one vaporizer in operation and prevents operating two vaporizers simultaneously.
- The problems are; the chances for leak or block to the flow of gases.

Interlock System
- When more than one vaporizer is mounted on the back bar of the machine, there is every chance of accidentally opening two vaporizers simultaneously.
- The interlock system will permit only one vaporizer to be 'ON' at a time.
- Once one vaporizer is turned 'ON', a stout pin from this vaporizer projects out and presses the corresponding pin of the neighboring vaporizer **(Fig. 7.25)**.
- This automatically locks the other vaporizer and it cannot be turned 'ON' unless the operating vaporizer is turned 'OFF'.
- There are many such mechanical devices used to inactivate the control knob of the vaporizers that are not in use.

Filling Systems
- Different filling systems are available in various vaporizers for filling the right agent in the vaporizer.
- The commonly used systems are *Funnel filling, Keyed filling, Quick-fil, Easy-fil,* and *Desflurane filling system.*

American Society for Testing Material (ASTM) recommends that vaporizers should be designed for a single agent fitted with a permanently attached agent specific device to prevent accidental filling with a wrong agent.

Funnel Filling (Anti-spill)
- Bottle has a color-coded collar that cannot be removed.
- The filling adapter has a screw threaded cap and skirt with slot that match the projections on the bottle collar **(Fig. 7.26)**.
- This helps in filling the vaporizer without spilling the liquid.

Keyed Filling
- Vaporizer filling receptacle, filler socket, filler unit, fill and drain system are the names referring this.

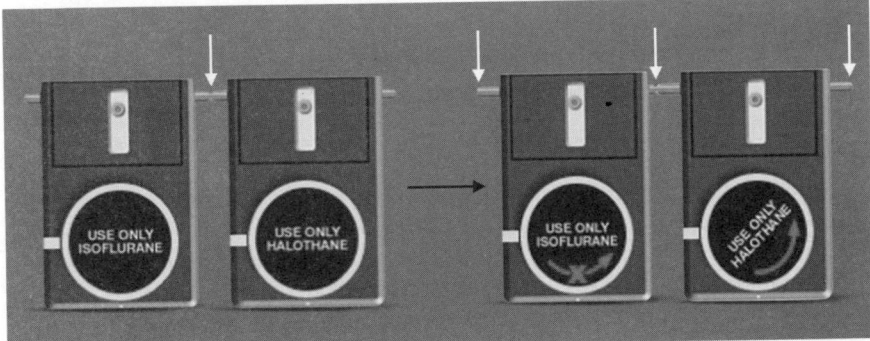

Fig. 7.25: Interlock system in vaporizer. • As seen from above- the dials of the vaporizers and the interlock pins • When the Halothane vaporizer is 'ON' the stout pin juts out to press the corresponding pin of the other vaporizer and locks it

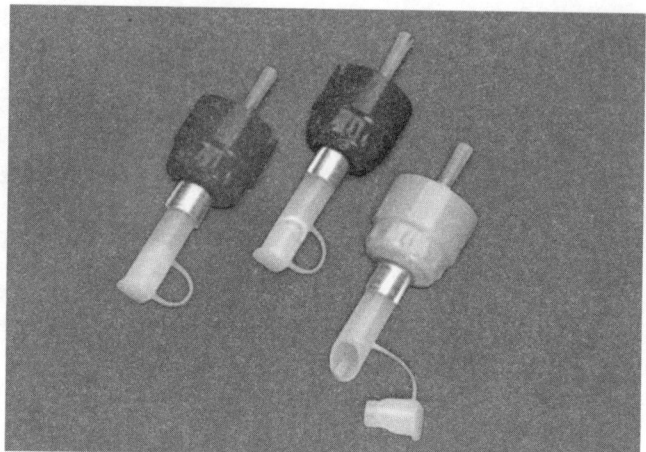

Fig. 7.26: Anti-spill Funnel filling device for halothane, isoflurane and sevoflurane

- The unit permits only the intended bottle's adapter to be inserted.
- Bottles have color-coded collar attached to the neck that cannot be removed **(Fig. 7.27)**.
- *Keyed filling adapter:* Adapter assembly is also color-coded. It is a short flexible tube. At one end, there is a connector with screw thread and skirt fitting on the bottle. The other end has a male connector that fits into the filler receptacle of the vaporizer **(Fig. 7.27)**.
- The male connector is a rectangle piece of plastic with a groove on one side. This is different for each agent. There are two holes on one surface; one larger hole for filling or draining the agent, and the other smaller hole for air to leave the chamber (vent).
- For filling, the vaporizer is turned 'OFF'. After screwing, the adapter to the bottle, the plug is removed. Filler connector is inserted and retaining screw is tightened. Filler valve (air vent) is opened and the bottle is raised. Now the liquid enters the vaporizer.

Quick-fil

This is used for Sevoflurane only.

Easy-fil

This is used in all TEC 7 vaporizes **(Fig. 7.28)**.

Desflurane-filling System

- The bottle has a crimped on adapter that has a spring-loaded valve that opens when the adapter is pushed into the filling port.
- The bottle is fitted to the filling port and pushed against the spring. Then, it is rotated upwards and held in that position for filling.
- After filling, the bottle is rotated downwards and the bottle removed.

Splitting Ratio

The ratio of bypass flow to the vaporizing chamber is referred to as 'Splitting ratio'.

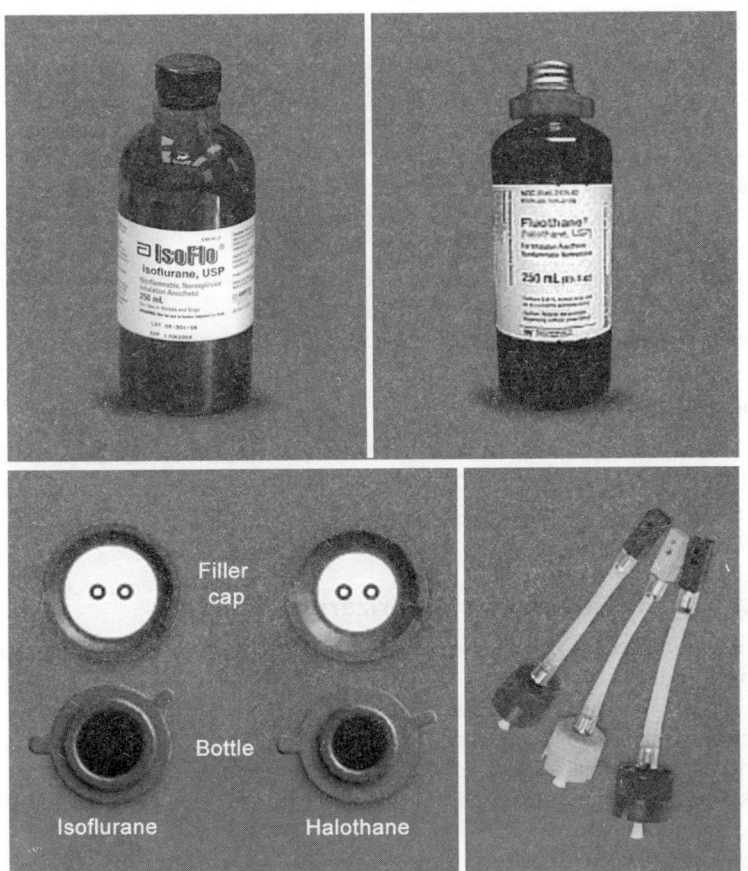

Fig. 7.27: Keyed filling adapters and the bottle collars • Bottles with agent specific color-coded collar and the color-coded filler cap that fits only on the specific collar

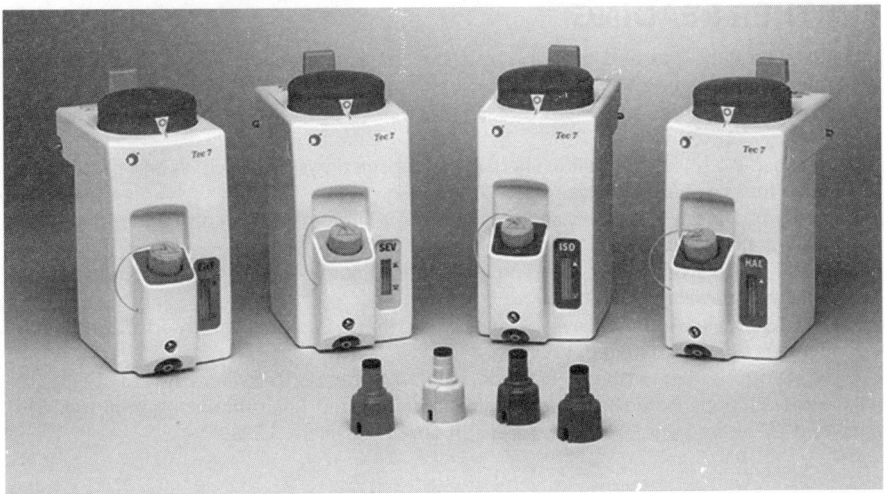

Fig. 7.28: Easy-fil filling system for TEC 7 vaporizers

Pumping Effect

During anesthesia when IPPV is applied, the positive pressure is transmitted back into the machine through the common gas outlet. This back pressure causes compression of gases inside the vaporizing chamber and picks up more volatile agent. When pressure is released, the gas which has picked up a higher concentration enters the breathing system and increases the inspired concentration of anesthetic agent. This is known as *Pumping effect*. The effect is more pronounced when low flow rate is used.

Various modifications in vaporizer design were attempted to correct this problem. If a unidirectional valve is incorporated in the outlet, the 'pumping effect' is prevented. TEC 5 vaporizer has this provision (Back pressure compensation).

Pressurizing Effect

This effect is usually seen with high flow rates. This again is due to the compression of gases in the chamber. When the pressure is released, the volume expands and the effect of the added vapor is diluted and there is no change in the output concentration.

Safety Features in Modern Vaporizers

Modern vaporizers (e.g. *Datex-Ohmeda Tec 5, 6 and 7*) have several safety advantages over their predecessors:
- An interlock to isolate vaporizers not in use
- A clear indication of liquid level
- A non-spill reservoir with up to 180° of allowable tilt
- A keyed-filler or pour-fill systems prevent filling with an incorrect volatile agent and minimize leaks
- An increased wick capacity

Recent innovations have included injection of volatile agent into the fresh gas stream, at a rate calculated (by computer) to produce the desired concentration.

FURTHER READING

1. Al-Shaikh Baha, Stacey Simon. Essentials of Anaesthetic Equipment, 1st edn. London, Churchill Livingstone, 1995.
2. Chakravarti S, Basu S. Modern Anaesthesia Vapourisers. Indian J Anaesth. 2013;57(5):464-71.
3. Dhulkhed V, Dhulkhed P, Naik S, Shetti A, Vapourisers: Physical principles and classification. Indian Journal of Anaesthesia. 2013;57(5):455-63.
4. Dorsch JA, Dorsch SE, Understanding Anaesthesia Equipment, 4th edn. London. Lippincott Williams and Wilkins, 1999.
5. Dorsch JA, Dorsch SE, Understanding Anaesthesia Equipment, 5th edn. London. Lippincott Williams and Wilkins, 2008.
6. John TB Moyle, Andrew Davey. Ward's Anaesthetic Equipment, 4th edn, London: WB Saunders Company Limited, 1998.
7. Lee's Synopsis of Anaesthesia, 11th edn, London. Butterworth-Heinemann Ltd., 1993.
8. Morris LE. Copper Kettle Revisited, Classic Papers Revisited. Anaesthesiology. 2006;104:881-4.
9. Ward CS. Anaesthetic Equipment, 2nd edn. London: Balliere, S;1985.

Anesthetic Breathing Systems

chapter 8

Though anesthetic breathing systems are part of the anesthesia machines, considering the intricate detail of the subject, it is discussed in a separate chapter.

HISTORY

- *1846: WTG Morton* in 1846 devised an inhaler for ether which was a globular glass container with sponge soaked in ether kept inside. There was a provision for air inlet and a mouthpiece for breathing with a non-return valve **(Fig. 8.1)**.
- *1867: Junker Bottle* for insufflation technique for chloroform.
  Ferdinand Ethelbert Junker designed this apparatus in 1867 in London. Fresh air is driven by hand bellows through the liquid itself. It was introduced by Benjamin Ward Richardson
- *1890: Schimmelbusch mask* for open drop anesthesia with ether or chloroform. This device was invented by Curt Schimmelbusch in 1890, and was used until the 1960s though it is still being used in some developing countries.
- *1920: Sir Ivan Magill* in *1920* popularized the breathing system he designed, and it is in extensive use even today popularly known as *Magill's breathing system*. It is actually Mapleson A.
- *1954: Mapleson* in *1954* described the various modes of assembling a breathing system with five similar components occupying different positions and the components being *fresh gas flow inlet, reservoir bag, facemask, corrugated breathing hose* and *expiratory valve*. He had classified it from A to E.

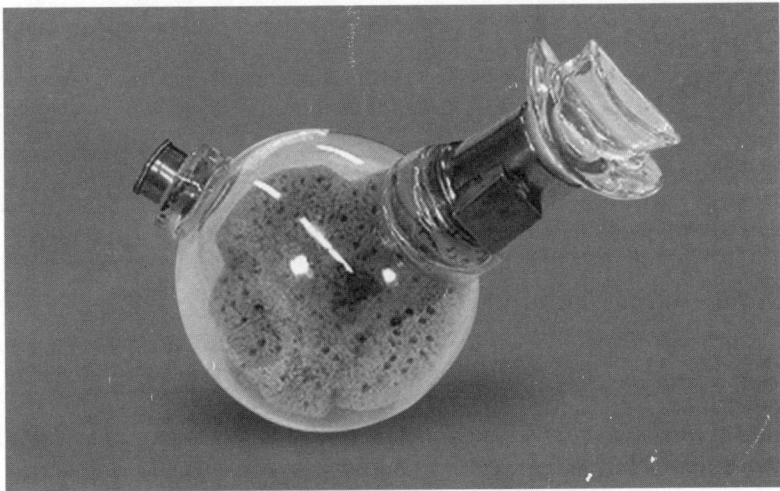

Fig. 8.1: A model of ether inhaler used by WTG Morton

- *1975: Jackson-Rees modification* on E was added by *Willis* in *1975*, called as Mapleson's F.

The part of the anesthesia machine through which the anesthetic gas mixture from the 'common gas outlet' of the machine is delivered to the patient's airway is known as the anesthesia breathing system or circuit.

The name 'breathing circuits' is no longer in use because not all the breathing systems are circuits.

Anesthetic gas mixture of inhalational anesthetic agents—both gases and vapors of volatile anesthetic agent—has to be delivered to the respiratory tract. There it has to be conducted to the alveoli from where it is taken up by the blood for anesthetic action in central nervous system.

In earlier days when ether or chloroform was used as a sole anesthetic agent, various methods of vaporizing the agent in atmospheric air as carrier gas were developed. Out of all that open drop method using a "Schimmelbusch" mask became popular and was in use till recent years.

Later the system was improved slowly where oxygen and nitrous oxide also were used as carrier gases instead of atmospheric air. Anesthesia machines with the gas cylinders came into use.

Since then generating *anesthetic gas mixture* in the machine and delivering it through the 'breathing systems' were developed.

The desired anesthetic gas mixture is generated by setting *three variables* by the anesthesiologist.

1. *Flow rate of gases*: Flow rate of each gas used is set in the flow meter in such a way that it gives the total gas mixture (L/minute).
2. *Percentage of oxygen:* Whatever be the constituents of the mixture, it is mandatory that at least 30% oxygen is present in gas mixture delivered. Flow rates are set accordingly.
3. *Concentration of volatile anesthetic agent:* The desired concentration is set on the vaporizer.

The anesthetic gas mixture thus formed is transmitted to the 'common gas outlet' of the machine to which the *'Anesthetic breathing system'* is attached.

DEFINITION

Anesthetic breathing systems are delivery systems to transport and deliver the anesthetic gas mixture from the common gas outlet of the anesthesia machine to the patient's respiratory tract.

All delivery systems are not circuits.

But some of the delivery systems are circuits.

So the term Anesthetic circuit is no longer scientifically correct.

Definition in the Modern Terms

An Anesthetic breathing system is the assembly of tubes, valves and reservoirs through which the anesthetic mixture is conveyed from the anesthetic machine to the patient's respiratory tract.

All 'Anesthetic breathing systems' start from the 'common gas outlet' of the anesthesia machine.

CLASSIFICATION

In the 169 years since the first clinical anesthesia was demonstrated, a large number of different breathing systems have been developed, many of which differ from each other only in minor details. Various classification systems have been developed to aid understanding of how the systems operate.

Open, Semi-open, Semi-closed, and Closed Systems

- This most basic classification of breathing systems divides them into open, semi-open, semi-closed or closed.
- It is based on the method of vaporization the volatile agent, the equipment used and the carrier gas used.
- Unfortunately, in different parts of the world, the same terminology is used for different systems causing confusion.
- Now this classification has become obsolete as open and semi-open methods are no longer in use today and only semi-closed and closed systems are in use.

For the sake of completion, the 'open' and the 'semi-open' systems are briefly discussed below.

Open System

- *Examples:* Open drop ether anesthesia with Schimmelbusch mask; Insufflation technique with Junker bottle for chloroform.
- No reservoir bag, No rebreathing or negligible rebreathing.

Advantages

Simple and inexpensive.

Disadvantages

- Unpredictable inspired concentration of the agent
- Dilution of anesthetic concentration by ambient atmospheric air
- Environmental pollution.

Semi-open System

- It is similar to the open system, but loss of concentration and air dilution are reduced.
- A rectangular gamgee pad with a longitudinal slit that allows only the nose and mouth of the patient exposed into the Schimmelbusch mask is placed in between the mask and face.
- This occludes the gaps between the uneven surface of face and the rigid mask so that patient breaths through the mask only. No air enters through the sides of the mask to cause air dilution and loss of concentration is also prevented.
- Incidentally, it protects the eyes from the ether falling in.
- Sometime a tubular metal frame "Ongston's frame" is fixed on the mask. This frame is encircled with lint cloth that channelizes the flow of air through the frame and keeps the concentration within the frame without being lost into the atmosphere.

Modern Classification

In current anesthesia, practice only semi-closed system' and 'closed system' are in use. Hence the classification of breathing system comprises of only two.

Semi-closed System

- *Non-rebreathing system* (Absolute)
  This requires a non-rebreathing valve like 'Rubens non-rebreathing valve' and sufficiently high flow rate. Intermittent flow with a demand valve may be used. Not in common use because there is no special advantage.
- *Non-rebreathing system* (Partial rebreathing–physiologically insignificant)
  All the semi-closed systems in common use belong to this category.
  Hence, the non-rebreathing systems discussed in this chapter belong to this group.

Closed System

- Rebreathing system
  - To and Fro system
  - Circle system

Analysis of the above classification makes it clear that all the breathing systems can be grouped into three classes. Out of the three *Nonrebreathing* (Absolute), is not popular on practical and economical considerations and is not in common use and are not discussed here.

Hence, all the systems that are in common use can be grouped as follows.

Non-rebreathing System (Semi-closed) and Rebreathing System (Closed)

The classification of nonrebreathing versus rebreathing systems is less open to confusion.
- *Nonrebreathing systems:* In this system, the exhaled gases containing carbon dioxide is vented out to atmosphere from the system.
- *Rebreathing systems (Closed systems):* In this system, carbon dioxide from the exhaled gases is removed by sodalime in the system and so the same gas mixture is breathed repeatedly. This does not cause CO_2 accumulation in the patient's system.

1. Non-rebreathing System (Partial Rebreathing) Semi-closed System

- Patient's respiratory tract is connected to common gas outlet through the breathing system which is virtually closed
- Only during expiratory pause, a spring-loaded expiratory valve (APLV) opens to vent expired gases out into atmosphere.

2. Rebreathing System: Closed System

- Patient breathes within the system which is totally closed.
- Exhaled CO_2 is absorbed by the sodalime present within the circuit.
- It may be *'To and Fro'* closed-breathing system or *'Circle'* closed-breathing system.

Criteria for an Ideal Breathing System

Before going into the details of construction of any breathing systems, it is necessary to consider some *principal criteria* required for the breathing systems to fulfill the anesthetic requirements and physiological requirements of the patient's breathing as well. These are required for effective and safe functioning of the breathing systems.
- Predictable inspired oxygen concentration
- Predictable inspired anesthetic concentration
- Permit adequate elimination of carbon dioxide
- Minimal resistance to breathing
- Provision to assist or control the ventilation of the lung if needed.

Apart from the essential criteria, there are some *secondary criteria*. These are related to factors that are not as vital as principal criteria.
- Simple in design to use in all clinical situations
- Economy of equipment and drugs
- Less pollution to the theater environment
- Ease of cleaning and sterilization.

Non-rebreathing System (Semi-closed)

- *Examples*: Magill's breathing system—Mapleson A, Jackson Rees modification of Ayer's T-piece—Mapleson F.
- Practically during the inspiratory phase and up to the end of expiration the system is closed.
- But during the expiratory pause, it is mostly open to the atmosphere through an expiratory valve (APL Valve) to allow the expired gases to go out to the atmosphere. That is why it is known as *Semi-closed System*.
- If properly used with adequate fresh gas flow, there will be no rebreathing.
- The characteristic feature of non-rebreathing system is that elimination of carbon dioxide is accomplished by removing all expired gases from the system and venting them to atmosphere.
- This is normally achieved by using sufficient fresh gas flow from the anesthetic machine and the expired gases are allowed flow out of the system though a valve (an expiratory valve).
- Inspired concentration of volatile anesthetic agent is as fixed by the anesthesiologist.
- Usually, non-rebreathing systems provide good control of the inspired gas concentrations, since during each breath, for every inspiration fresh gas is delivered from the anesthetic machine.
- However, they are less economical in use than rebreathing systems because the fresh gas flow equal to the minute volume of patient (or more) must be supplied to prevent rebreathing.
- They contribute more to the problem of atmospheric pollution with anesthetic agents.
- There is a risk of operator error since an inadequate fresh gas supply will result in rebreathing.

In *1954, Mapleson* classified the semi-closed breathing system into 5 types as from A to E.

Mapleson's Classification of Non-rebreathing Systems

- The Mapleson's classification of breathing systems necessarily needs the common gas outlet of an anesthesia machine for attaching.

Mapleson's Classification of Non-rebreathing Systems

- Mapleson's classification divides nonrebreathing systems into functionally similar groups, based on the fresh gas flow required to prevent rebreathing and the ease with which intermittent positive pressure ventilation may be performed.
- The five components are:
  1. Fresh gas flow (Machine end)
  2. Reservoir bag
  3. Corrugated tube
  4. Expiratory valve
  5. Facemask (Patient end)
- This classification is based on the positions of the five components and five such configurations were described as Mapleson's A to E. In 1975, Jackson Rees modification of E was done and is named as Mapleson F **(Fig. 8.2)**.
- Mapleson   **A**: Magill's breathing system

  B: Lack's system

  C: A modified version of this is "Water's to and fro" closed system.

  D: Bain's coaxial system

  E: Ayre's T-piece system

  F: Jackson Rees modification of Ayre's T-piece
- All the available breathing systems fall in to this classification.
- The only exception is the circle-breathing system.

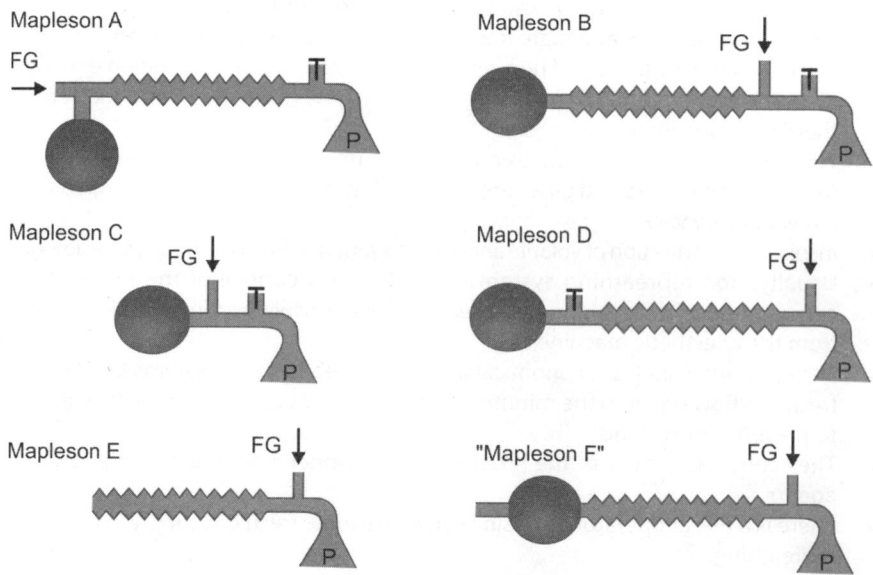

FG = Fresh gas, P = Patient

Fig. 8.2: Mapleson's classification of non-rebreathing systems. • The configuration of the five components namely fresh gas flow, reservoir bag, expiratory valve, facemask and corrugated tube, determine the classification from A to F

Magill's Breathing System (Mapleson's A System)
Semi-closed Breathing System

- Most commonly used system for spontaneous breathing popularized by *Sir Ivan Magill*.
- This system connects the patient's respiratory tract to the machine through which the patient breathes the anesthetic mixture in and out.
- For all practical purposes, this is a closed system because "from the patient's airway to the machine's common gas outlet 'No' part of this system is open to the atmosphere throughout the respiratory cycle except during the expiratory pause.
- During expiration, the expired gases released out into the atmosphere through a device known as *Heidbrink's expiratory valve*. This expiratory valve opens to release the expired gases and closes immediately.
- This system is closed, opens only to release the expired gases to the atmosphere is called as a *semi-closed system* **(Figs 8.3 to 8.5)**.
- The fresh gas enters from the common gas outlet to the "T" tube (Bag Mount), where the reservoir bag is attached. The reservoir bag has a capacity of 2 L.
- The other end of bag mount opens into the corrugated breathing tube.
- The tube is 100 cm long with 22 mm diameter in corrugation and 25 mm outside.
- The volume of the corrugated breathing hose is about 550 mL which is a little bigger than the average tidal volume. This prevents rebreathing.
- The end of corrugated breathing tube is attached to the Heidbrink's spring-loaded expiratory valve. From this through an elbow connector, it is connected to the facemask.
- FGF must be 70–90% of the minute volume.
- Apparatus deadspace consists of the volume from the APL to the endotracheal connector.
- Rebreathing is physiologically insignificant.

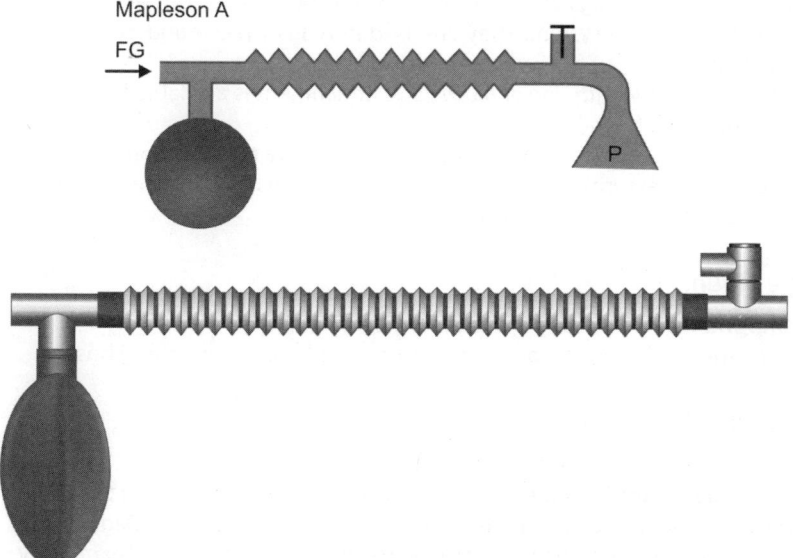

Fig. 8.3: Magill's breathing system

Components of Magill's Breathing System

- It starts from the *common gas outlet* of the Machine (Machine end).
- Consists of the following components; *Fresh gas flow inlet, bag mount, reservoir bag, corrugated breathing hose, expiratory valve, angle mount* and *facemask*.

Bag Mount

- The bag mount is a metal attachment and has three ends **(Fig. 8.4A)**.
- It is a 'T' tube with the side limb.
- One end of the straight tube is 22 mm male connector attached to the common gas outlet.
- The other end is 23 mm female connector receives the 22 mm angle connector of corrugated tube.
- The third end at right angle to these two faces downwards (Side limb of the 'T' tube) to which a 2 L reservoir bag is attached.
- Bag is attached to the mount with the help of a hard rubberbush known as 22 mm 'Bush Neck'.
- There is a lever for closing or opening of gas entering the Bag.

Reservoir Bag

- 2 L capacity antistatic rubber bag **(Fig. 8.4B)**.
- The mouth of the bag has 22 mm Bush neck for Magill breathing system (Adult).
- The bag is made of antistatic rubber.
- Synthetic rubber bags (latex free) are also available.
- 'Antistatic rubber' is a mix of 20% 'acetylene black' in latex rubber.
- Ordinary latex rubber (natural rubber) is non-conductive and accumulates 'static electric charges' which may cause 'static spark' leading to fire.
- Acetylene black is very fine carbon particles that offers electrical conductivity to the rubber so that 'static electric' charges are dissipated, not accumulated.
- 1/2 L, 1 L, 1.5 L bags available with 15 mm bush neck, but are never used in Magill's breathing system. They are used in 'Ayres T-piece' and other systems for children.
- Bag with *Rat tail with ring or bleed valve* attachment is available for Jackson Rees modification of Ayre's T-piece.
- During normal manual ventilation, by compressing a reservoir bag, it is not possible to create a pressure of more than 30 mm Hg (40 cm H_2O). Hence it is very unlikely that barotrauma is caused by this way.

Angle Mount

- One end fits into the bag mount assembly **(Fig. 8.4C)**.
- The other end connects one end of corrugated rubber-breathing hose.

Corrugated Rubber Breathing Hose

- This is also made of antistatic rubber **(Fig. 8.4D)**.
- An 'Angle mount' is connected to the proximal end of corrugated tube. The angle mount through the 22 mm male connection is attached to the Bag mount.
- Other end of corrugated tube receives Heidbrink's spring-loaded expiratory valve.
- Corrugations are for non-kinking quality. Corrugations have inner diameter is 22 mm and the outer diameter is 25 mm.

Anesthetic Breathing Systems

- Normally, the length is 104 to 110 cm and 550 mL internal volume. At the two ends, 2 cm plain tube is provided for 22 mm metal or rubber bush neck.
- PVC tubes measuring 160 cm are available.

Heidbrink's Spring-loaded Valve

- A variable tension spring-loaded valve for venting the expired gases (APL) (Heidbrink's expiratory valve) **(Figs 8.4E and H)**.
- This is also known by the other names. Adjustable pressure limiting (APL) valve, Pop-off valve, dump valve, expiratory valve (Less commonly used name)
- It has a spring-loaded disc that opens by increased pressure during expiration.
- The distal end of Heidbrink's valve gives attachment to the angle mount (right angle) which is again fixed on to the facemask.
- It causes a resistance of 5 cm H_2O at the flow rate of 25 L/min flow rate (Acceptable limit).

Right Angle Mount

One end fits into the Heidbrink's valve (22 mm male connectors) and the other end fits into the facemask **(Fig. 8.4F)**.

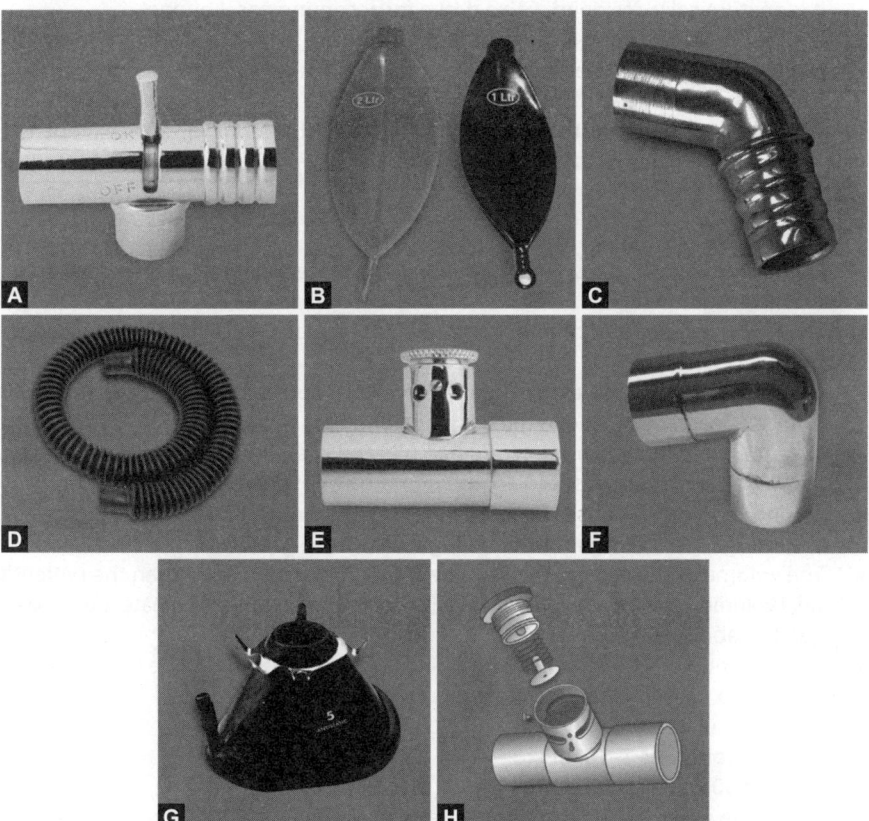

Fig. 8.4: Components of Magill's breathing system. • Bag mount, reservoir bag, angle mount, corrugated breathing tube, Heidbrink's valve, right angle mount, facemask • The disc, spring and the adjusting device of Heidbrink's valve are shown in exploded view

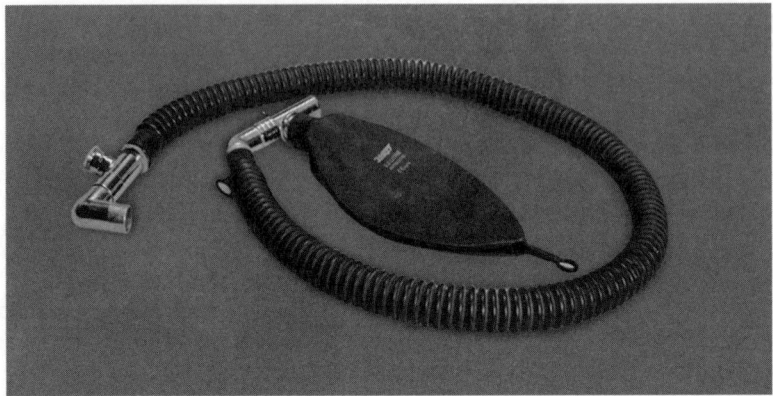

Fig. 8.5: Magill's breathing system. • From left to right: angle mount for mask, Heidbrink's expiratory valve, corrugated breathing hose, angle mount, bag mount

Facemask

- This piece of equipment is also of antistatic black rubber **(Fig. 8.4G)**
- It has a tough malleable body and a rim of air-inflatable cushion
- It is anatomically designed with a grove for accepting nasal bridge
- Rim of air cushion gives an airtight fir on the face.
- Adult mask size 5 has deadspace of about 75 mL. This can be measured by inverting the mask and filling with water.

'Magill's breathing system' assembled with all the components except the face mask is shown in **Fig. 8.5**.

Functioning

- During inspiration, the spring-loaded valve is closed; patient breathes fresh gas from corrugated tube.
- The fresh gas from the common gas outlet of the machine collects in the reservoir bag.
- During expiration, the expired gases enter the corrugated tube; the fresh gas from the machine is filled in the bag and continues to fill.
- Towards the end of expiration, the bag fills and pressure rises to open the valve, allowing the expired gases to escape into the atmosphere.
- During expiratory pause, fresh gas washes the entire expired gases from the breathing tube (corrugated) and filling it with fresh gas for the next inspiration.
- The volume of the reservoir (corrugated) tube must be greater than the patient's tidal volume; otherwise, expired gas will enter the bag and contaminate the inspired gas. It is about 550 mL.
- For preventing rebreathing, the fresh anesthetic gas flow has to be set as equal to that of the patient's minute volume.
- This is calculated this way:
  - Tidal volume is 7–10 mL/kg.
  - For a 50 kg patient, tidal volume is 10 × 50 = 500 mL.
  - Minute volume = Tidal volume × Respiratory rate, i.e. 500 mL × 12 = 6000 mL
  - Fresh gas flow rate is set around 7–8 liters/minute.

Respiratory Requirements to be met by the Breathing Systems

In clinical practice, two major concerns are to be satisfied:
1. To deliver oxygen to the respiratory epithelium
2. Removal of carbondioxide, which has diffused into alveoli.

In an average adult, weighing *70 kg* the following facts are carefully considered.
- Oxygen consumption is 240 mL/min
- During anesthesia the requirements are reduced 15–30%. So the value is 200 mL/min
- Total Capacity of the lung is 6 liters
- Maximum amount of air that can be exchanged (Vital Capacity) is 4.8 liters
- Residual Volume (that cannot be exchanged) is 1.2 liters
- Tidal Volume is 500 mL
- When the tidal volume enters the lung there is already 2.2 liters of gases containing carbon-dioxide and this is functional residual capacity (FRC)
- FRC = Residual Volume + Expiratory Reserve Volume
- The mean alveolar carbon-dioxide tension is 40 mm Hg (5.2%)
- The oxygen uptake is 200 mL/min
- The carbon-dioxide production is 160 mL/min. This 160 mL of carbondioxide is diluted in FRC
- To maintain the alveolar carbondioxide at 5% an alveolar ventilation of 3.2 liters is required.
- Tidal volume is 500 mL.
- About 1/3rd of tidal volume is in anatomical deadspace (130 mL).
- The part of the gas which occupies the dead space is 1/3rd of the tidal volume, so, the first part of the tidal volume which enters the alveoli is the gas belonging to the last part of previous expiration
- So to produce 3.2 liters of alveolar ventilation 4.8 liters of minute volume is needed (Ve – Expired minute volume)
- To this anatomical dead space a small volume of apparatus dead space must be added
- In designing the breathing system, this dead space must be reduced to the minimum
- Anatomical dead space is approximately halved by intubation

The Purpose of Reservoir Bag in Magill's Breathing System

Flow requirements in breathing system
- In each respiratory cycle, the inspiration takes 1/3 of the time.
- Expiration along with expiratory pause takes remaining 2/3 of cycle **(Fig. 8.6)**.
- In a continuous flow machine, if there is no reservoir bag available, during inspiration fresh gas can flow into lungs (1/3 time).
- But during expiration part of the expired gases will pass into the corrugated tubes and when the pressure builds up adequately to lift the spring-loaded valve the excess gas escapes into atmosphere. For next inspiration the expired gases from the corrugated tube will enter the lung.
- This results in rebreathing within the corrugated rubber tube.
- If this to be avoided, three times the minute volume of the patient (about 21 L/min) has to be set as flow rate and delivered, so that throughout the respiratory

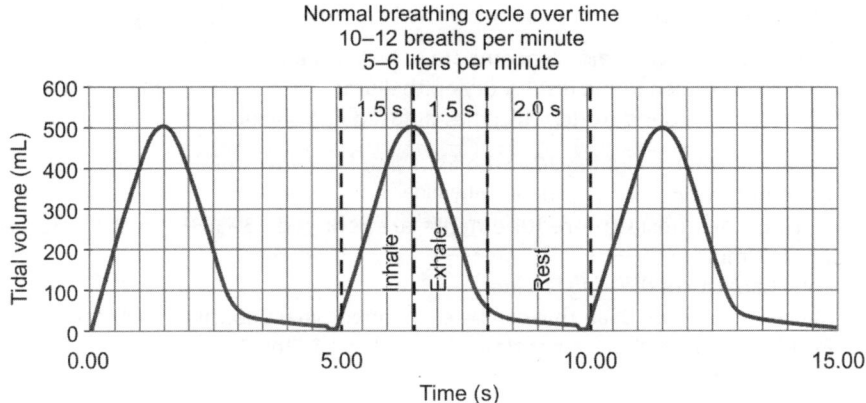

Fig. 8.6: Respiratory cycle

cycle there will be fresh gas available for the patient to inspire and the excess gases will be wasted by lifting the expiratory valve open continuously.
- Even then, there is another problem. The peak inspiratory flow rate cannot be supplied by this flow rate of 21 L/min.
- During the peak of inspiration, flow rate of gases in the respiratory tract is around 30 L/min.
- This is the speed with which gases are drawn *during the peak of inspiration* which is a momentary need.
- Many times it may not be possible to give this flow rate with normal flow meters. This status is highly detrimental.
- By adding a reservoir bag, all these problems are eliminated.
- The peak inspiratory flow rate in anesthetized patients never exceeds 30 L/min.
- The average value is 20 L/min.
- The flow meter allows a steady flow rate that does not meet this value; usually 8 L/min is fixed. (Nitrous oxide – 5 L/min and Oxygen – 3 L/min).
- As inspiration occupies 1/3 of the respiratory cycle, the reservoir bag collects the fresh gases from the machine during expiratory phase—the remaining 2/3 of the cycle.
- For each inspiration fresh gas is drawn from the reservoir bag.
- Transiently increased rate of flow during peak of inspiration is easily drawn from it.
- So it is necessary to incorporate *a Reservoir Bag* which accommodates this *volume of gases for momentary high flows* needed during peak of inspiration.
- This will prevent rebreathing, and the peak inspiratory flow of 30 L/min can be drawn from the bag without any resistance.

Resistance in Breathing System

At this point, it is necessary to discuss about the resistance offered by the breathing systems
- All the breathing systems impose some amount of increased resistance to the respiratory gas flow. It must be kept as minimum as possible.
- Usually, resistance is caused by tubes, orifices and valves. These are known as resistors to flow.
- When gases pass through these there will be a pressure drop between the upstream and downstream of the resistor.

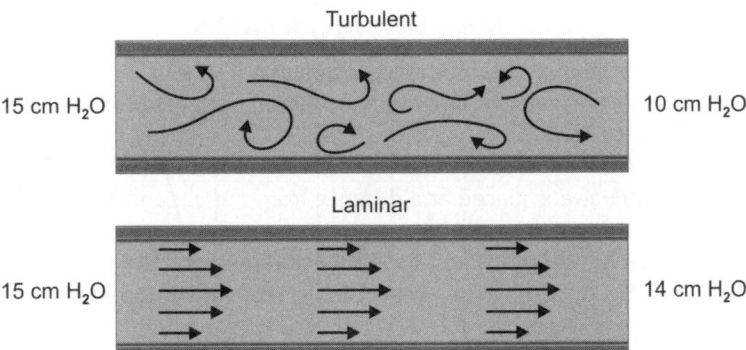

Fig. 8.7: Turbulent Flow and Laminar flow pressure difference

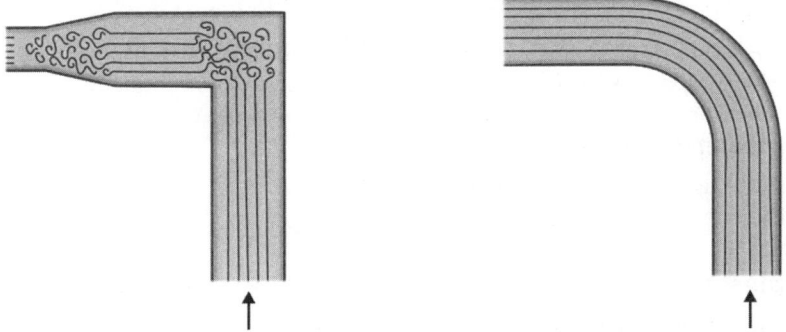

Fig. 8.8: Flow in Rowbotham's connector and Magill's connector

- Two types of flow of gases are possible in air passages. They are *Laminar Flow and Turbulent Flow* **(Fig. 8.7)**.
- In *laminar* flow, there is minimum resistance – *Viscosity* will modify this
- In *turbulent* flow, there is increased resistance – *Density* will modify this
- Any *acute angles, branches, sudden narrowing, rough walls, projections* and all such things present in the breathing system will increase the resistance. So all these have to be avoided or minimized in the construction of a breathing system.
- For example, Rowbothem's endotracheal tube connector is a right angle connector with a tapering end which causes turbulent flow at the angle and the narrowing. Whereas Magill's endotracheal connector is a smooth-curved connector with uniform lumen that permits laminar flow **(Fig. 8.8)**.
- Resistance to flow is measured as the pressure drop across the resistor. For example, orifices, tubes, valves, etc.
- The highest permissible resistance to respiratory gas flow is 2 cm H_2O of water pressure difference when the flow rate is 20 L/min.
- Heidbrink's valve (APL) – the resistance is 5 cm of H_2O at 25 L/min flow rate.
- In a 9 mm endotracheal tube, the resistance is below 1 cm H_2O.
- In Corrugated rubber tubing, it is extremely low.
- Corrugated rubber hose (Elephant tube) is in use for the past 90 years.
- The internal diameter is 20 mm. The outer diameter of corrugation is 22 mm. The corrugation causes a rough lumen and may increase the resistance. But it is used for preventing kinking.

Lack's System

- This is a modification of Mapleson' A configuration **(Fig. 8.9)**.
- It is a coaxial system with the inner tube is 14 mm diameter and the outer tube is 30 mm diameter
- The inner tube is the expiratory tube.
- The expiratory valve is placed at a distance from the patient end nearer to the machine end through a long tube.
- The difference between this and the Bain's system is that the outer tube is the inspiratory tube and exhalation occurs through the inner tube which ends up in an APL valve near the machine end.
- The reservoir bag is also near the machine end.
- Two versions, one co-axial and the other parallel are available
- There is no advantage, but enormous increase in the expiratory resistance is the major disadvantage.
- Fresh gas flow (FGF) of 70 mL/kg used for spontaneous ventilation.
- Not suitable for controlled ventilation.

Mapleson B System

- Not in use—No advantage **(Fig. 8.10)**
- High degree of rebreathing.

Mapleson's C System

- The difference between B and C is the absence of the corrugated tube **(Fig. 8.11)**.
- Same disadvantage of rebreathing is present.
- Mapleson C is modified by interposing a sodalime canister between the fresh gas flow and the reservoir bag makes the "Water's To and Fro closed system".

Mapleson D System

Mapleson D is modified as Bain's breathing system **(Fig. 8.12)**.

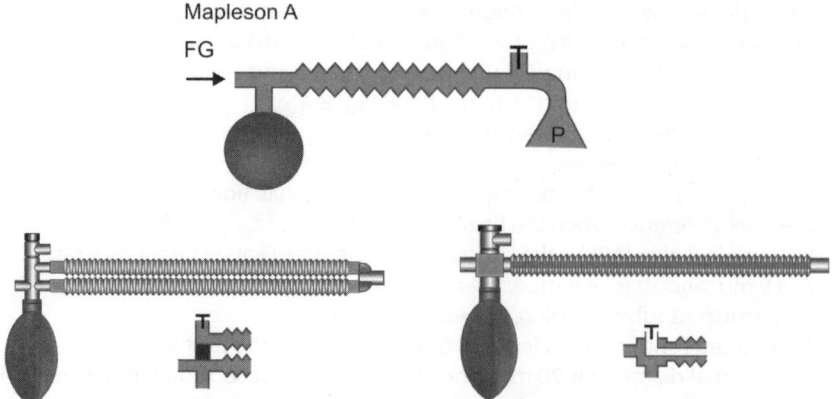

Fig. 8.9: Mapleson A 'Lack' breathing system—parallel and coaxial

Coaxial Systems

These are partial rebreathing systems.

Commonly used systems are:
1. *Bain's co-axial system*; it has a modified version also—*Bain's parallel system*.
2. *Lack's co-axial system*; this also has a modified version called *Lack's parallel system*. Lack's co-axial and parallel systems are discussed in page 184 **(Fig. 8.9)**.

Bain's Breathing System (Mapleson D)

- This system was introduced by Bain and Sporrel in 1972.
- Modification of Mapleson D system; It is actually a modified T-piece.
- It is a coaxial breathing system. This means a tube inside a tube having the same axis. It has two channels but one axis.
- Available in three lengths:
  1. *180 cm* for routine use
  2. *270 cm* for head and neck surgeries—machine is kept away at the foot end.
  3. *540 cm* for MRI room examination—machine is kept far away from magnetic field.

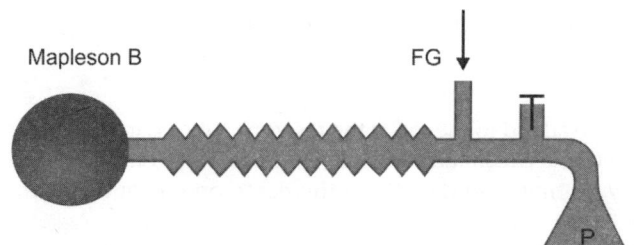

Fig. 8.10: Mapleson B system

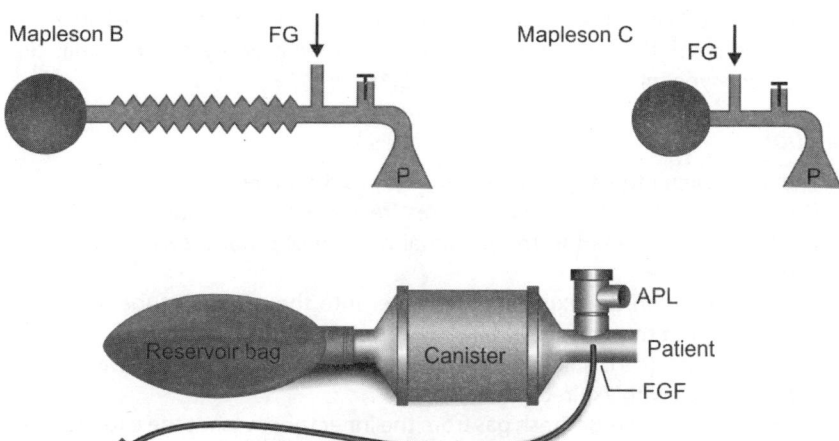

Fig. 8.11: Mapleson C system. • Mapleson B and C are compared and the difference is the absent corrugated tube • This is modified as a closed system by interposing a sodalime canister in between the fresh gas flow and reservoir bag

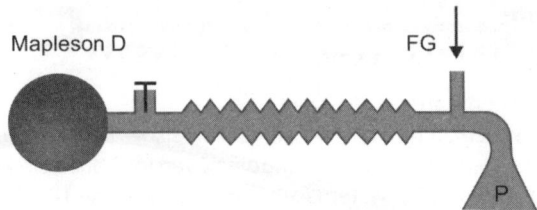

Fig. 8.12: Mapleson D system

Construction

- The fresh gas flow (FGF) flows through a 6 mm narrow tube that enters at the proximal end of the outer tube (exhalational limb) lies in it all along its length to open near the patient end **(Fig. 8.13)**.
- A flange supports the inner tube at this point.
- The inner tube small tube (6 mm) carrying fresh gas (F) pierces the outer corrugated tube (R), at the machine end, travels inside throughout the length, and opens near the patient end (P).
- Catheter mount and endotracheal tube is connected at this end.
- The reservoir bag and the adjustable pressure limiting (APL) valve are situated at the proximal end of exhalation tube **(Fig. 8.14)**.

Modifications

- A bag may be added to the tail of the reservoir tube, as in the T-piece.
- Alternatively, the circuit may be attached to a block assembly with an expiratory valve may be mounted directly to the common gas outlet of the anesthesia machine.
- At this mount, there is provision for attaching a reservoir bag.
- This arrangement facilitates scavenging and intermittent positive pressure ventilation **(Fig. 8.15)**.
- Another modification—the so-called *'Parallel Bain'* system is also available.
- In this system, the inner and outer tubes are replaced by conventional circle-absorber-type tubing and Y-piece **(Fig. 8.16)**.

Function

- The Bain's circuit functions in the same way as the T-piece.
- During inspiration, the patient inspires fresh gas from the inner tube and also the fresh gas collected in the proximal portion of outer reservoir tube during expiratory pause.
- During expiration the expired gases enter into the reservoir tube (outer tube) and vented out through the expiratory valve.
- Although fresh gas is still flowing into the system at this time, it is wasted as it is contaminated with expired gas.
- During *expiratory pause,* fresh gas from the inner tube washes the expired gas out of the reservoir tube, filling it with fresh gas for the next inspiration.
- *Fresh gas flow*:
  - *Spontaneous ventilation*   -   90 to 150 mL/kg body weight
  - *Controlled ventilation*   -   75 mL/kg (normocarbia)
  -   -   100 mL/kg (hypocarbia)

Anesthetic Breathing Systems

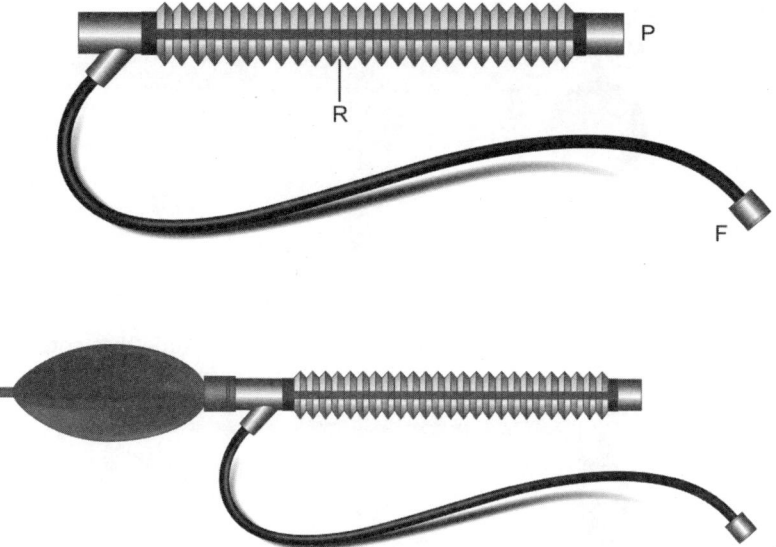

Fig. 8.13: Bain's breathing system. • F: Fresh gas flow continues through the inner tube; R: Corrugated outer tube (reservoir tube or breathing tube); P: Patient end for connecting to endotracheal tube. • Modification with a bag attached without expiratory valve

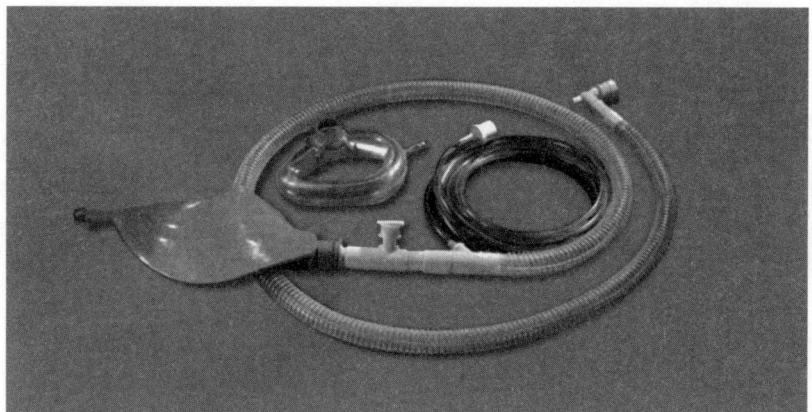

Fig. 8.14: Bain's breathing system with a bag, expiratory valve and mask

Advantages

- Light weight, portable, convenient, and reusable, can be sterilized easily.
- Can be used in all age groups.
- Can be used for spontaneous breathing and control ventilation.
- Since the overflow valve is located far away from the patient, expiratory gases may be readily scavenged.
- Ideal for head and neck surgery.
- There is some warming of the inspired fresh gases by the exhaled gas present in the outer tubing.

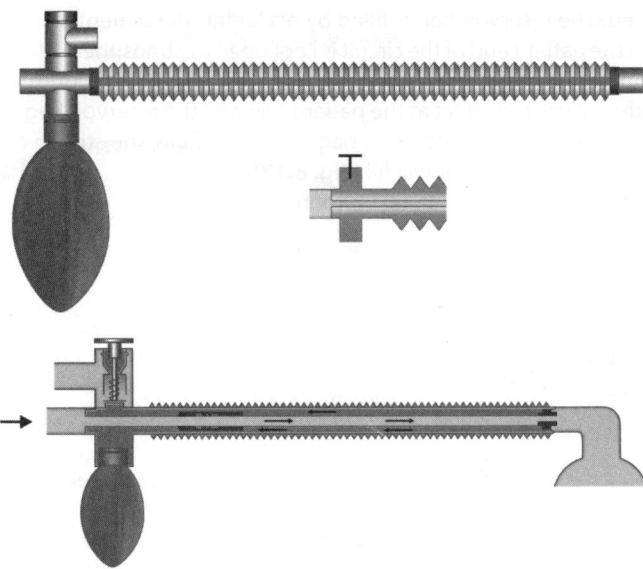

Fig. 8.15: Bain's system with block assembly and gas flow pattern

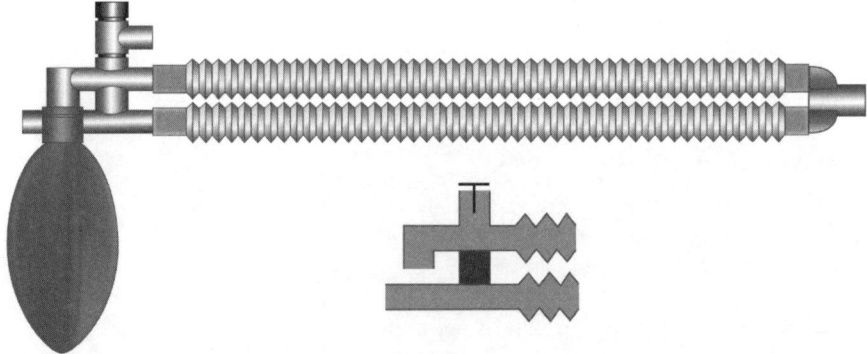

Fig. 8.16: Parallel Bain's system

Disadvantages
- Capnography gives a peculiar wave form that does not touch the inspiratory base line indication that rebreathing is present.
- As with other coaxial systems, if the inner tube may become disconnected or broken.
- Then the entire breathing tube becomes dead-space, leading to severe alveolar hypoventilation.

Two Tests for checking the integrity of inner tube:
1. A flow meter is set on with flow 500 mL/min. The little finger is inserted into the distal end of the outer hose occluding the inner tube. If the inner tube is intact the bobbin in the flow meter will be depressed by the back pressure when the inner tube is obstructed.

2. *Pethick test:* The reservoir bag is filled by occluding the patient end of outer tube and then the patient end of the circuit is kept open to atmosphere. Now the oxygen flush (emergency oxygen) is opened. High flow of gas through the inner tube will produce a venturi effect at the patient end and the reservoir bag will collapse. If the inner tube is damaged, then bag will not deflate, the stream of gas will be directed into the bag and it will fill **(Fig. 8.17)**.
Among the two the occlusion test is more reliable.

Mapleson's E

Ayre's T-Piece

- Designed by Philip Ayre in 1937 as no valve breathing system for pediatric patients **(Fig. 8.18)**.
- This is truly Mapleson's E. Most commonly used breathing system for pediatric patients.
- The only system imposing the *least resistance for breathing* because *there are no valves*
- Most commonly used breathing system for spontaneous respiration in pediatric age group of patients.
- Used mainly in pediatric patients up to 25–30 kg.
- The volume of the reservoir tube must be equal to the patient's tidal volume. If it is less, it will permit atmospheric air entering the system causing dilution of anesthetic mixture (air dilution). If it is more, it will result in rebreathing.
- A number of different designs of T-piece are available, which function in essentially the same way **(Fig. 8.18)**.

Construction

- T-piece comprise of three parts, namely, *inspiratory limb, expiratory limb* and *side limb*.
- Inspiratory and expiratory limbs may be any one of the axial limbs. *The side limb is always for fresh gas flow.*
- A three-way T-tube whose limbs are connected to: The side limb of the 'T' is connected to the fresh gas flow (F) from the machine.
- Among the other two, one is *inspiratory limb* connected to endotracheal tube (P) (Patient).
- The other *expiratory limb* is connected to a corrugated reservoir tube (R) **(Fig. 8.19)**.

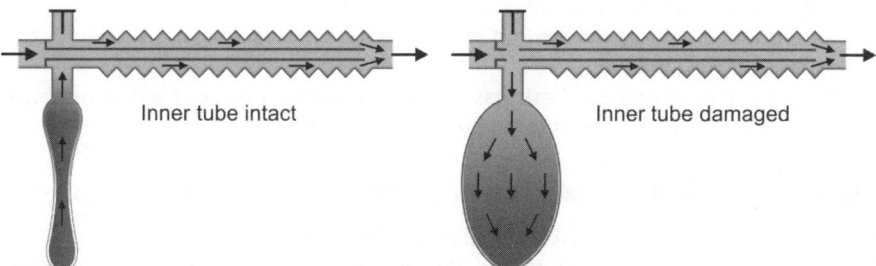

Fig. 8.17: Test for identifying broken inner tube

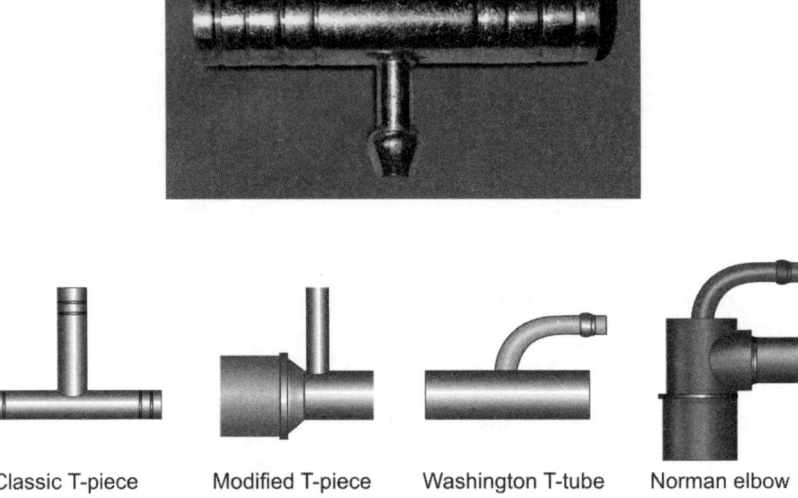

Classic T-piece   Modified T-piece   Washington T-tube   Norman elbow

Fig. 8.18: Ayr'e T-piece. • The T-piece designed by Phillip Ayre and subsequent modified versions

- The volume of the reservoir tube must be equal to the patient's tidal volume. If it is less, it will permit atmospheric air entering the system causing dilution of anesthetic mixture (air dilution). If it is more, it will result in rebreathing.
- If the total fresh gas flow is fixed as *a little more than twice the minute volume,* and then we can ignore the volume of the expiratory limb.
- *Fresh gas flow—150 mL/kg*—for spontaneous breathing.
- Minimum flow rate must be 4 liters per minute.
- Intermittent positive pressure ventilation may be performed by intermittently occluding the end of the reservoir tube.
- Controlled ventilation can be done with intermittent occlusion of the expiratory limb or by *adding a reservoir bag with rat tail and bleeder valve* having a capacity of 500 mL or 1 liter.
- T-piece can be connected to ETT for O_2 enrichment in a spontaneously breathing patient in ICU.

Functioning

- During inspiration, the patient inspires fresh gas from the reservoir tube.
- During expiration, the expired air enters into the reservoir tube.
- Although fresh gas is still flowing into the system at this time, it is wasted as the expired air contaminates it.
- During expiratory pause, fresh gas washes the expired gas out of the reservoir tube, filling it with fresh gas for the next inspiration.

Mapleson's F System (Jackson Rees Modification of Ayre's T-piece)

- Introduced by Willis 1975, it is called as Mapleson's F
- A *0.5 liter reservoir bag with rat tail and bleed valve* is attached to the expiratory limb of T-piece (This is the modification) **(Fig. 8.20)**.

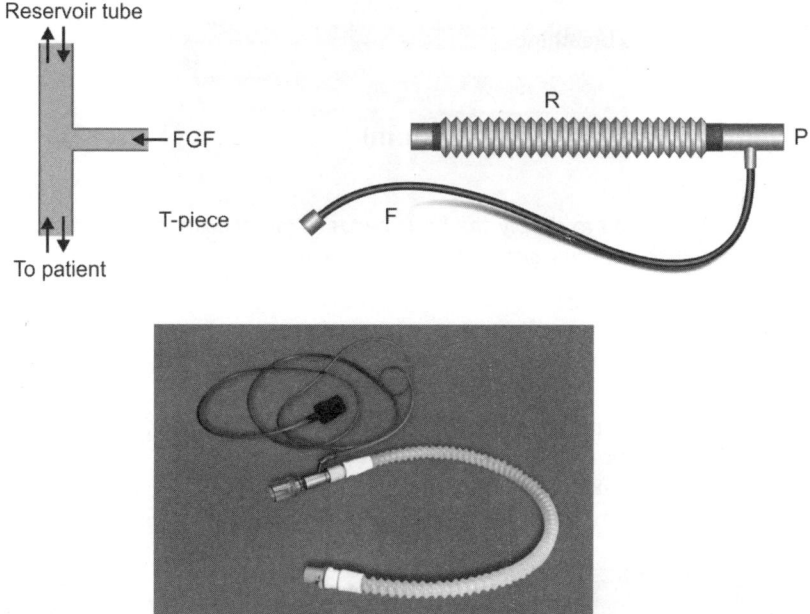

Fig. 8.19: The three limbs of T-piece—configuration to make the breathing system

- The capacity of the bag may be 500 mL or 1000 mL according to the weight of the patient.
- Rebreathing can occur, but a bag helps in monitoring and assisting the ventilation.
- For spontaneous breathing, fresh gas flow of 150 mL/kg to prevent rebreathing.
- For controlled ventilation, 100 mL/kg flow rate with a minimum flow of 3 L/min.
- This allows respiratory movements to be more easily seen and permits intermittent positive pressure ventilation (IPPV), if necessary.
- The bag is, however, not essential to the functioning of the system.
- Intermittent positive pressure ventilation may be performed by occluding the tail of the bag between a finger and thumb and squeezing the bag.
- Alternatively, a *Bag-tail valve* or a *Bleeder valve*, **(Fig. 8.20)**, which employs an adjustable resistance to gas flow, may be attached to the bagtail.
- This causes the bag to remain partially inflated and so facilitates one-handed performance of IPPV.
- Jackson Rees modification causes some amount of continuous positive airway pressure (CPAP).
- Another aid to IPPV is the Kuhn bag **(Fig. 8.20)**, which has the gas outlet on the side of the bag, rather than the tail. This allows the outlet to be occluded with the thumb during IPPV, but leads to difficulties in scavenging the waste gases.
  - Modern T-pieces incorporate 15 mm fittings for the reservoir bag, tube and endotracheal adapter.

Advantages of T-piece Systems

- Compact
- Inexpensive
- No valves

- Low dead space
- Low resistance to breathing
- Economical for controlled ventilation.

Rebreathing System (Closed System)

Principle

If sufficient O_2 is added to supply the basic needs of metabolism and exhaled CO_2 is efficiently absorbed, the same gas mixture can be breathed repeatedly.

Functioning

- Patient's respiratory tract is connected to common gas outlet through the breathing system.
- At no phase of respiration, the system opens to the atmosphere, and so it is called as *closed anesthetic breathing system.*
- As the same gas mixture is re-breathed in a closed system, elimination of CO_2 into the atmosphere is not possible.

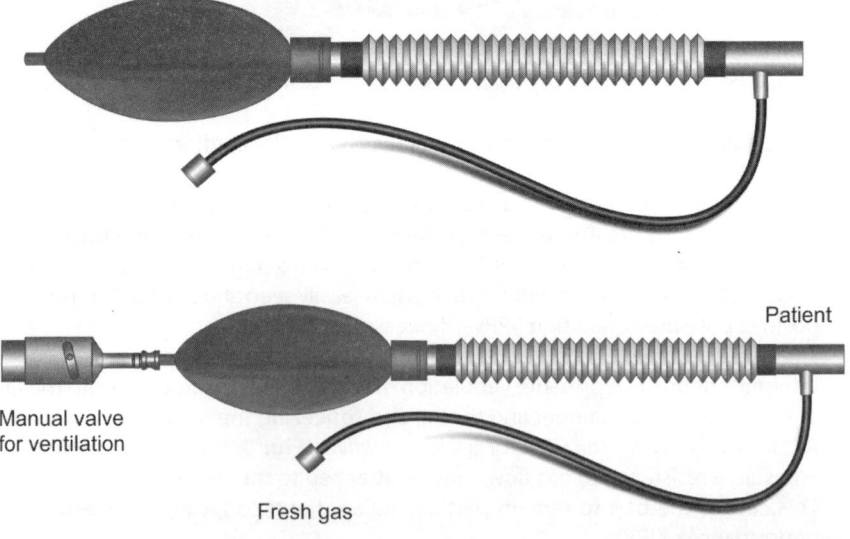

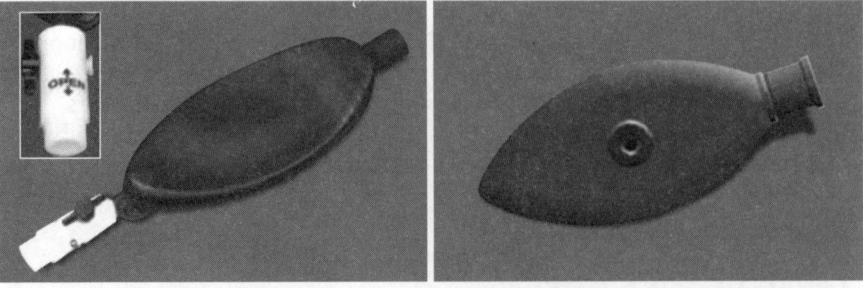

Fig. 8.20: Jackson Rees modification of Ayre's T-piece. • System assembly is seen with rat-tailed bag. • Rat-tailed bag with bleeder valve. • Kuhn bag with a side opening for IPPV

- So, there must be a provision for absorption of exhaled carbon-dioxide within the system.
- Exhaled CO_2, absorbed by sodalime/Baralyme contained in a canister in the system.
- When the expired gases pass through the space among the sodalime granules (inter-granular space), the CO_2 is efficiently absorbed.
- The remaining exhaled gas free from CO_2 is then inspired again without the problem of carbon dioxide retention.
- As same gases are re-breathed, the fresh gas flow has to be considerably reduced.
- There is a likelihood of pressure building up in the system, so an adjustable pressure limiting (APL) valve must be incorporated to release the built up pressure.
- There must be a provision for controlling the respiration.
- To prevent hypoventilation and maintain adequate ventilation, the respiration is taken over and controlled.
- Usually to achieve this, ideally the patient is paralyzed with the use of muscle relaxants.

Advantages

- Economy of anesthetic consumption.
- Warming and humidification of the inspired gases.
- Reduced atmospheric pollution.

A caution with closed-breathing systems when N_2O and O_2 are used:
- Because N_2O is rapidly absorbed from the alveoli into the bloodstream and after a period of time N_2O is saturated in all the tissues. Since that time very little or negligible amount of N_2O is taken up from the alveoli. So, the concentration of N_2O starts building up in the breathing system.
- Highly perfused tissues such as brain heart and kidney will be saturated with N_2O in about 25 to 30 minutes. Moderately perfused tissues such as muscles take about another 30 minutes for getting saturated with N_2O. Poorly perfused tissues like fat may take up N_2O very slowly for a long time. So after about 1 hour, the uptake of N_2O from the breathing system is negligible.
- Whereas O_2 from the breathing system is continuously absorbed and part of it, about 200 to 250 mL/minute is continuously used up—expended in the basal metabolic process.
- If oxygen flow rate is 500 mL/minute, after continuous removal of 200 mL for basic metabolic utilization the remaining 300 mL re-circulates in the breathing system.
- It is conventional that anesthetic mixture contains 30% O_2.
- When uptake of N_2O becomes negligible after a certain time, concentration of N_2O starts building up rapidly and encroaches into oxygen and dilutes it.
- N_2O builds up because no absorption and O_2 removed continuously; there is every chance that the anesthetic mixture contains O_2 less than that of air (21%) making it a hypoxic mixture.
- It is advised that in closed breathing systems at least 50% of O_2 is used to prevent hypoxia, particularly in long procedures.
- The barest minimum flow rate of O_2 in a closed system is 500 mL.

Carbon Dioxide Absorption

This is achieved by using sodalime in the canister of closed systems.

Sodalime

Composition

- Sodium hydroxide   5%
- Calcium hydroxide   94%
- Potassium hydroxide   1% (Acts as a catralyst)
- Traces of silica
- Moisture content   14–19%
- In modern, sodalime sometimes potassium hydroxide is not used.

Carbon dioxide absorption occurs by the following chemical reactions:
- Moisture is necessary for the reaction, as the CO_2 has to get dissolved in water before it reacts with sodalime.
- It is an exothermic reaction. The heat thus produced is known as 'heat of neutralization'.
- Temperatures up to 60° C have been recorded inside canisters.

There are two main steps of reaction:
- Sodium hydroxide reacts with carbon-dioxide to form sodium carbonate and water, releasing heat.
- The sodium carbonate thus formed reacts with calcium hydroxide to form sodium hydroxide and calcium carbonate.
- This sodium hydroxide formed continues the cycle of reaction.

$$CO_2 + 2NaOH \rightarrow H_2O + Na_2CO_3 + Heat$$
$$Na_2CO_3 + 2Ca(OH)_2 \rightarrow 2NaOH + CaCO_3$$

A small amount may be absorbed in the following way:

$$CO_2 + Ca(OH)_2 \rightarrow CaCO_3 + H_2O + heat$$

- This reaction requires (water) moisture since the carbon dioxide must be dissolved before it can react.
- The moisture is present in the granules 14–19% and also provided by the patient's exhalation.
- Too much of moisture will cause 'caking'
- Less moisture will cause reduced reaction and poor CO_2 absorption.
- Completely dry sodalime will not absorb carbon dioxide.
- It is an exothermic reaction and liberates heat (heat of neutralization)
- Carbon dioxide combines with sodium hydroxide to form sodium carbonate and water.
- Sodium carbonate thus formed reacts with calcium hydroxide to form sodium hydroxide and calcium carbonate. This sodium hydroxide combines with CO_2 again to continue the cycle.
- Thus calcium hydroxide provides the main capacity for carbon dioxide absorption of sodalime.
- Potassium hydroxide is added to accelerate the rate of absorption (as a catalyst).
- A pH sensitive dye indicates when exhaustion of the sodalime occurs.
- Silica is to preserve its granularity (Hardness).
- Sodalime comes in airtight containers **(Fig. 8.21)**.

Other Features

- *Hardness number:* 75–80
- *Granule size:* 4 – 8 mesh (6.2–3.1 mm)
- Various indicator are used to indicate exhausted sodalime; Ethyl violet, Methyl orange, phenolphthalein
- Now continuous CO_2 monitoring—Capnography—makes the indicator insignificant.
- Intergranular space must be equal to or more than the tidal volume. If it is lesser than the tidal volume, then CO_2 absorption will be inadequate.
- Removal of carbon dioxide is very fast—contact with sodalime for 0.16 seconds is enough to bring down 5% CO_2 to 0.5%
- Sodalime can absorb CO_2 equal to 20% of its own weight (100 gm can absorb 25 liters of CO_2.
- But invariably, as the efficacy varies and the channelling causes variable absorption, considerable reduction in the absorption capability occurs, and the value can be around 10 liters of CO_2/100 g.
- Highest permissible level of CO_2 in any breathing system is 0.2%.
- Exothermic reaction of absorption may raise the temperature of the canister up to 60° C.
- Sodalime regenerates on standing.

Indicators

- Used to identify the exhaustion of sodalime.
- Methyl orange, ethyl violet, and phenolphthalin are some of the indicators used.
- The indicators are not to be relied on fully and clinical assessment is needed. In case of doubt, change the sodalime.

Baralyme may be used as an alternative to sodalime.
- It has efficient absorption capability, but no regeneration.
- It contains 80% barium hydroxide (octohydrate) with 20% calcium hydroxide and no silica.
- It is more efficient that sodalime—absorbs 17 L of CO_2 per 100 g.
- It is less dusty and the dust is less alkaline than that of sodalime.

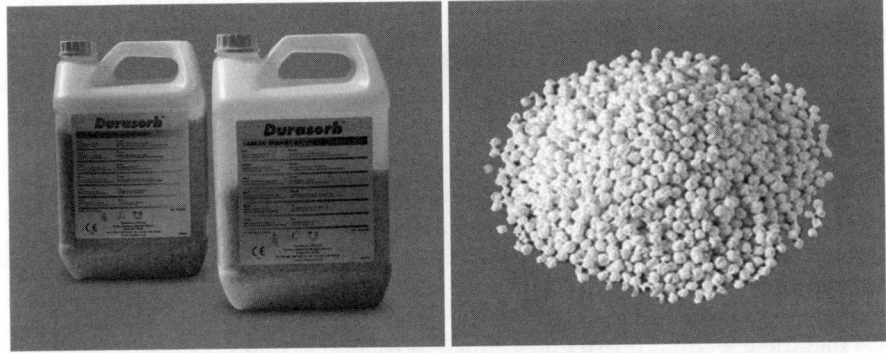

Fig. 8.21: Sodalime granules in airtight containers and loose granules

Caution about Sodalime

- The correct size granules (4–8 mesh size) must be used.
- Proper packing of granules should be done. Too tight packing will reduce the space for absorption; too loose packing will cause channeling.
- Inappropriate size granules (smaller than 8 or bigger than 4 as specified) should not be used, as it will result in poor absorption.
- Powder should never be used as it increases the resistance to gas flow, reduces the inter-granular space, and cause channeling resulting in poor CO_2 absorption.
- Sodalime should never be allowed to become dry, as it will badly affect CO_2 absorption. For effective functioning, it must have a moisture content of 14–19%.
- There are two types of sodalime in use, one of which turns from white-to-purple when it is exhausted, the other changing from pink-to-white upon exhaustion, which may result in confusion.
- Since the color change disappears when sodalime is left to stand, it should be changed immediately exhaustion occurs.

Clinical Indicators of Exhausted Sodalime

- Increase in BP (systolic hypertension)
- Increase in pulse rate and bounding pulse
- Increased sweating
- Warm and moist extremities
- Increased oozing from surgical wound.

Hardness Number

- This number indicates the hardness of the granules from braking into powder.
- A specific quantity of sample is kept on a rocking tray with 15 steel balls of a fixed diameter and rocked for 30 minutes.
- Then the granules are placed on a 40 mesh sieve and again shaken for three minutes.
- The amount retained on the screen should not be less than 75% of the original and is described as hardness number.
- If it is more CO_2 absorption will be less.
- If it is less, granules get crumbled and become powder and cause caking and reduction in inter granular space.
- The hardness number is directly related to the amount of moisture present and to a lesser extent to silica.

Granule Size

- In preparation, the mixture is fused into sheets and then allowed to harden.
- After this, it is fragmented and graded according to the size of the granules.
- The optimum size required for effective absorption with maximum surface area and minimal resistance is 4–8 mesh.
- For this purpose, a wire mesh screen is used as a sieve. A 4-mesh screen means that there are four quarter inch square opening per one square inch (approximately 6.2 mm square openings per 25 mm square); an 8-mesh screen signifies eight openings per one square inch (3.1 mm per 25 mm square).

- Fragmented sodalime is sieved through 8 mesh sieve first so that all sizes smaller than 8 mesh will pass through and that is discarded.
- Then it s sieved through a 4-mesh sieve which allows all sizes from 8–4 mesh to pass through, and is collected and stored. The bigger size granules are retained on the sieve.

For Efficient CO_2 Absorption

- Sodalime must be fresh
- Tidal exchange must be adequate
- There should be no channeling—vertical canister prevents channeling.
- Highest concentration of CO_2 permissible in any breathing system must be less than 0.2%, which can be identified by a capnography.
- Exothermic reaction of CO_2 absorption may raise the temperature of canister to 60°C, which may cause trilene and sevoflurane decomposition.

Methods to Find Out Exhaustion of Sodalime

- Change of color of the indicator. It should never be relied on fully.
- Increased $EtCO_2$ in a capnography, progressively rising baseline.
- Tachycardia and hypertension.
- Increased oozing in the field of surgery.
- Sweating.
- When in doubt, change the sodalime.

Rebreathing Systems

This system (closed system) is available are in two forms:
1. To-and-fro system
2. Circle system.

To-and-fro System

- This is actually a modified *Mapleson's C* where a sodalime canister is incorporated in between the reservoir bag and fresh gas flow (FGF) **(Fig. 8.22)**.
- Here the anesthetic gas mixture flows between the patient's respiratory tract and the reservoir bag of the system in a *to-and-fro* pattern where a canister containing sodalime (Water's canister) is interposed to absorb the CO_2 from the exhaled mixture.

Water's to-and-fro Closed System

Sir Ralph Milton Water introduced this system in 1920.
- The original Water's canister was made of brass metal.
- Cylindrical structure, measures 13 cm long and 8 cm diameter.
- Water's canister containing sodalime
- It can hold 1 pound of sodalime granules—1 lb canister.
- There are no unidirectional valves. But an APL valve is present.
- 400–450 mL of intergranular space that equals an average tidal volume.
- Fresh gas flow (FGF) enters near the patient end.
- At the patient end, there is a spill valve and catheter mount. It is to be connected to the endotracheal tube.

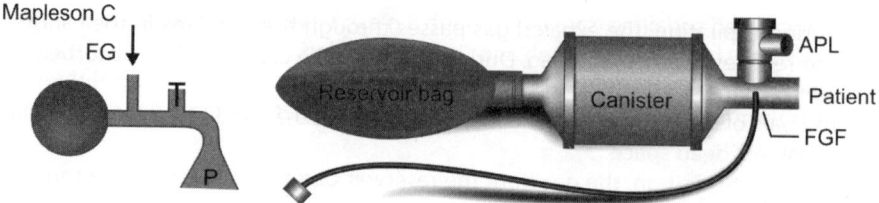

Fig. 8.22: Mapleson's C is modified as Water's closed system. • Incorporating a sodalime canister in-between fresh gas flow and the reservoir bag make the modification

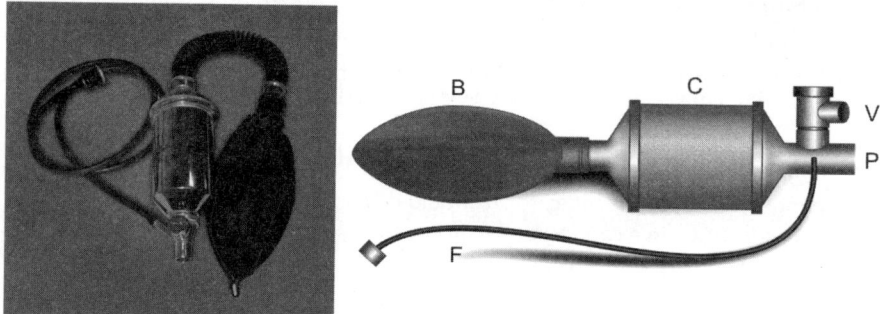

Fig. 8.23: Water's 'To and Fro' breathing system. • The original Water's 'To and Fro' system made of brass and the newer version made of acrylic; • Five components; F: Fresh gas inlet; B: Reservoir bag; C: Sodalime canister; V: Expiratory valve; P: To Facemask

- On the other end, there is a bag mount where reservoir bag is fixed.
- There are no unidirectional valves, so the gases pass to-and-fro to the bag during inspiration and expiration through the sodalime.
- The sodalime gets exhausted from the distal end (patient end).
- Can be continuously used for 90 minutes; intermittently can be used for 2–3 hours.
- Cheap and can be sterilized by any method when used in an infected case.
- For children smaller canister; ½ lb canister may be used.

Construction

All the five components; fresh gas flow, sodalime canister, reservoir bag, APL, and patient's connector are assembled in the proper way as shown in **Figure 8.23**.

Operational Requirements

- The volume of the reservoir bag must be greater than the patient's inspiratory capacity.
- This is usually estimated at 30 mL/kg body weight.
- Since sodalime contains 50–70% air around the granules, then volume of the absorber canister should be more than the tidal volume of the patient for optimal efficiency.

Functioning

- Fresh gas flow enters the system near the patient end.
- During inspiration fresh gas enters the respiratory tract.

- During expiration, the exhaled gas passes through the sodalime in the canister and reaches the reservoir bag. During this time, the exhaled CO_2 is absorbed by the sodalime.
- The part of sodalime nearer the patient end gets exhausted and this adds to the appararus dead space.
- For next inspiration, the gas from the reservoir bag passes through the canister to the patient.
- This way the gas makes a 'To-and-fro' movement during inspiration and expiration.
- Excess gas is vented when necessary via the pressure-relief valve-APL.

Advantages

- Portable and inexpensive.
- Most of the parts can be autoclaved, if used in an infected patient.
- There is no loss of moisture.

Disadvantages

- The canister close to the patient's head is a major inconvenience. Fixing the canister is difficult.
- Exhaustion of sodalime starts from the patient end and will add on to the apparatus dead space. Progressively increasing apparatus dead space **(Fig. 8.24)**.
- As it is horizontal, channeling is a problem, if not well packed.
- As it is close to the respiratory tract caustic alkaline dust may reach the respiratory tract.
- Resistance to breathing may be increased.
- Heat retention may be caused in prolonged use.
- Not suitable for head and neck surgery, because it causes drag on endotracheal tube.

Channeling

- One problem with the original horizontal canister is that, unless it is tightly packed, the sodalime tends to settle and leave an empty space above.
- As gas flow takes the passage of least resistance, preferential flow of gases occurs through this space not through the sodalime. This preferential flow of gas is called 'channeling' **(Fig. 8.25)**.
- Channeling will lead to substantial rebreathing and CO_2 retention.
- This problem can be avoided by ensuring that the sodalime is tightly packed using nylon retainers at the ends.

Circle System

- The circle system can be used for any patient weighing more than 25 kg (Tidal Volume >175 mL).
- In this system, there are two unidirectional valves that direct the gas flow in two different breathing hoses (one is inspiratory limb and the other is expiratory limb) in a circular fashion.
- Exhaled gases pass through expiratory limb and enter the inlet of a large sodalime canister usually with two compartments.
- Exhaled gases after passing through the sodalime is free from CO_2 collect in the reservoir bag along with the fresh gas flow from the machine.

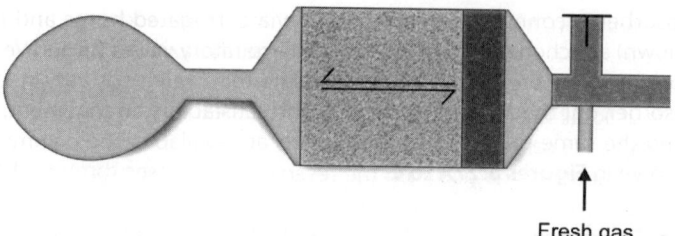

Fig. 8.24: Exhaustion of sodalime in 'To-and-fro' canister. • The sodalime at the patient end of canister is used up and exhausted first (Shaded area); • This will add to the apparatus dead space.

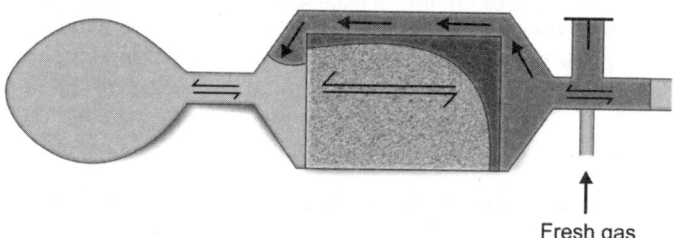

Fig. 8.25: Channeling in a loosely packed canister. • Channeling occurs above the sodalime granules with rebreathing; • Shaded area shows the exhausted sodalime

- During the next inspiration, the gases from the reservoir bag open the inspiratory valve and pass through the inspiratory limb to the patient.
- Unidirectional valves direct the flow of gases in a circular fashion.
- Now almost universally the circle system is used for its advantages **(Figs 8.27A to C)**.
- The flow pattern of gases is indicated in **Figure 8.26.**

Advantages of the Circle System

- This system is convenient as the canister is away from the patient.
- Economy of anesthetic consumption
- Warming and humidification of the inspired gases
- Reduced atmospheric pollution
- This can be used continuously for 6–8 hours.
- No channeling occurs as it is a vertical canister.
- More efficient use of sodalime than in Water's canister.

Construction

The essential components of the circle absorber are:
- Fresh gas flow (FGF) line supply
- Two unidirectional valves—inspiratory and expiratory
- Two corrugated breathing hoses—inspiratory and expiratory—with 'Y' piece
- Sodalime canister (usually 2 kg or Twin canister 1 kg each)
- A reservoir bag
- Pressure-relief valve (APL)
- A and A' Indicate positions of expiratory valves to let out excess gases
- V and V' are unidirectional valves.

- The absorber is connected to the patient via corrugated hoses and a Y-piece (not shown) attached to the inspiratory and expiratory valves (Vi and Ve).
- The position of the breathing bag and pressure-relief valve may vary in relation to the absorber, but the above is a common and satisfactory arrangement.

Applying the same principle various models are available. The commonly used model is shown in **Figures 8.27A to C**.

Sodalime Canisters

- 2 kg canister with 2 compartments.
- Canister has capacity of 2100 mL with inter granular space of 900–1000 mL.
- Usually, it is a transparent cylindrical acrylic drum and fixed vertically.
- It has three baffles (sieve-like separators)—one fixed at the middle to divide it into two compartments **(Fig. 8.27B)**.
- The other two are at the end, with rubber washers, which can be removed for filling sodalime.
- Sodalime can be filled only up to the line marked on the canister otherwise leaks may be caused.
- ON and OFF lever for isolating the Canister for removing and charging canister or inverting it.
- Exhaled gas from the patient enters through the lower compartment and so the lower compartment is exhausted first.
- The *Inlet and Outlet ports* of Canister are connected to corrugated rubber tubes of the circle breathing system.
- Canister has two unidirectional valves to make the flow of gases in a circular fashion.
- These valves are *"disc on knife edge"* valves which offer minimum resistance.
- There is a spill valve present on the top of canister to release the expired gas mixture when needed.
- It is situated near the inlet of the canister so that the released gases are only expired gases.

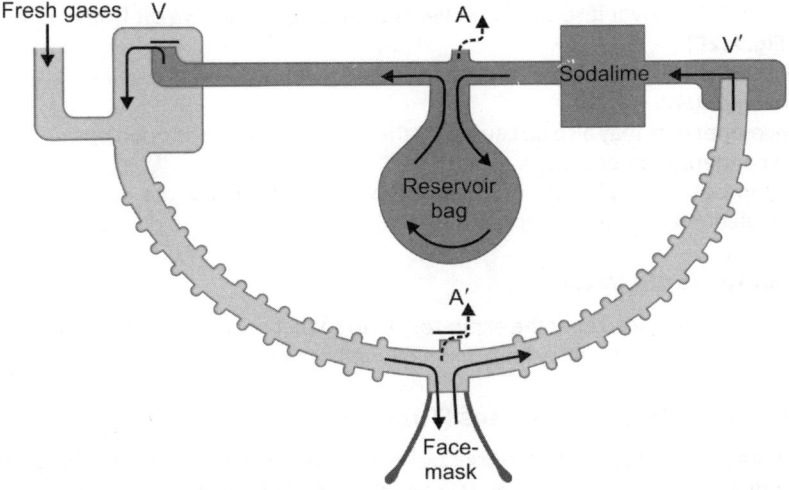

Fig. 8.26: Gas flow pattern in circle-breathing system

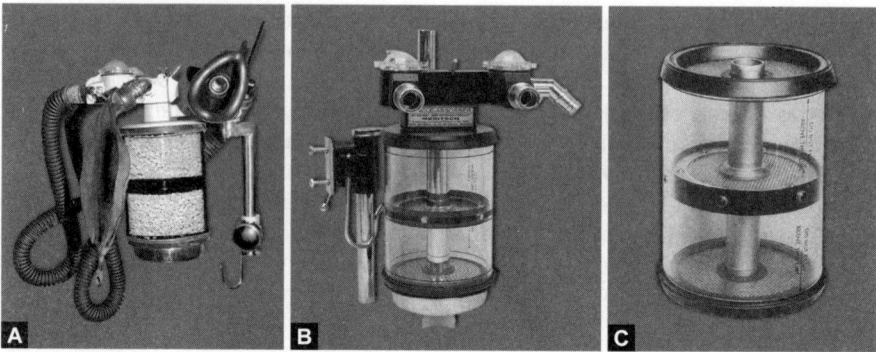

Figs 8.27A to C: "Circle absorber" assembly and 2 kg sodalime canister. • The circle absorber assembly with breathing hoses, reservoir bag and mask; • The circle absorber assembly without the breathing hoses shows the canister, unidirectional valves, 'inlet and outlet' of the canister and the attachment for reservoir bag; • The canister is larger so that it can be used continuously for many hours. • Canister has three baffles, which divide it into two compartments that can be inverted, if needed or can be filled independently

- The canister can be inverted, if the sodalime in the lower compartment is exhausted.
- Fresh gas flow must enter the system near the inspiratory limb.
- The spill valve (airway pressure release valve—APRV) must be positioned near the expiratory limb so that the gases wasted will be only expired gases.

Unidirectional Valves

- The unidirectional inspiratory and expiratory valves in most circle absorbers are of the turret type (Disc on knife-edge), in which the pressure generated by the patient's breathing causes the disc to rise and allow gas to pass in one direction only **(Fig. 8.28)**.
- The knife-edge is to make the disk to seat well without leak.
- Most valves have transparent dome so that the operation of the valve may be observed.
- The disc material may be mica, ceramic or plastic. Usually a cage or protector is provided to cover it so that it prevents the disc being blown off from the seating **(Fig. 8.28)**.
- Plastic is less expensive, but tends to warp and allow the valve to become incompetent.
- Incompetence may also be caused by the valve sticking in the open position owing to condensation of water vapor.
- Incompetent inspiratory or expiratory valves will reduce the efficiency of gas circulation and result in rebreathing and consequent carbon dioxide retention.

APL Valve (Spill Valve)

- It should be placed near the expiratory limb so that only the exhaled gas is vented.
- If placed near inspiratory limb, fresh gas will be vented out.

Corrugated Breathing Hoses (Tubing)

- There are two corrugated rubber hoses known as breathing hoses. The proximal ends are connected to the canister and the distal ends connected to a swivel with expiratory valve and connector for catheter mount.

- The absorber is connected to the patient by means of inspiratory and expiratory corrugated tubes and a Y-piece or "Wye" piece with a release (expiratory) valve.
- The corrugated tubes may be made of black rubber, neoprene, silicon rubber or more recently plastic **(Fig. 8.29)** *(108 cm long and 25 mm diameter)*.
- Each corrugated tube has an internal volume of about 500 mL.
- Corrugations are essentially for preventing kinking of the tube.
- There is another angle mount with 1 meter corrugated rubber tube fitted with a reservoir bag close of the outlet of the canister for controlling the ventilation.
- Recently, the so-called universal F circuit has become popular. This is a coaxial system, the inspiratory tube running inside the expiratory limb.

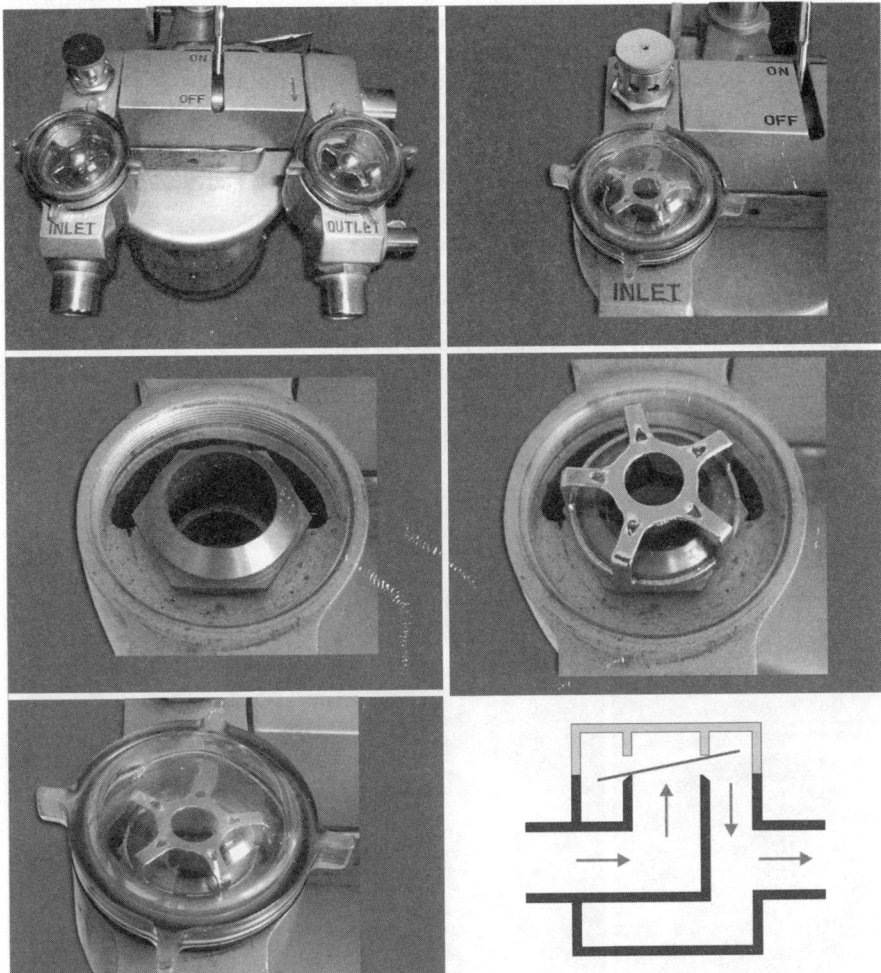

Fig. 8.28: Circle absorber with two unidirectional valves and APL. • It has an 'ON' 'OFF' lever to isolate the canister for dismantling during work; • Two unidirectional valves—for inlet and outlet; • APL is placed near the expiratory limb (inlet); • Unidirectional valve of circle absorber (Disc on knife edge type); • Schematic diagram of unidirectional valve; • Knife-edge of valve ring, disc with protector and transparent dome to cover; • The disc is lifted by flow in one direction and closes when the flow is in opposite direction

Functioning

During Inspiration

The expiratory valve closes and gas flows from the breathing bag to the patient via the inspiratory limb of the system.

During Expiration

- The inspiratory valve closes and gas flows via the expiratory limb into inlet of the canister
- The exhaled gas containing CO_2 will reach the bottom of the canister and form there flows up through the canister.
- When the gases ascend up through the sodalime the CO_2 is fully absorbed. Hence, the lower compartment of the canister gets exhausted first.
- The gases from which CO_2 is removed collect in the reservoir bag along with the fresh gas flowing from the common gas outlet of the machine.
- When the reservoir bag is compressed during the next inspiration, the expiratory valve closes, the inspiratory valve opens and this gas mixture free from CO_2 will flow through the inspiratory limb to the patient.
- The excess gas is vented when necessary via the pressure-relief valve situated near the expiratory limb.

Advantages

- Can be continuously used for more than 6 hours.
- 1 pound (450 g) will last for 1 hour when used continuously and 2 hours when used intermittently.
- Sodalime dust will not enter into the patient's lungs as the canister is far away.
- Heat retention will not be caused.
- No channeling of gases, as it is a vertical canister.

Disadvantages

- Resistance to breathing will be twice that of 'To and Fro' closed breathing system.

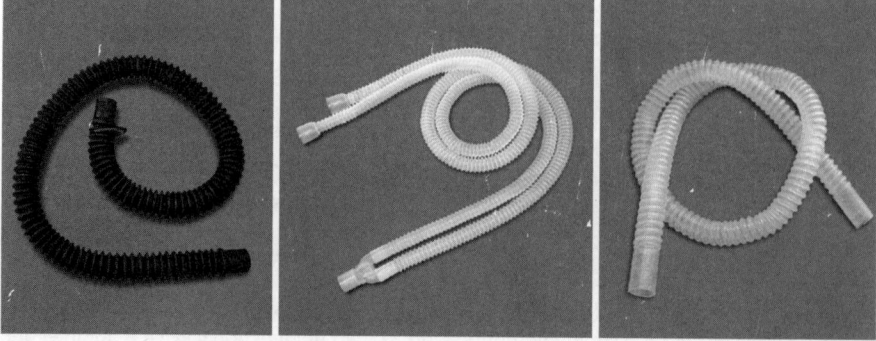

Fig. 8.29: Corrugated breathing hoses. • Antistatic black rubber breathing hose; • Plastic corrugated tubes with "Y" piece for use in circle absorber; • The knot put on the corrugated tube does not kink it because of corrugations.

Anesthetic Breathing Systems

- Volatile anesthetics may be left as residue in the sodalime and rubber parts that may cause contamination to the next patient. This needs flushing before use for another patient.
- Temperature of the canister may rise to 60° C as the carbon-dioxide absorption is an exothermic reaction.
- If the corrugated tubes are older, there will be *a considerable expansile volume* in the corrugated tube that will reduce the effective tidal volume.
- Moisture loss will be there as the water vapor from the expired gases will condense in the corrugated tubes exposed to atmospheric temperature, on the way to canister.

Methods to Check the Integrity of Circle Absorber

Leak Test

Set the flow meter of O_2 at 5 liter per min, occlude the outlet the swivel mount of the circle system tightly and allow the circle system to be filled with O_2 so that the reservoir bag becomes tense. Then close the flow meter and compress the bag repeatedly to see whether there is any considerable loss of gas.

Flow Test

- To test the integrity of the unidirectional valve
- Disconnect the swivel mount and through the inspiratory limb, we must be able to inhale but not exhale. Through the expiratory limb, we must be able to blow in but not inhale.

Other Important Facts

- When not in use, the soda lime canister can be closed by using the 'ON' 'OFF' lever present on the top **(Fig. 8.28)**. This prevents the sodalime getting dried up faster.
- 2 kg canisters have large intergranular spaces >1500 mL and when not in use it is filled with atmospheric air. Because of this, when low flow rates are used, initially the air in the inter-granular space will dilute the anesthetic gases particularly oxygen and is likely to cause hypoxia in the beginning. So to compensate this, initially a little higher percentage of inspired oxygen concentration and higher flow rate to flush this air in the inter-granular space and breathing tubes has to be used.
- When low flow rates are used in a closed system, a constant amount of oxygen, 200–250 mL/min is utilized for metabolism. So the remaining oxygen will re-circulate for rebreathing. Nitrous oxide in the initial phase will be rapidly taken up and saturation of highly perfused organs will be achieved in about 20 minutes (Brain, heart and kidney). Other moderately perfused tissues may take another 30 minutes for saturation. Subsequent to that very negligible amount of N_2O will be taken up by the blood stream particularly after one hour. This will allow almost all the N_2O delivered into the system to re-circulate whereas O_2 is constantly taken up for the basal metabolic needs. In this situation, the excess N_2O will dilute the oxygen resulting in a hypoxia mixture.
- As the body tissues are already saturated with N_2, the nitrogen in the canister will not be absorbed from the alveoli. It has to be eliminated by venting through the spill valve in the 'circle absorber'.

- With low flow rates, elimination of N_2 from the system takes longer time. For example; with 500 mL/minute flow rate, 20% of N_2 will be present in the system after one hour.
- N_2O uptake declines from 462 mL/minute to 110 mL/minute after 2 hours.
- Possibly after 4 hours of anesthesia the uptake of N_2O is likely to be negligibly small.
- This will result in accumulation of N_2O in the breathing system.
- The O_2 uptake and utilization is about 220 mL to 250 mL/minute continuously.
- If a flow rate of 500 mL of O_2 is used, then after 4 hours the accumulation N_2O will dilute the O_2 and reduce it to less than 25%, causing hypoxia.
- This clearly indicates that the FiO_2 must be at least 50% in long anesthetic procedures lasting more than 2 hours.
- If the flow rate of oxygen is only 250 mL/minute, the ventilation perfusion mismatch will not permit all the 250 mL of oxygen to be taken up into the blood stream.
- To compensate this at least double the basal requirement must be supplied in the closed system.
- The lowest flow rate of O_2, which can be maintained in any absolutely closed system, should not be less than 500 mL/minute though the basal requirement of oxygen for metabolism is 250 mL/minute.

The above analysis offers two cautions in practice.
- The lowest flow rate of O_2 in any closed breathing system should not be <500 mL (at least double the basic need must be given). Ideally it must be 1000 mL.
- After compensating the ventilation-perfusion mismatch, which normally occurs in anesthesia, the basic need of 250 mL O_2 could be taken up from the alveoli.
- For longer surgical procedures, lasting more than an hour, as the percentage of N_2O is likely to build up in the system, minimum 50% of oxygen must be used, and otherwise hypoxia will ensue inevitably.

Double-Canister Absorbers

- Many absorbers designed for use in human patients employ two canisters placed in series.
- The top canister is exposed to the expired gases first and removes most of the carbon dioxide **(Fig. 8.30)**.
- Any remaining carbon dioxide is then removed by the bottom canister.
- When the top canister is exhausted, the absorbent is discarded, the bottom canister is placed in the top position and a canister with fresh absorbent is inserted underneath it.
- This arrangement provides optimal efficiency and economy in carbon dioxide absorption.
- However, these absorbers are bulkier, heavier and more expensive than single-canister models.

Caution

- If this type of absorber is used, it is a false economy to fill only one of the two canisters.
- The sodalime will be exhausted at the same rate, efficiency of absorption will be reduced, and the greater volume of the circuit will delay equilibration of the gas in the circuit with the fresh gas supplied from the anesthetic machine.

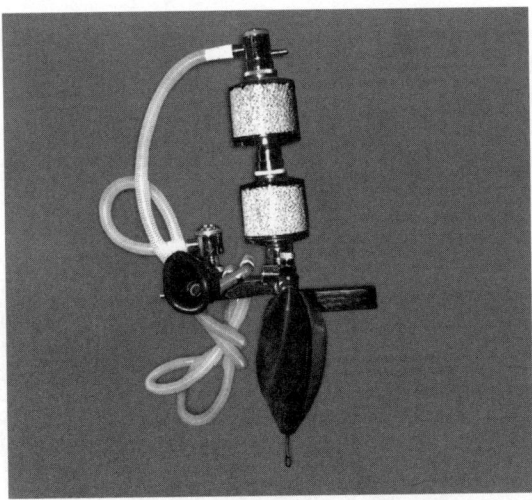

Fig. 8.30: Circle absorber with double canister

Universal "F" Circuit

- This is a co-axial tube (tube inside a tube) for use in circle closed-breathing system
- The inner tube differently colored is the 'inspiratory' limb and the outer tube is the 'expiratory' limb **(Fig. 8.31)**.
- Near the machine end, the outer tube is connected to the inlet of the canister through a short corrugated tube
- This arrangement aids in warming and humidification of the inspired gases at the expense of an increase in inspiratory resistance to breathing.
- One problem with this system, as with other coaxial circuits, is that, if the inner tube breaks or becomes disconnected at the absorber end (which may not be noticed on casual inspection), the entire volume of the tube becomes apparatus dead space.
- It should also be noted that, in all other aspects, this system is identical in function to a conventional, dual-limb system, and does not provide an economical alternative to the Bain system.

FACEMASKS

Facemask is the device which allows administration of anesthetic gases to the patient from the breathing system without introducing any instrument into the patient's mouth.
- Facemasks are integral part of the breathing systems.
- The facemask can be connected to the distal end (patient end) of a breathing system to deliver the anesthetic mixture to the patient.
- There are many types available but no single type is suitable for all patients.
- The facemasks should fit snugly on the face without leak and must be comfortable for the patient without undue pressure.
- Facemask increases the apparatus dead space.
- Dead space can be approximately measured by inverting it, filling it with water and measuring the volume.
- Most of the masks fit the face without much leak.
- This is achieved by an air-inflatable cushioned rim.

210 Anesthetic Equipment Made Easy

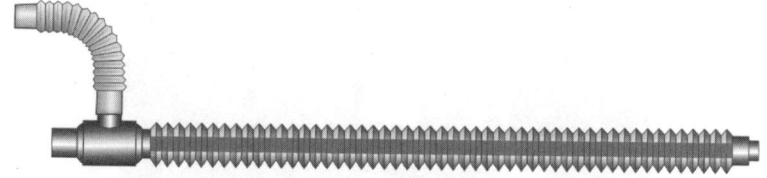

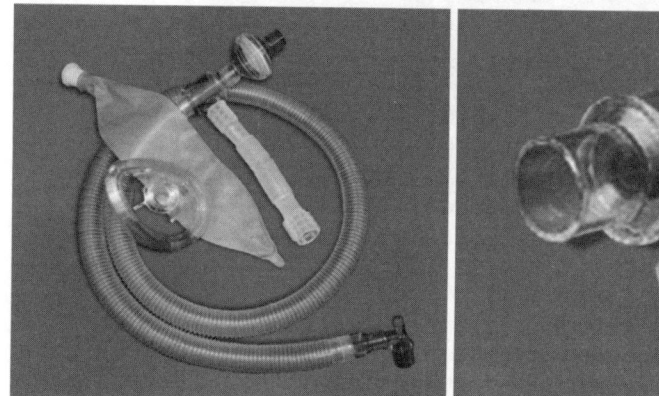
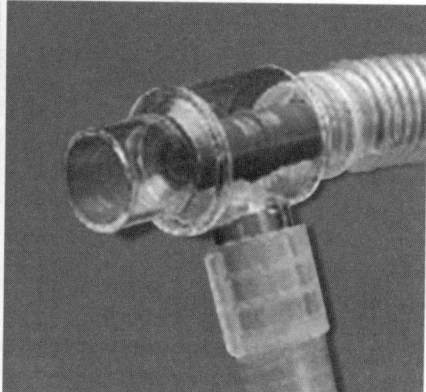

Fig. 8.31: Universal 'F' breathing system. • This is a co-axial tube (tube inside a tube) for use in circle closed breathing system; • The inner tube differently colored is the 'inspiratory' limb; • The outer tube is the 'expiratory' limb; • Near the machine end, this is connected to the inlet of the canister through a short corrugated tube

- It has three parts—the mount, the body and the rim or edge.
- The body may be made of malleable firm rubber which can be moulded a little. It may made of neoprene, plastic, polycarbonate or silicon rubber.
- The mount is usually 22 mm female taper, which accommodates the "elbow" bend of Magill's breathing system or any other connector.
- Usually facemasks are made of antistatic black rubber with brim of *inflatable air cushion,* commonly known as *'anatomical facemasks'* (**Fig. 8.32**).
- The air cushion has a special contour that suits the face, with a sharp notch for nose and a curved section for chins to fit well.
- It is available in 0, 1, 2, 3 sizes for pediatric patients and 4, 5, 6 sizes for adults.
- For average, adult size 5 and big adults size 6 will suit.
- Rubber masks cannot be autoclaved so masks made of other material are available.

Polycarbonate and Silicon Masks

- Facemasks made of transparent polycarbonate with brim of inflatable air cushion made of silicon rubber are available (**Fig. 8.33**).
- Similar transparent polycarbonate masks with *flap rims* made of silicon rubber are available (**Fig. 8.34**).
- Transparent mask permits observation of the patients mouth and nose for any pressure and also to look for secretions or vomits'.
- Opaque silicon masks are also available.
- These masks stand autoclaving. The cuff must be deflated before autoclaving.

Anesthetic Breathing Systems 211

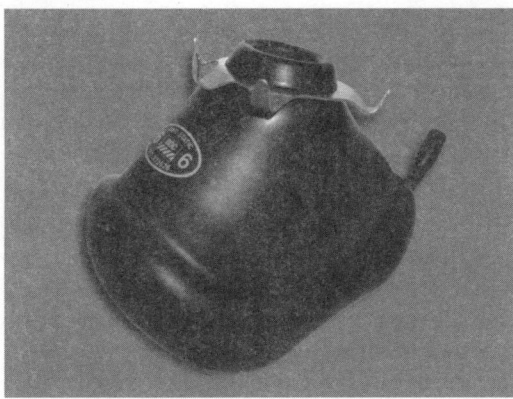

Fig. 8.32: Antistatic black rubber anatomical facemask with air cushion rim. • Anatomically shaped mask gives a very good fit on the face. • Available from 0 size for infants to 6 size for big adults; • Can be washed with detergents for decontamination; should not be autoclaved

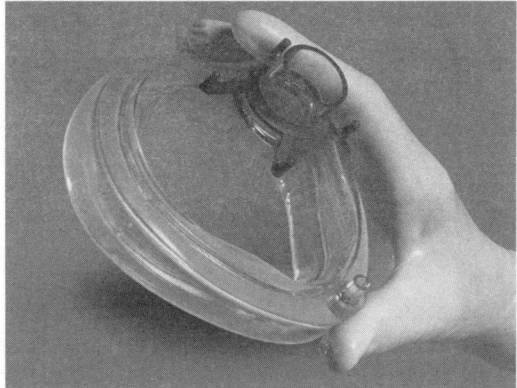

Fig. 8.33: Polycarbonate transparent mask with inflatable rim. • Body is made of polycarbonate and the inflatable rim is made of silicon rubber; • Can be autoclaved after deflating the cuff

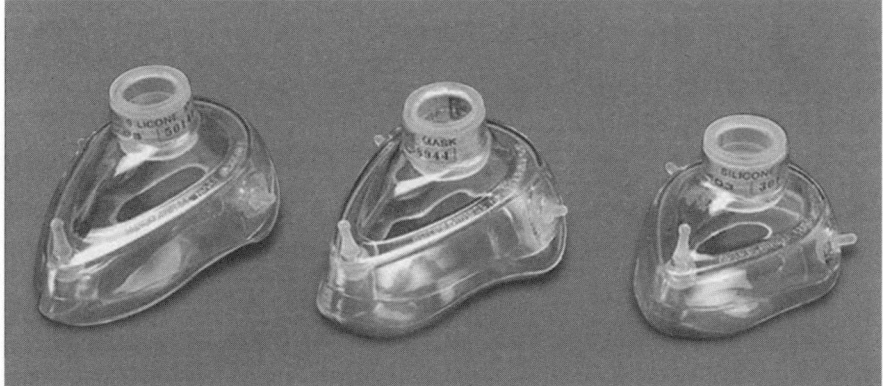

Fig. 8.34: Polycarbonate facemasks with flap rim. • The body is made of polycarbonate and the flap is made of silicon; • Available from 3 to 6 size for bigger children to big adults; • Anatomically shaped gives a good fit on the face. • Can be autoclaved

Latex-free Mask

- For patients with history of latex (natural rubber) allergy, special masks made of *synthetic rubber* (usually in green color) are available.
- In appearance, these masks are very similar to the antistatic black rubber anatomical masks with inflatable air cushion **(Fig. 8.35)**.

Pediatric Masks

- Pediatric patients have relatively flat face without any prominences and so conventional design of mask may increase the apparatus dead space enormously.
- Usually, these masks are pliable and round in shape that can easily accommodate the nose and mouth without undue pressure.
- These masks are available in black rubber, in sizes from 0 to 3.
- Similar opaque silicon rubber masks are available **(Fig. 8.36)**.

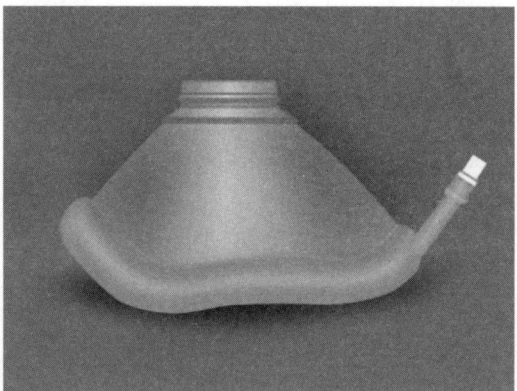

Fig. 8.35: Latex free anatomical facemask. • Made of synthetic rubber (usually in green color) for patients with latex allergy; • Similar to other anatomical mask with inflatable cushion; • Cannot be autoclaved

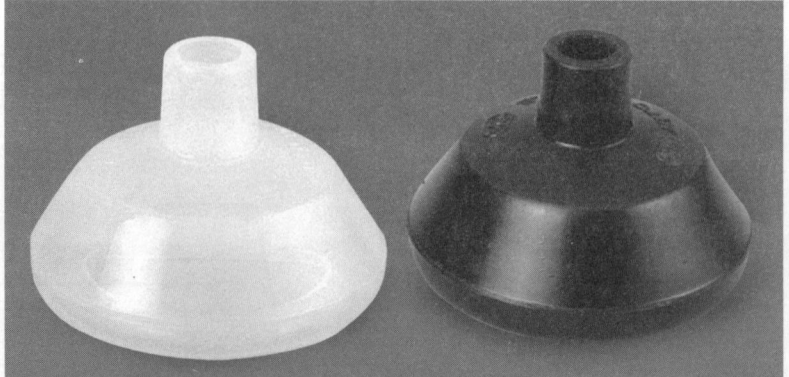

Fig. 8.36: Circular facemasks antistatic black rubber, silicon rubber. • Available for children - sizes from 0 to 3; • No aircushion but only flap rim; • Gives a reasonably good fit on the face; • Can be washed with detergentsl • Rubber mask cannot be autoclaved; Silicon mask can be autoclaved

- Round masks made of soft transparent silicon rubber are available for pediatric use **(Fig. 8.37)**.
- Silicon masks can be sterilized by autoclaving.

Rendell-Baker-Soucek Mask (For Neonates)

- These are specially designed masks for use in neonates and infants less than 1 year of age.
- Silicon rubber and black rubber masks are available **(Fig. 8.38)**.
- Special advantage is that it has a shallow mask cavity that suits the flat contour of the neonate's face.
- So the dead space is minimal. Three sizes are available, small medium and large. Have 2 mL, 4 mL and 6 mL of dead space.

Advantages

- Fits well on the neonate's face which has a flat contour without much projections.
- Minimal dead space. Neonates have tidal volume of 7 mL/kg. Hence, a neonate with 21 mL tidal volume addition of 4 mL dead space is significant.

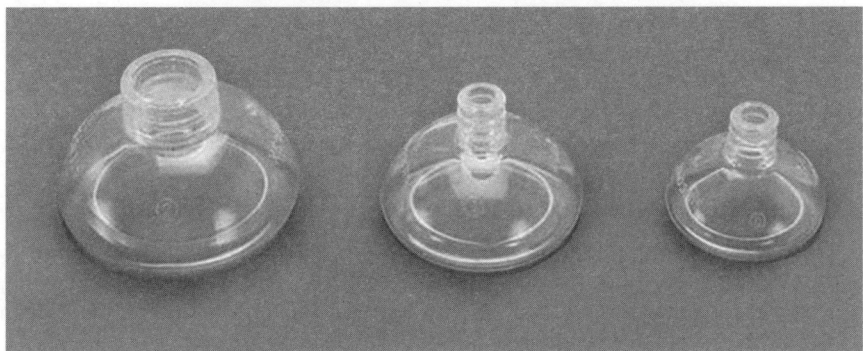

Fig. 8.37: Soft silicon round facemasks. • Available from 0 to 3 sizes for children; • Relatively soft to make good fit on the face; • Can be autoclaved

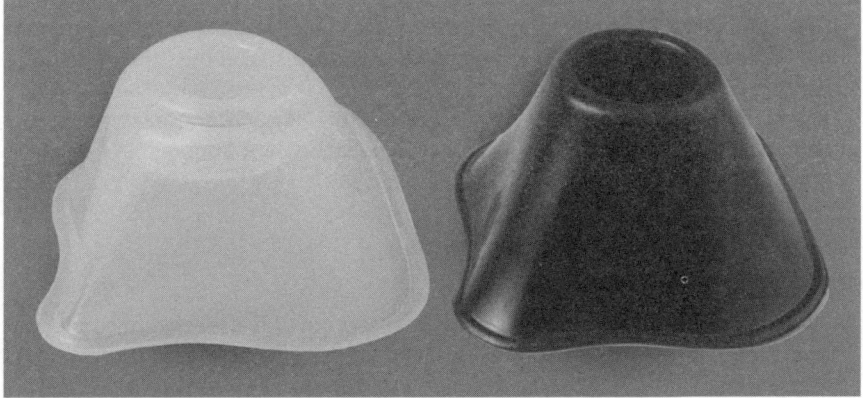

Fig. 8.38: Rendell Baker mask for neonates

Problems

- When IPPV is needed, it *does not give an airtight fit*
- Now transparent air-cushioned neonatal masks are available made of polycarbonate and silicon rubber.

Quick Review

Facemask

Black Antistatic Rubber Facemask with Air-cushioned Rim

- Body is made of malleable hard rubber.
- Brim is formed by the inflatable air cushion to fit on to irregular contour of the face.
- There can be prongs in the proximal end to attach 5-tailed harness, to fix the mask without holding it.
- *Dead space is reasonably high which can be measured by filling the inverted mask with* water and assessing the volume.
- In Adult mask the dead space is approximately - 75 mL.

Sizes

0	-	Infant and Smaller child
1	-	Smaller children
2 and 3	-	Bigger children
4 and 5	-	Adults
6	-	Extra Large

Catheter Mount and Connectors

- Once the patient is intubated, the breathing system has to be connected to the endotracheal tube.
- *Catheter mount* is the piece of equipment that makes a connection between the endotracheal tube and the breathing systems.
- The conventional catheter mount used in Boyle's machine has one 22 mm male metal base connecting to the 23 female end of Heidbrinks valve of Magill's breathing system **(Fig. 8.39A)**.
- A short piece of rubber tube is connected to this to which the Magill's metal connector is fixed. The Magill's connector is introduced into the endotracheal tube.
- As the catheter mount adds to the apparatus dead space, this tube must be as short as possible.
- The Magill's connectors may be oral connectors or nasal connectors. The 'oral connectors' have smooth obtuse angle, whereas the 'nasal connectors' have acute angle **(Figs 8.39A and B)**.

Plastic Catheter Mounts (Non-swivel, Single Swivel, Double Swivel)

- Plastic catheter mount (PVC) is meant for accepting universal 15 mm connectors.
- *Non-swivel:* One end fits well with standard 15 mm connectors of the tube **(Fig. 8.40A)**
- The other end fits well with 22 mm outlet of the breathing system.
- The 15 mm connector end has a "Swivel" which allows 360° rotation without leak.

- Some catheter mounts have "Double Swivel" (axial and circular) which rotates 360° on two axes **(Fig. 8.40B)**
- The swivels prevent twisting and kinking of the endotracheal tube.
- There is a provision of "Suction port" covered with a rubber stopper.
- A set of 15 mm universal endotracheal connectors (1.5–11 mm) is available with 15 mm adapter with double swivel **(Fig. 8.41)**.
- Present day catheter mounts have 'Double swivel' which rotate 360° at two axes.
- The length of corrugated tube can be reduced by 'concertina effect' to reduce the dead space **(Fig. 8.40C)**.

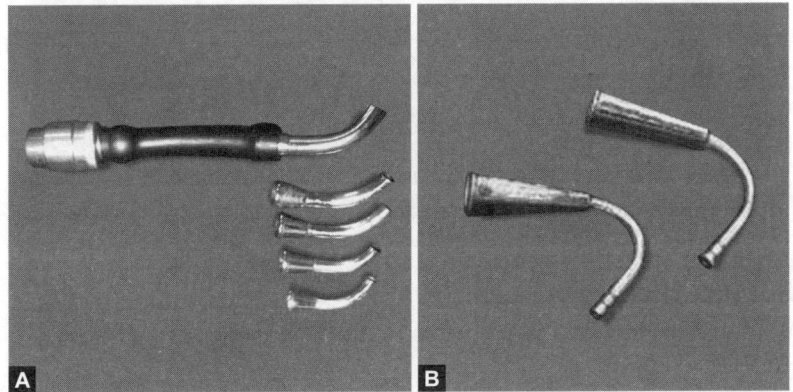

Figs 8.39A and B: Catheter mount with Magill's connector. (A) Catheter mount with Magill's metal oral connectors fixed; (B) Magill's nasal connectors showing acute bend

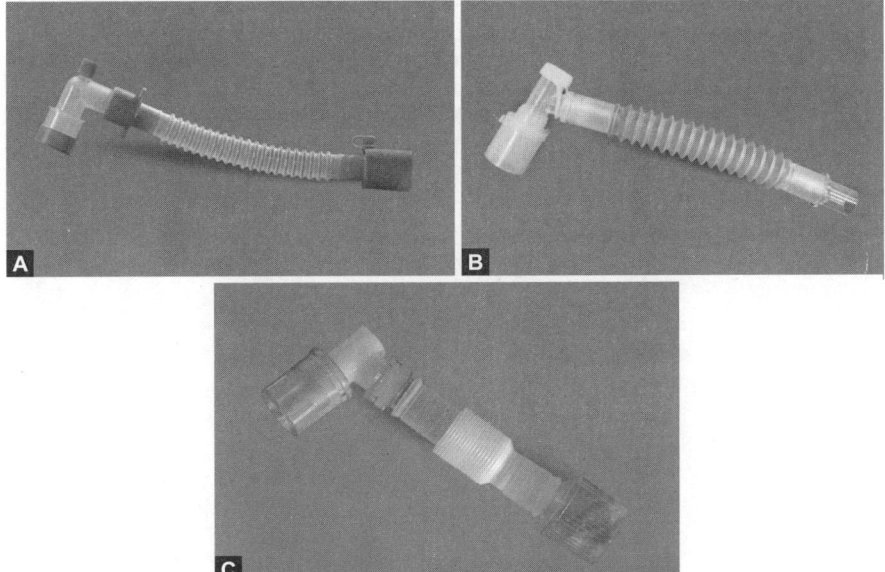

Figs 8.40A to C: Plastic catheter mounts. (A) Non-swivel catheter mount; (B) One way swivel mount with 'concertina tube'; • Single swivel mount with single swivel and 'concertina tube'; • There is a suction port covered by a rubber stopper; (C) Two ways swivel mount—axial swivel and circular swivel combined; • The two swivels can rotate 360° in two axes; • No drag on the ETT; • The length of corrugated tube is reduced by concertina effect

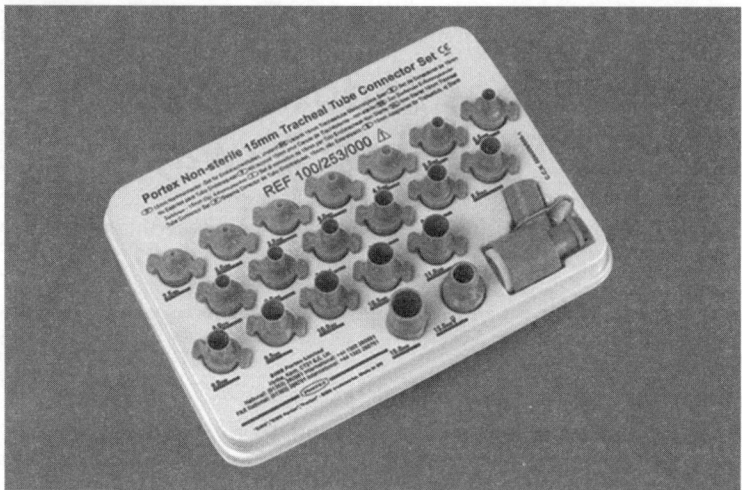

Fig. 8.41: 15 mm universal connectors (1.5–11 mm) with a swivel mount

FURTHER READING

1. Al-Shaikh Baha, Stacey S. Essentials of Anaesthetic Equipment, 1st edn. London: Churchill Livingstone, 1995.
2. Dorsch JA, Dorsch SE. Understanding Anaesthesia Equipment, 4th edn. London: Lippincott Williams and Wilkins, 1999.
3. Dorsch JA, Dorsch SE. Understanding Anaesthesia Equipment, 5th edn. London: Lippincott Williams and Wilkins, 2008.
4. Kaul TK, Mittal G. Mapleson's Breathing Systems, Indian J Anaesth. 2013;57(5):507-15.
5. Lee's Synopsis of Anaesthesia, 11th edn, London: Butterworth-Heinemann Ltd., 1993.
6. Moyle JTB, Davey A. Ward's Anaesthetic Equipment, 4th edn. London: WB Saunders Company Limited, 1998.
7. Ward CS. Anaesthetic Equipment, 2nd edn. London: Balliere, S;1985.

Laryngoscopes Endotracheal Tubes and Airways

chapter 9

LARYNGOSCOPES

History

1854: Manuel Garcia invented the first laryngoscope
1895: Alfred Kirstein made the direct vision laryngoscope
1943: Sir Robert Macintosh designed the first curved blade laryngoscope which is still in use worldwide for more than 7 decades.

- Laryngoscope is the instrument for visualizing the larynx. (Scope- visualizing instrument).
- Mainly used for visualizing the larynx (and adjacent structures) for the purpose of intubation of trachea with an endotracheal tube. Rarely used for removing a foreign body from the hypopharynx or larynx.
- It has two parts namely the 'handle' and the 'blade'.
- The handle contains the batteries for powering the bulb in the blade, which illuminate the larynx for intubation.
- The handle has rough surface for improved grip.
- The blade is hinged to the handle in such a way that when the handle is opened to right angle the light is switched on.
- The blade is used to lift the mandible and the tongue to visualize the larynx (after proper positioning of the head and neck)
- The handle is used for applying suitable leverage to the blade.
- There are two types of blades–straight blade and curved blade.
- *MacIntosh laryngoscope* has curved blades **(Fig. 9.1A)**
- Usually, it comes with four sizes of blades, infant size, child size, adult size and extra-large size for bigger adults. Sometimes there is a neonate size also included **(Fig. 9.1B)**.
- Straight blade laryngoscopes are available in various versions, but they are not commonly used.
- For pediatric patients, because of the anatomical difference, it is preferred to use a special design straight blade laryngoscope.
- *Miller straight blade pediatric laryngoscope* is the common type used. Sizes of blade 0–4 are available **(Fig. 9.2)**.
- Another model is *Sheila Anderson laryngoscope*. The blade is straight like Miller and has the tip as a spatula that lifts the epiglottis.

Fiberoptic (Green Coded)

- These are different from the conventional laryngoscope in the mechanism of illuminating the larynx.
- The lamp is within the handle.

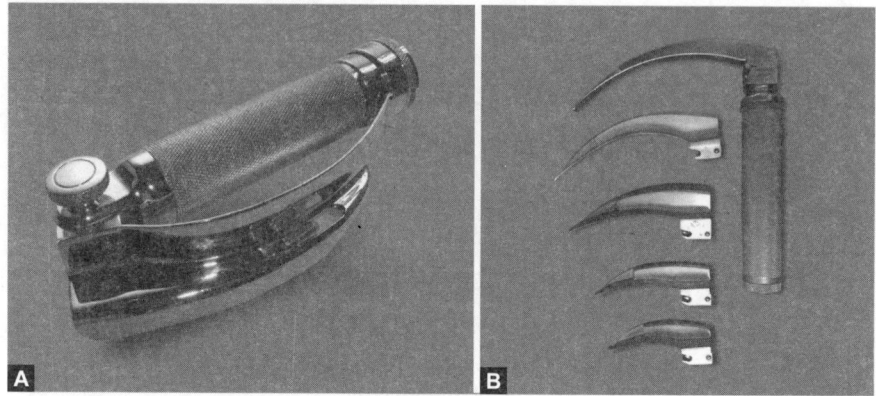

Figs 9.1A and B: (A) Traditional screw type laryngoscope with adult size blade illuminated by a bulb at the tip; (B) Hook on type fiber-optic laryngoscope with five blades; neonate, infant, child, adult and extra large sizes. The green band on the distal end of the handle indicates that it is fiber-optic instrument (Green coded)

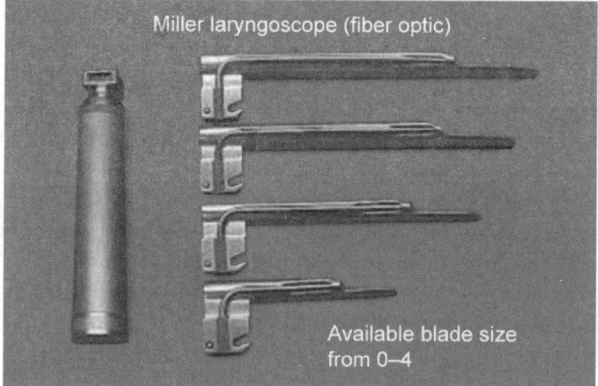

Fig. 9.2: Miller straight blade laryngoscope

- The handle at the distal end has the bulb which is switched on once the blade is hinged on to the handle.
- From this source, fail proof light is transmitted to the tip of the blade through fiberoptic light bundle fixed in the blade.
- As there is no electrical circuit within the handle, failure of light during laryngoscopy does not occur.
- These laryngoscopes are identified by the green band on the distal end of the handle **(Figs 9.1B and 9.2)**.

Technique of Laryngoscopy

The head and neck are positioned in such a way that oral cavity and the larynx are brought to lie in a straight line for the best possible view of larynx.

Position: Optimal position for most patients is *'sniffing position'* **(Figs 9.3A and B)**.
- Flexion of lower cervical spines 25 to 35°
- Extension of head at atlanto-occipital joint 85 to 90°

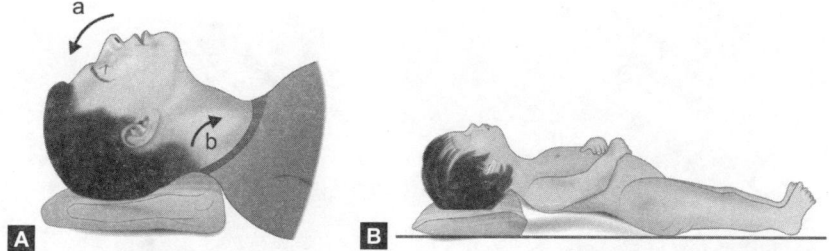

Figs 9.3A and B: Position of head and neck for intubation; adult and child

- Pillow to a height of 4" under the head.
- For children it may not be necessary to flex the lower cervical spines.
- For neonates a small pad is kept under the back (shoulder blades) to elevate the shoulder as the head is larger.

Steps

- Laryngoscope is held in the left hand with the thumb at the junction of the handle and blade.
- Optimum opening of the mouth is done the right thumb and index finger.
- Introduce the tip of the blade into the mouth without engaging lips and teeth.
- As half of the blade enters the oral cavity, sweep the tongue to the left.
- Advance the blade along the side of the tongue till right tonsillar fossa is seen and then move the blade to the midline.
- Advance the blade behind the base of the tongue and pulling the handle along its axis will make the epiglottis visualized.

From now on there is a different technique for *curved blade* and *straight blade*.

Curved blade **(Fig. 9.4A)**
- Blade is advanced until the tip fits into the vallecula (glosso-epiglottic recess).
- Traction applied along the axis of the handle moves the base of the tongue and epiglottis forward and glottis will be visualized well.

Straight blade **(Fig. 9.4B)**
- The blade is advanced till epiglottis its identified.
- The tip of the blade is advanced posterior to the epiglottis.
- The blade is lifted anteriorly elevating the epiglottis directly and the glottis is visualized.

Anatomical Differences in Neonates and Infants

- Large head, large tongue, small oral cavity, mandibular angle 140° (obtuse).
- Epiglottis is narrow, floppy, longer, 'U' shaped and angled backwards.
- Larynx is at the level of C3–C4 forms an acute angle with the base of the tongue.
- Straight blade (Miller) designed to pass beyond epiglottis and elevate it.

Other Types of Laryngoscopes

Though numerous types of laryngoscopes were introduced over the past 7 decades, not all of them became popular or claimed superiority in performance. Some of the

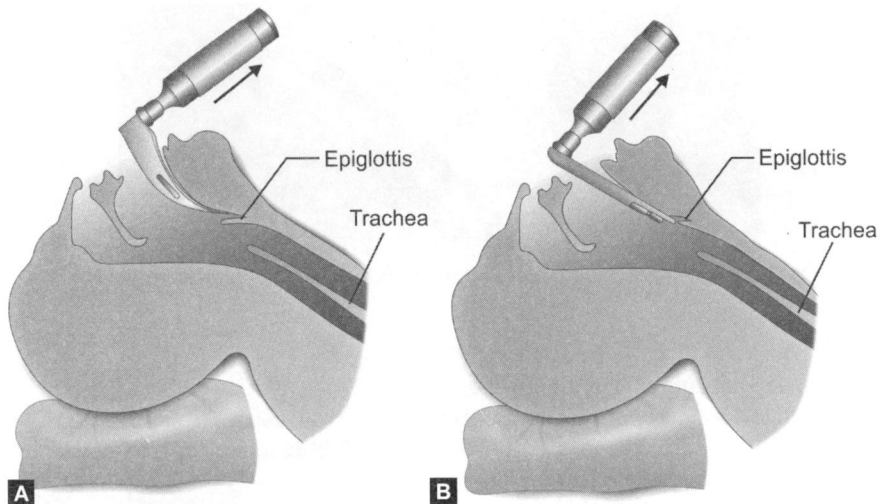

Figs 9.4A and B: Position of laryngoscopy: (A) Macintosh blade (curved blade); the tip of the blade is at vallecula; (B) Miller blade (straight blade); the tip of the blade is posterior to epiglottis and lifts it

laryngoscopes were modifications in the existing one to overcome certain types of difficulties in intubation.

McCoy Laryngoscope

- The hinged tip of the blade is controlled by a lever attached to the proximal end of the blade **(Figs 9.5A and B)**.
- When the lever is pushed towards the handle, the tip is flexed to a maximum of 70°.
- This flexion of the tip further elevates the epiglottis and enhances the view of the larynx.
- Advantages; less force is required, less trauma and ideal for difficult intubation.

Howland Lock

- The Howland lock is an additional block that has the provision for conducting the light and hooking on features.
- Howland lock is hooked on to the handle and the laryngoscope blade can in turn be hooked on to the lock and thus changes the angle of the handle allowing for a natural lifting action that simplifies visualization of larynx.
- By adding the Howland lock any conventional laryngoscope's angle can be reduced to 45° **(Fig. 9.6A)**.
- For conventional laryngoscope the lock has continuity of electrical circuit for the bulb **(Fig. 9.6A)**.
- For fiber-optic laryngoscopes, the block has continuity of optical conduction of light **(Fig. 9.6B)**.
- In 'difficult intubation' situations such as receding chin, anteriorly placed larynx, protruding teeth, 'Bull neck', facial contractures, decreased jaw mobility, etc. the use of Howland lock may make the procedure easier.

Laryngoscopes Endotracheal Tubes and Airways

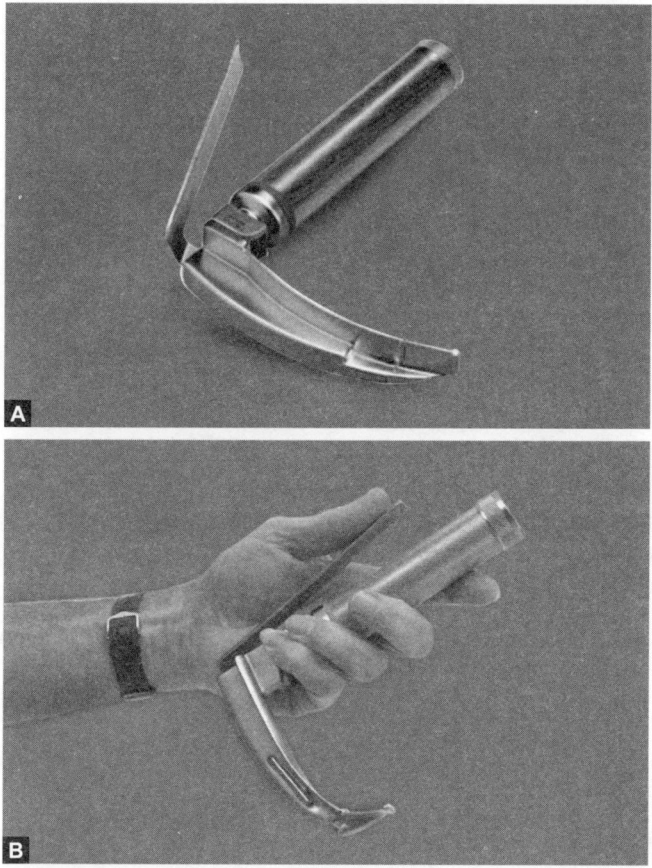

Figs 9.5A and B: (A) Flexi-tip laryngoscope (McCoy); (B) The tip of McCoy laryngoscope during use

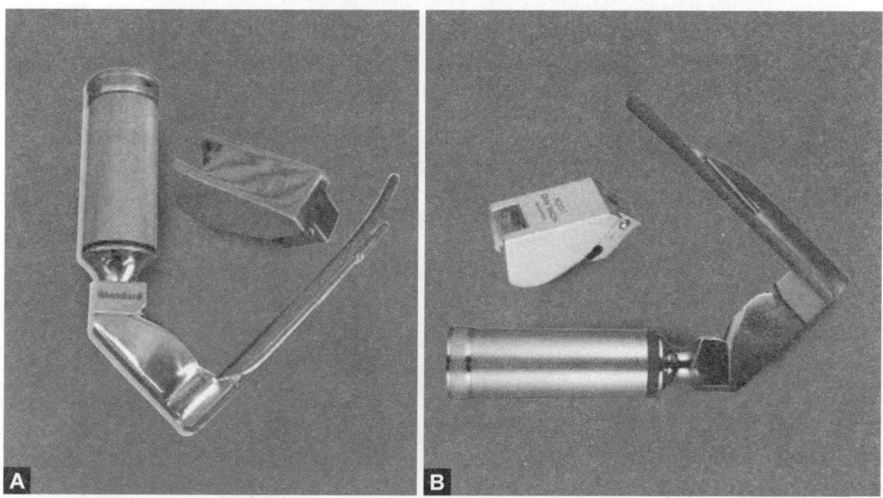

Figs 9.6A and B: Howland lock: (A) Howland lock on conventional laryngoscope; (B) Howland lock on fiber-optic laryngoscope

Polio Laryngoscope

- Originally designed to incubate patients on iron lung negative pressure ventilation during polio epidemic.
- The blade is mounted at 135° to the handle **(Fig. 9.7)**.

Patil-Syracuse Laryngoscope

- Designed by Dr Vijayalakshmi Patil and colleagues in 1983 at the State University of New York at Syracuse.
- Has an adjustable handle which can be set and locked in 4 angles; 45°, 90°, 135° and 180°
- These positions mimic the Howland Lock and polio blade as well as the conventional arrangement **(Figs 9.8A and B)**.

Bullard Fiberoptic Laryngoscope

- It is an indirect fiberoptic laryngoscope designed by Dr Roger Bullard.
- Rigid metal fiberoptic laryngoscope that is shaped to fit the anatomical contour of the oropharynx and epiglottis **(Figs 9.9A and B)**
- This comes in three sizes; *pediatric, pediatric long* (8–10 yrs) and *adult (more than 10 years and adults)*.
- There are three channels; a *light bundle* on the left, *image bundle* on the right and the *working channel* on the center.
- The working channel extends from body of the cope to the point where the light bundle ends at the tip.
- Proximally the working channel divides into two; one with Luer-lock and the other for passing a stylet.
- This working channel can be used for suctioning, insufflation of oxygen, instillation of local anesthetic or saline.
- The light source may from an adaptor of cold light source **(Fig. 9.9A)** or a battery loaded handle which can be attached **(Fig. 9.9 B)**.
- It may be used as a passage for airway exchange or jet ventilation.
- *Advantages*: Difficult situations like cervical spine injury where movement of spine may be dangerous, Pierre Robin syndrome, upper body burns, etc.
- *Disadvantage*: The operator must have sufficient experience.

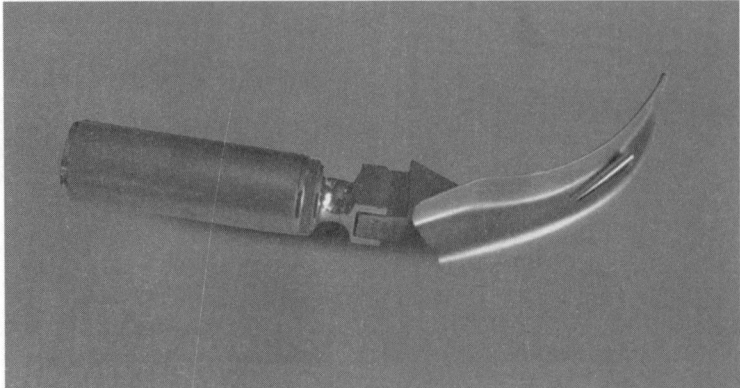

Fig. 9.7: Polio laryngoscope

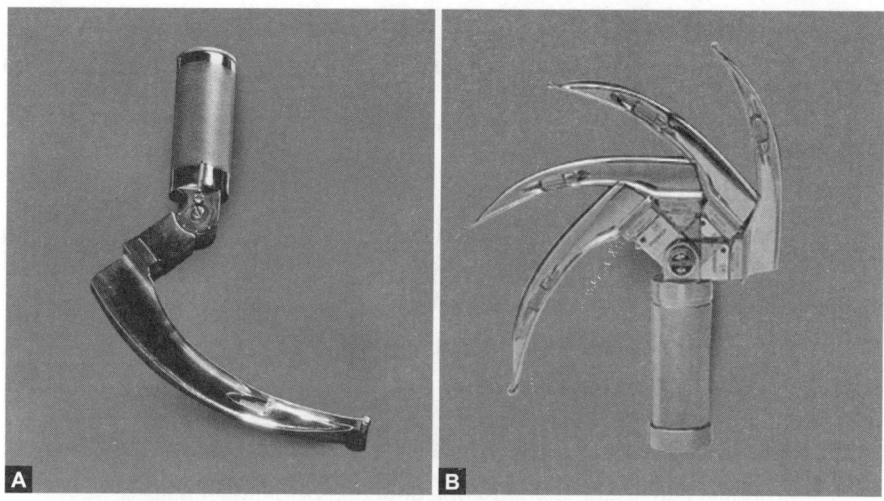

Figs 9.8A and B: (A) Patil-Syracuse laryngoscope; (B) Same blade shown in the 4 positions; 45°, 90°, 135° and 185°

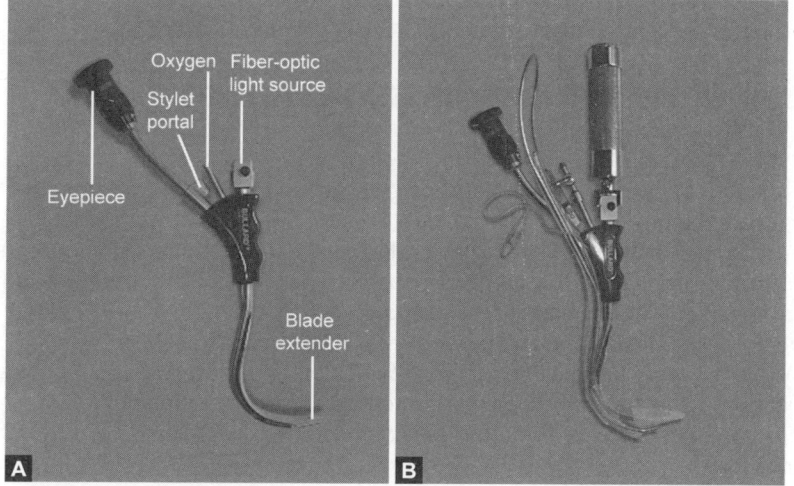

Figs 9.9A and B: (A) Bullard laryngoscope; (B) Bullard laryngoscope with battery attached

Video Laryngoscopes

- These are new generation laryngoscopy techniques.
- The image of the glottis is visualized in a clear better and magnified way that the intubation is done easily.
- The image from the end of the scope is carried directly to the attached screen or through optic cable to a distant screen **(Fig. 9.10)**.

Advantages

- Better visualisation of the glottis is possible.
- Less mouth opening and extension of neck is needed for intubation.

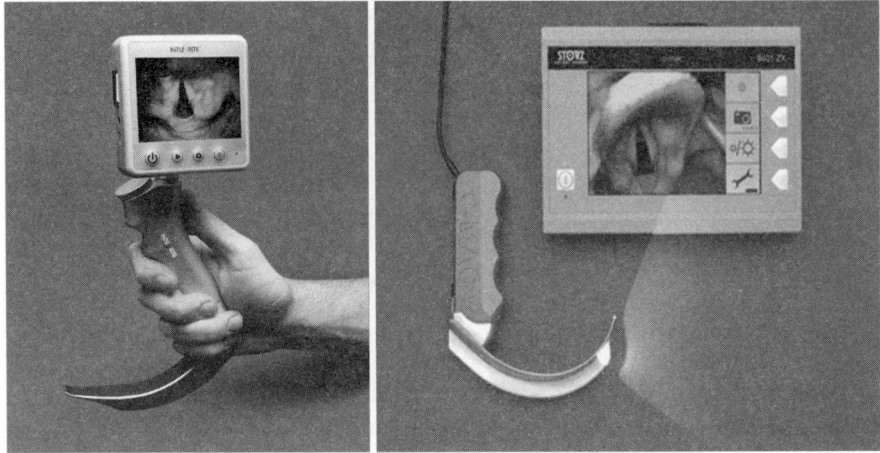

Fig. 9.10: Video laryngoscopes: Two versions; with an attached screen and a distant screen

- Ideal for difficult airway management.
- Assisting technician also can visualise the glottis and help easily.
- The two versions; with an attached screen and a distant screen.

FIBER-OPTIC INTUBATING BRONCHOSCOPE

History

In 1967, Dr P Murphy used a Choledochscope passed through an endotracheal tube to intubate the trachea.

The flexible bronchoscope is a device that can be used for direct laryngoscopy for endotracheal intubation. It is particularly useful when direct laryngoscopy is difficult or impossible, or would be dangerous. For awake intubation, flexible bronchoscopy is better tolerated than laryngoscopy with a standard laryngoscope.

While the term "flexible fiberoptic intubation" has been used for this technique in anesthesia, newer bronchoscopes no longer use fiberoptic technology.

This technique has become the gold standard for the management of difficult laryngoscopy.

Principle and Design

- The fundamental principle in 'Fiberoptic" is "Total internal reflection".
- The pathway for carrying light and the image consists of thousands of very fine glass fibers of 10 microns diameter.
- Each fibre is made of a central glass core surrounded by a thin cladding of another type of glass with a different refractory index.
- As a result of the differences in the refractory indices, the light entering the glass fiber at one end undergoes 'total internal reflection' along the length of the fiber to be transmitted and emerge out of the other end.
- For image transmission, the arrangement of fibers must be identical in relation to each other at either ends of the bundle. This is essential as each fiber caries a tiny bit of the overall image and any fault in it will result in distortion of image. This is known as 'Coherent Bundle' **(Fig. 9.11)**.

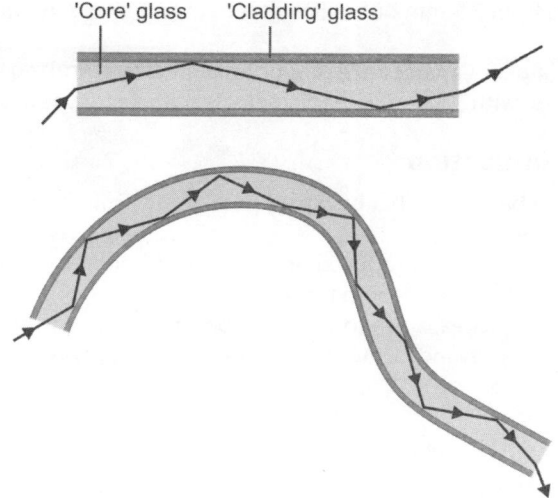

Fig. 9.11: Principle of fiber-optic—'Total internal reflection'

Parts of the Fiberoptic Laryngoscope

- It has a powerful external light source—'Cold light source' which prevents tissue damage by radiant heat.
- The scope has two parts; A handle and a flexible insertion portion.

The insertion portion has the following components:
- Two light bundles
- One image bundle
- One working or biopsy channel
- Two angulation wires that control the flexible tip of the scope
- All these components are bound together by a spiral stainless steel wrap.
- This is further protected by a stainless steel 'braid' and covered with a water proof material.
- This gives a rigid cross section while permitting overall flexibility **(Fig. 9.12A)**.

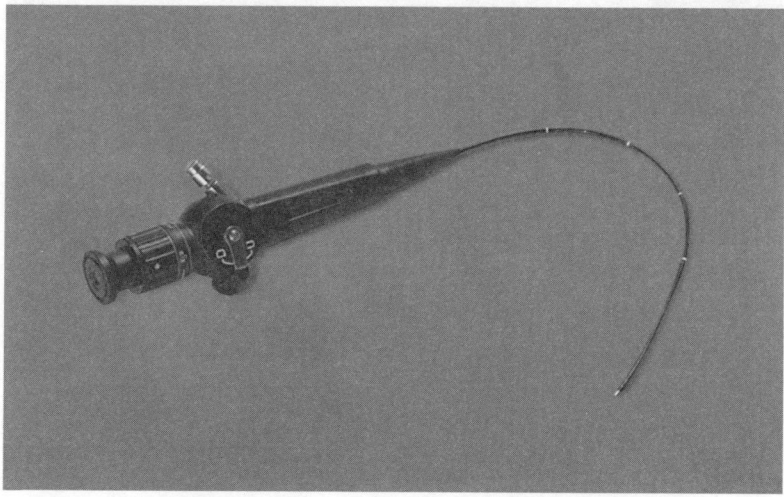

Fig. 9.12A Fiber-optic intubating laryngoscope

- Sizes ranging from 2.5 mm outer diameter to over 6 mm outer diameter scopes are available.
- Scopes with larger diameter have proportionately larger working channel.
- A laryngoscope with 3.5 mm outer diameter is suitable for use in adult patients.

Technique of Intubation

- Intubation can be done either by oral or nasal route. Oral route is a little difficult than nasal route.
- The fiberoptic scope is introduced and advanced behind the tongue to reach larynx and further advanced into the larynx.
- Once inside the trachea, an endotracheal tube which has been previously loaded on to the scope is advanced into the trachea and the scope is withdrawn.

Advantages

- Reliable technique in difficult airway situations
- Facility for recording and reviewing and also for documentation.
- Record review will help to improve the learning process.

Disadvantages

- Expensive and fragile equipment
- Technically more difficult and time consuming than direct laryngoscopy
- Needs experience for operating.

Single use Flexible Intubating Bronchoscope

- Now single use flexible intubating devices are available. It does not have fiberoptic cable, instead has a small camera at its tip illuminated by an LED. The image is transmitted through a slim cable in the device to a reusable screen. *Example*: Ambu a Scope **(Fig. 9.12B)**.
- Available in sterile pack, handy and is cheaper compared to the cost and maintenance of conventional fibreoptic equipment.

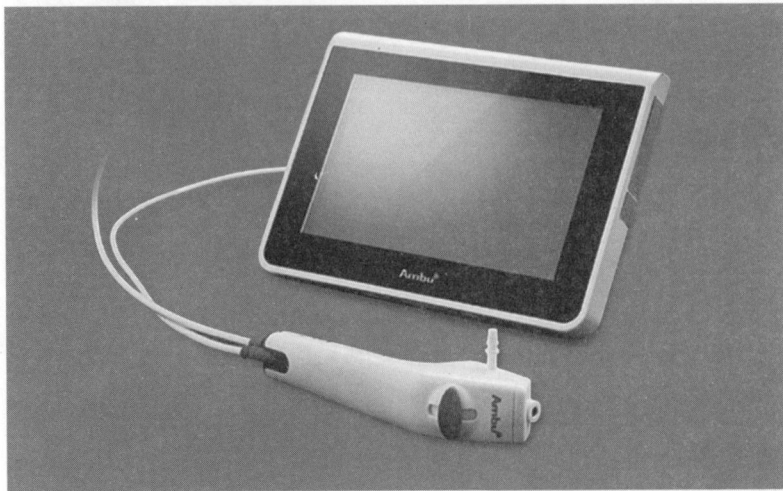

Fig. 9.12B Disposable flexible intubating bronchoscope with reusable screen

ENDOTRACHEAL TUBES

History
- C. Kite of Gravesend described oral and nasal intubation for resuscitation of the apparently drowned in 1788.
- Historically, tracheostomy was preferred to intubation because it was believed that a laryngeal tube will not be tolerated.
- In 1871, Friedrich Trendelenburg developed a cuffed catheter for insertion though a tracheostomy to prevent soiling of lungs during operation in upper airway.
- In 1878, William Mac Evan, a surgeon of Glasgow, placed a metal tube into the trachea by manual palpation through mouth and administered chloroform anesthesia.
- Edgar Stanley Rowbotham and Ivan Whiteside Magill first used endotracheal anesthesia by passing a gum elastic tube in trachea.
- The first blind nasal intubation was performed by Stanley Rowbotham.
- Magill published his results of blind nasal intubation with a wide bore rubber tube in 1928.
- Inflatable cuffs were used even earlier, but reintroduced in 1928 by Ralph Milton Waters and Arthur E Guedel.
- Before the days of muscle relaxants, blind nasal intubation under deep inhalational anesthesia was in practice.
- Use of muscle relaxant to facilitate intubation was pioneered by Bourne.
- In 1950s, the use of cuffed endotracheal tube became the standard of anesthesia practice.

Indications for Intubation of Trachea
- In situations where it may not advisable to administer anesthesia with a face mask.
- When there is a need for the use of muscle relaxant and positive pressure ventilation.
- For maintaining the airway in unconscious patients.
- Preventing aspiration of secretions or regurgitated gastric contents and protecting the respiratory tract with a cuffed tube.
- For sealing the respiratory tract and breathing circuit.
- For mechanically ventilating patients in ICU.

Tubes
- Traditional tubes for either oral or nasal intubation were 'Magill endotracheal tubes'.
- These tubes were made of mineralized rubber to keep them retain their shape and lumen are relatively firm without collapsing.
- The tip of the tube is obliquely cut facing left side called 'bevel' that facilitates the insertion into the glottis.
- Oral tubes have thicker walls and are firm with a short bevel (35°).
- Nasal tubes are relatively softer with a long bevel (45°) for easy negotiation in the nasal cavity.
- Their size is mentioned in mm, 8 mm, 8.5 mm, etc. indicate the internal diameter of the tube.
- These specially designed tubes can be passed into the trachea for delivering anesthetic mixture into the respiratory tract.

- Laryngoscopy is done for visualizing larynx to be intubated.
- The tube may be passed, depending upon the necessity, either through the nose (Naso-tracheal intubation) or through the mouth (Orotracheal intubation).
- The procedure of passing an endotracheal tube into the trachea is called as "endotracheal intubation" shortly known as "intubation".

Magill's Endotracheal Tube

Red Rubber Tube

- Latex rubber is impregnated with minerals—'mineralized' rubber-to make it hard and retain the shape.
- It is colored red to indicate that as a medical product.
- There is a preformed (built in) curvature that helps in easy intubation
- Available as plain tubes (non-cuffed) or cuffed tubes **(Figs 9.13A and B)**.
- The cuff is made of soft latex rubber and is *small volume, high pressure* type.
- These 'low volume—high pressure' cuffs may cause pressure on the submucosal vessels leading to mucosal ischemia.
- There are different tubes meant for orotracheal and nasotracheal intubation.

Differences between *oral* and *nasal* tubes

	Oral tubes	Nasal tubes
• Curvature	14 cm radius	18 cm radius
• Bevel	45° short bevel	35° long bevel
• Texture	Relatively rigid	Relatively soft

Nasal tubes are softer with long bevel for negotiating the nasal cavity without causing injury to turbinates. Red rubber tubes cause irritation to the mucosa and prolonged use may cause laryngeal granulomata.

Plastic Endotracheal Tubes

- These are transparent tubes are available as plain (noncuffed) and cuffed tubes.
- Available in sizes from 2 mm to 11 mm sizes.
- Most of the tubes come with 'Murphy's safety eye'. **(Figs 9.14A to C)**

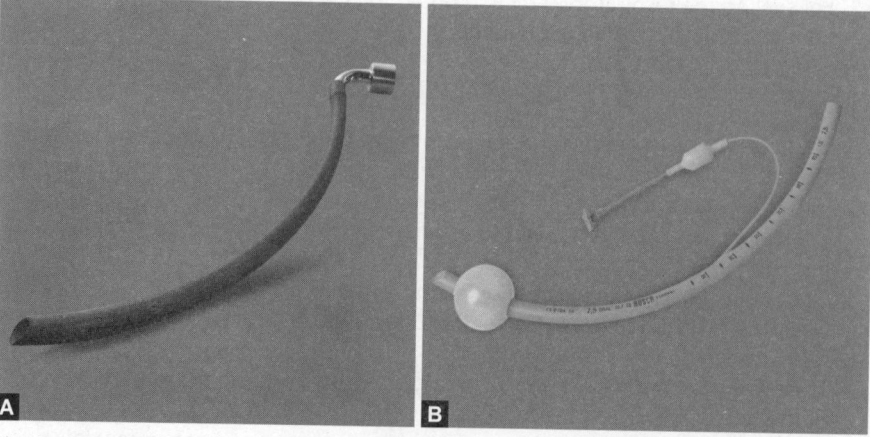

Figs 9.13A and B: Magill' red rubber endotracheal tube—noncuffed and cuffed (A) Oral tubes have the short bevel of 35° and arc of 18" radius; (B) Small volume high pressure cuff

- Murphy's eye is an oval hole on distal end of endotracheal tube on the opposite side of the bevel.
- This functions as a vent, and prevents the complete obstruction of the patient's airway, should the primary distal opening of an ETT become occluded.
- Relatively nonirritant and have large volume low pressure cuffs that give an airtight seal for normal airway pressures.
- The cuff can be inflated with air using a plastic syringe through a tube "cuff inflating tube with pilot balloon.
- Cuff inflating tube is embedded in the anterior wall of the tube and it extends out for a length and end in a pilot balloon with spring loaded self-sealing valve.
- The large volume low pressure cuffs do not cause pressure on the submucosal vessels to produce ischemia. Cuff pressure should not exceed 25 cm of H_2O.
- Different types are available depending upon the need. They are; fusiform, globular, elliptical, and square cuffs **(Figs 9.15A to D)**.
- For better seal with low pressure a square cuff is ideal.
- There is a radio-opaque blue line throughout the length on the posterior aspect of the tube for radiological confirmation of the position of the tube.

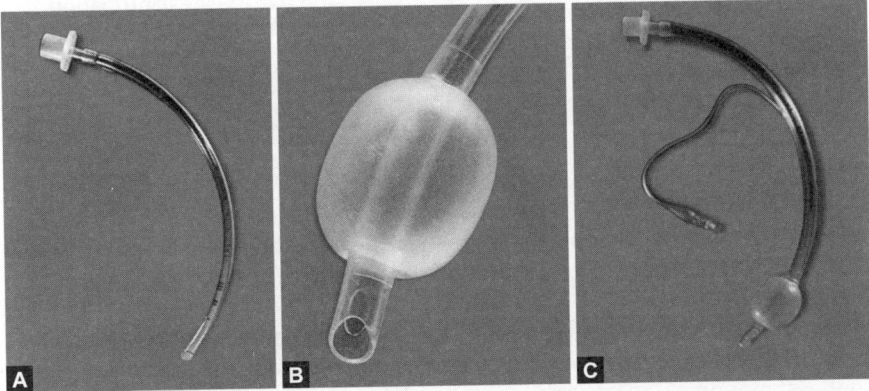

Figs 9.14A to C: (A) PVC endotracheal tube noncuffed; (B) High volume-low pressure cuff and Murphy' safety eye at the tip; (C) PVC cuffed tube

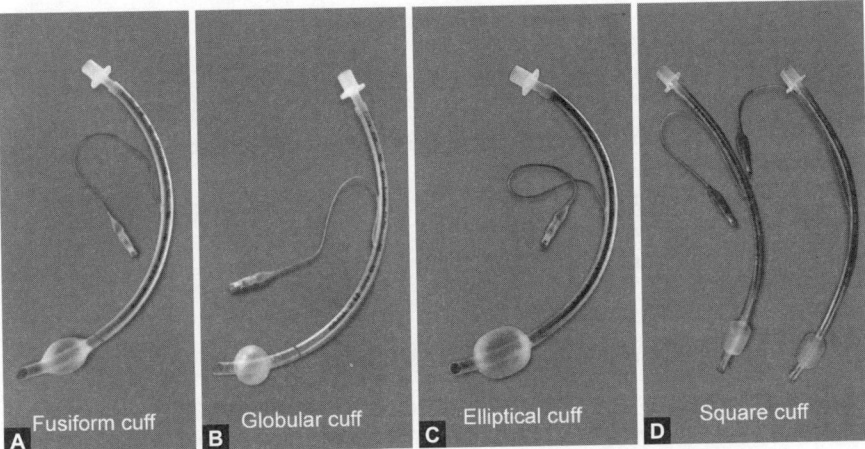

Figs 9.15A to D: Different types of high volume low pressure cuffs

Information present on the tube:
- Manufacturer's name
- Oral/nasal
- Internal diameter (ID)—large letters
- External diameter (ED)—small letters
- Z 79—Implantation test for tissue toxicity. As per ANSI standard.
- Length in cm—markings from the tip.
- Radio-opaque blue or black line on the posterior wall for radiological confirmation of the position of tube.
- A black ring proximal to the cuff—guides the position of the cuff just below the glottis.
- Pilot balloon has the size of the tube marked on it.

Different Types of Cuffs
- Small volume, high pressure cuff (usually rubber cuffs)
- Large volume, low pressure cuff **(Figs 9.14 and 9.15)**
  - Fusiform
  - Elliptical cuff
  - Globular
  - Square cuff
- Square cuff ensures more airtight seal with less pressure
- For a tracheostomy tube, the cuff is shorter and square.

Murphy's Safety Eye
Some tubes have an oval opening on the wall near the tip of the tube opposite to the bevel. It is an opening for an alternate passage for gas, if the tip of the tube is blocked **(Fig. 9.14B)**.

Modern endotracheal tubes are made of material other than rubber such as *plastic* (PVC), *polyurethane*, or *silicon rubber* and these tubes are less irritant. Silicon rubber stands heat sterilization.

Cuff Pressure
- It is desirable that the cuff seals the airway without causing undue pressure on the tracheal mucosa.
- With a pressure of 30 cm H_2O, the perfusion in the vessels in the submucosa is compromised.
- With 50 cm H_2O the perfusion completely ceases and leads to ischemic necrosis of tracheal mucosa.
- It is recommended that the intra cuff pressure is maintained between 25 and .30 cm H_2O to prevent ischemic necrosis.
- Cuff pressure should be monitored with a cuff pressure gauge during prolonged anesthesia.

Size of Endotracheal Tube
- The correct size of endotracheal tube needed for the patient must be used.
- Too small a tube needs very high pressure for seal and may lead to leaks.
- Too big tube may cause pressure on the glottis and lead to edema after extubation.

- Ideally three tubes must be ready. Expected size, one size bigger and one size smaller.
- Average adult male—8.5 mm ID size may be suitable.
- Average adult female—7.5 mm ID size may be suitable.
- For children age is the criterion for choosing the size of the tube.
  - 3 months and less   - 3 mm ID
  - 3 to 9 months   - 3.5 mm ID
  - 1 year and older   - mm ID (16 + age in years/4)
  - Younger than 6 years   - mm ID (age in years/3 + 3.5)
  - More than 6 years   - mm ID (age in years/4 + 4.5)
- Infants
  - Below 1 kg   - 2.5 mm
  - 1 to 2 kg   - 3.0 mm
  - 2 to 3 kg   - 3.5 mm
  - 3 kg   - 3.5 or 4.0 mm
- The diameter of the tip of little finger of the patient roughly corresponds to the outer diameter of the endotracheal tube. It is an approximate estimate.

Other Recommendations

Age of patient	Size in ID
Premature neonate	2.5 to 3.0 mm
Full term neonate	3.0 to 3.5 mm
3 months to 1 Year	4.0 mm
2 years	4.5 mm
4 years	5.0 mm
6 years	5.5 mm
8 years	6.0 mm
10 years	6.5 mm
12 years	7.0 mm

Length of the Tube from Incisors

After intubation, the tube tip must be in the middle third of the trachea with the head in neutral position.

The calculation for assessing the length of the tube from the incisor teeth to the middle third of trachea:
- Age in years/2 + 12 cm
- Weight in kg/5 + 12 cm
- Height in cm/10 + 5 cm
- ID of the tube in mm × 3

In adults:
- The tube is passed until the cuff is 2.25 to 2.5 cm below the vocal cords.
- In average adults, 23 cm for male and 21 cm for female at the incisor level is correct. For nasal intubation 5 cm should be added to the above lengths to fix the tube at the nares.

Endotracheal Tubes for Special Purposes

Apart from the regular endotracheal tubes, there are several specially designed endotracheal tubes meant for certain special applications.

During certain surgical procedures (neurosurgical) or positions for surgery a (sitting position), it is possible that endotracheal tube is bent on itself and gets kinked resulting in partial or complete airway block.

In such situations a nonkinkable endotracheal tube is used, most common being the 'reinforced' or 'armoured' tubes':
- *Latex rubber tube* with metal spirals embedded—straight tube—reusable. (Flexo-metallic) highly flexible made of pure latex rubber.
- *Plastic tubes* with metal spirals embedded—with or without preformed curvature.

Latex Rubber Armoured Tubes—Metal Spiral Reinforced Tubes (Nonkinkable Tubes)

- These are the true nonkinkable endotracheal tubes, as it does not get kinked in any possible positions of the head and neck.
- Originally reinforced tubes were made of soft latex rubber, *reinforced with metal spiral* embedded in its wall, commonly known as flexo-metallic tubes **(Fig. 9.16A)**.
- The reinforcement spiral embedded in the wall may be either steel spiral or nylon spiral and is known as 'Armour'.
- This makes the tube virtually nonkinkable in spite of bending on itself or even making a knot. The lumen of the tube remains unaltered.
- The two layers of rubber are fused together in between the spirals to prevent sliding of spirals.
- The cuff inflating tube is not embedded in the wall. It enters the tube proximal to first spiral, runs through the side of the tube within the lumen of the tube and enters into the cuff. This prevents the tube getting caught in the spirals getting blocked.
- The distal end of the spiral is almost at the tip of the tube.
- The bevel is very short and small (less than 35°) to prevent the soft bevel folding inwards and causing obstruction of the tube.
- It is a soft rubber tube, does not retain preformed curvature as seen in red rubber or PVC tubes and is straight.
- It needs an introducer or malleable stylet for intubation.
- The spirals stop short of the proximal end leaving only latex rubber tube for inserting the connector.
- The connector must be inserted to touch the first spiral otherwise the soft tube may get kinked at this point.
- These tubes are used for head and neck surgeries, mainly neurosurgeries.

Plastic Armoured Tubes

Most of these problems have been solved in the modern reinforced tubes.
- Most of them are made of soft material that the tube is a straight tube **(Fig. 9.16B)**.
- Nonkinkable in any position, even with a knot on it or folded on itself **(Figs 9.16C and D)**.
- Need for a stylet for intubation and possibility of kinking at the connector level are still there.
- The tip is more firm provided with bevel and Murphy's eye.
- Some plastic tubes come with preformed curvature, does not require introducer.
- Disposable

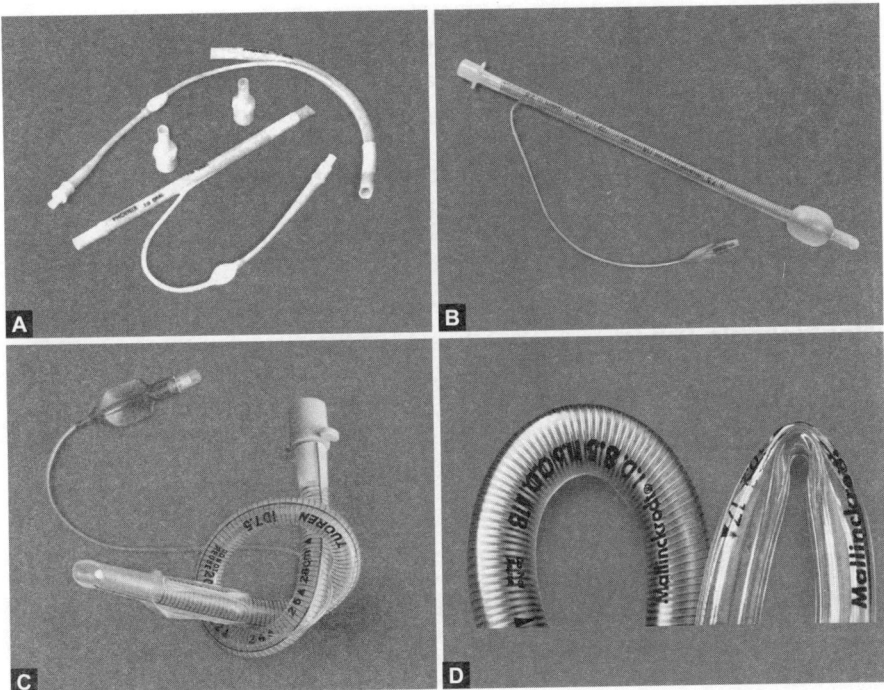

Figs 9.16A to D: Reinforced or armoured endotrachal tubes: (A) Latex rubber 'Flexometallic' tube—a straight rube—needs stylet for intubation; (B) Silicon rubber armoured tube—this also needs a stylet for intubation; (C and D) A knot on it or bending it on itself does not kink the tube; The connector should be inserted well to touch the first spiral

RAE Tubes (Ring Adair and Elwyn) Preformed Tubes

- These tubes are specially designed for use in head and neck surgeries particularly for facial surgeries and plastic surgeries.
- Also called as "preformed tubes" because of the special fixed curvature they have conforming to the natural passage to suit the use **(Figs 9.17A to D)**
- They are relatively nonkinkable and available as cuffed as well as noncuffed versions.
- *North Pole*: Towards head end–*nasal*
- *South Pole*: Towards foot end away from the field of surgery—*oral*
- Suction may be a little difficult.
- Short bevel.
- The nasal tube is called "North Pole" and the oral tube is called "South Pole".
- Double 'Murphy's eyes on both sides of the bevel.

Oxford Tubes

- These are right angled tubes specially designed for surgeries inside oral cavity.
- Very commonly used for "Cleft palate repair" surgeries and many other palate surgeries.
- These are relatively nonkinkable tubes because its preformed right angle portion fits well in the oropharynx **(Figs 9.18A to D)**.

234 Anesthetic Equipment Made Easy

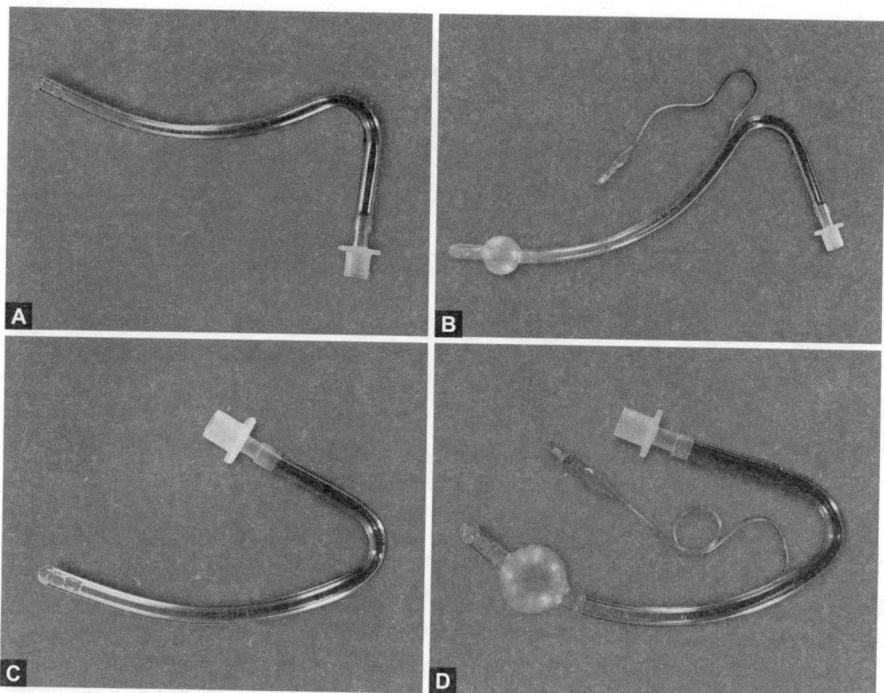

Figs 9.17A to D: RAE tubes: Nasal–plain and cuffed; Oral–plain and cuffed. (A) Nasal tube plain; (B) Nasal tube cuffed (North Pole); (C) Oral tube plain; (D) Oral tube cuffed (South Pole). Double 'Murphy's eyes are seen on both sides of the bevel

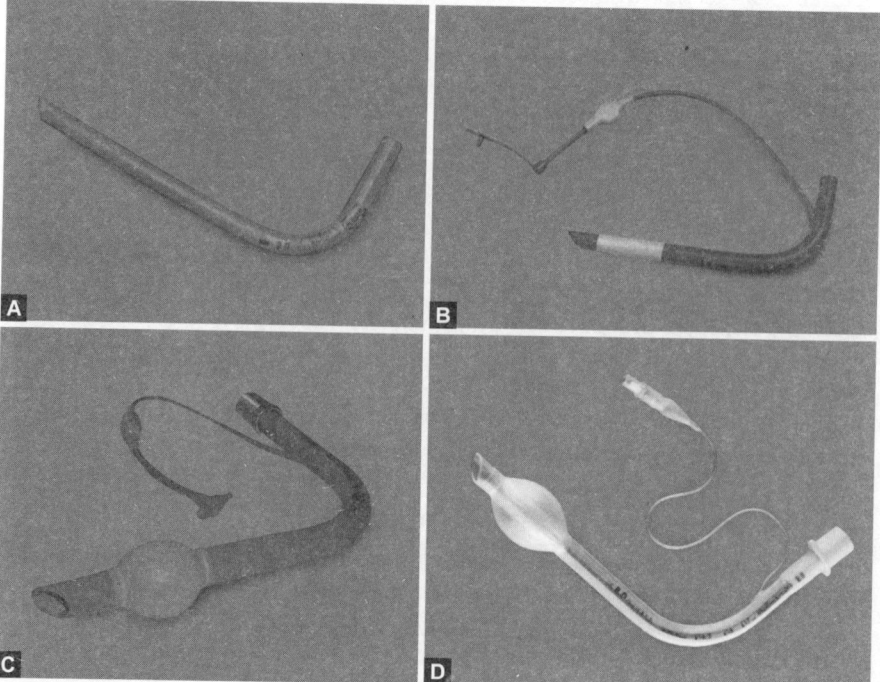

Figs 9.18A to D: Oxford tubes: Red rubber—uncuffed, red rubber cuffed and PVC cuffed

- Proximal end of the tube has bigger outer diameter whereas the distal end has smaller outer diameter. But, the inner diameter uniform and outer diameter is tapering. This is for easy insertion of the tube **(Fig. 9.18A)**.
- The bevel is short and faces posteriorly; to prevent accidental occlusion of the tip by opposing the anterior tracheal wall.
- After intubation, the tube will not protrude out of mouth but stops at the incisor tooth level.
- Hence, a special metal connector is introduced used for preventing the patient biting the tube and blocking the airway.
- The connector must be usually kept tightly fixed to the tube before intubation as after intubation connector cannot be fixed to the tube without dislodging the tube.
- For small children a right angled metal connector is used.
- Available in red rubber (reusable) and plastic (disposable).
- Noncuffed and cuffed versions are available.

Connectors for Oxford Tubes

- The right angled preformed curvature of the tube and the right angled connector form *"double right angle"* after application. This 'U' shaped passage will cause difficulty in passing suction catheter.
- Right angled connector—has hole or *fenestra (opening)* at the bend to facilitate suctioning which is covered with plaster.
- Connector must be sufficiently introduced into the tube so that when the mouth gag is applied, the tube is not compressed between incisor teeth and the tongue plate of mouth gag.

Endotracheal Tubes for Laser Surgeries

For surgeries in airway and neck using laser beam, standard endotracheal tubes are unsuitable as the laser beam striking at the tube may perforate or sever the tube leading to catastrophe. In the presence of oxygen it may ignite combustible material resulting in 'Airway fire'.

To prevent such dangers there are many tubes designed with the aim of reflecting the laser beams. Some of the tubes used are:

Norton: Spiral wound stainless tube

Bivona fome cuff: Aluminum spiral tube with silicon polyurethane foam cuff

Xomed Laser–Shield: Silicon elastomer tube containing metallic powder

Mallinckrodt Laser-Flex: Airtight stainless steel spiral wound tube with two PVC cuffs.

Out of the many available types of tubes, *Laser-Flex tube* has many advantages.

Laser-flex Tube (Manufactured by Mallinckrodt Medical Inc.)

- These are made of stainless steel spirals and are covered with PVC.
- The surface is rough for reflecting laser beam **(Fig. 9.19A)**.
- Non-cuffed tubes are available.

- The cuffed tube has two PVC cuffs and inflating lines which pass inside the lumen.
- The cuffs are filled with saline coloured with methylene blue.
- Proximal cuff is used first and if it is damaged by laser during work, the distal cuff can be inflated **(Fig. 9.19B)**.
- PVC tip with Murphy's Eye is provided.
- The laser beams strike at the metal will be reflected and will not damage the tube.
- The tubes are of thicker walls.

Double Lumen Endotracheal Tube

These are special tubes designed for one lung anesthesia, commonly employed for lung surgeries and any other thoracotomies to keep the lung down at will during surgery.
- There are two different lumens in the same tube for ventilating each lung separately.
- The lumens are 'D' shaped, proximally have two connecting pieces.
- For isolating the lungs, there are two cuffs, one in the bronchial portion (Bronchial cuff) and the other on the tracheal portion (Tracheal cuff).
- The pilot tubes and the balloons for inflating the cuffs are differently colored for easy identification.
- Right sided and left sided versions are available.

Carlen's Double Lumen Tube

- Originally double lumen tube was designed for bronchospirometry – was known as 'Carlen's catheter' and later only it was used for one lung anesthesia.
- *Carlen in* 1949 *designed this* for bronchospirometry to assess individual lung function.
- It is a left sided tube with left bronchial tube **(Fig. 9.20A)**
- It has a carinal hook that will rest on carina for proper positioning the tube **(Fig. 9.20B)**

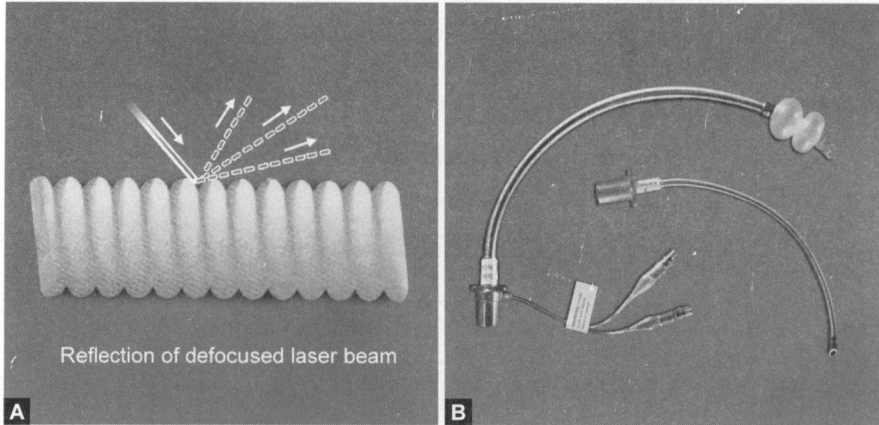

Figs 9.19A and B: Laser-Flex tube (Mallinckrodt Medical Inc). (A) Laser beam getting defocused and reflected on the surface; (B) Laser-Flex tube; Plain and cuffed

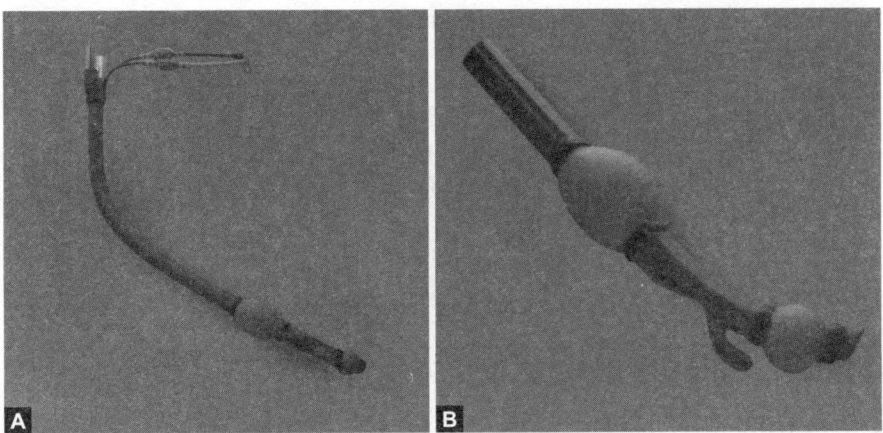

Figs 9.20A and B: (A) Carlen's double lumen tube; (B) The cuffs and 'carinal hook' are shown. The 'carinal hook' helps to position the tube in the right place

Green and Gordon's Right Endobronchial Tube

- Designed by Gordon and Green in 1955
- The problem of intubating the right bronchus without obstructing its upper lobe branch was solved.
- This tube has a right bronchial tube that lies in the right main bronchus.
- The tube with a slot on the bronchial cuff opposite the orifice of the right upper lobe bronchus ventilates the right upper lobe **(Fig. 9.21)**
- This is actually a right sided modified version of Carlen's tube with a 'carinal hook'.

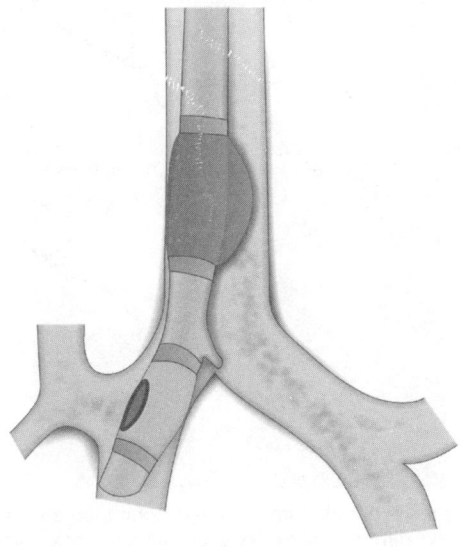

Fig. 9.21: Green and Gordon double lumen tube. • The bronchial cuff is in the right main bronchus; • The cuff has a opening opposite to upper lobe for ventilating the upper lobe

Robert Shaw Double Lumen Tubes for One Lung Anesthesia

- A modified Carlen's double lumen tube.
- Lumen is D shaped on cross section.
- Right and left side versions are available. No carinal hook.
- Right side version will have a slit on lateral aspect of bronchial cuff for ventilating the right upper lobe **(Figs 9.22A and C)**.
- This is the most commonly used tube.
- *Bronchial* cuff is *blue* and *tracheal* cuff is *red* with pilot balloons of corresponding colours
- Small, medium, large sizes were available. Now one more size extra small is added.

OTHER LESS COMMONLY USED TUBES

Cole's Tube

- Introduced for the purpose of preventing endobronchial intubation in neonates.
- Internal diameter is same throughout.
- Outer diameter is narrow near the tip to form a shoulder.
- When the tube is introduced, the shoulder rests on vocal cords so that only the narrow portion of the tube is inside the trachea and can't be introduced further.
- Distal portion measures 1.5 to 2 cm **(Fig. 9.23)**.

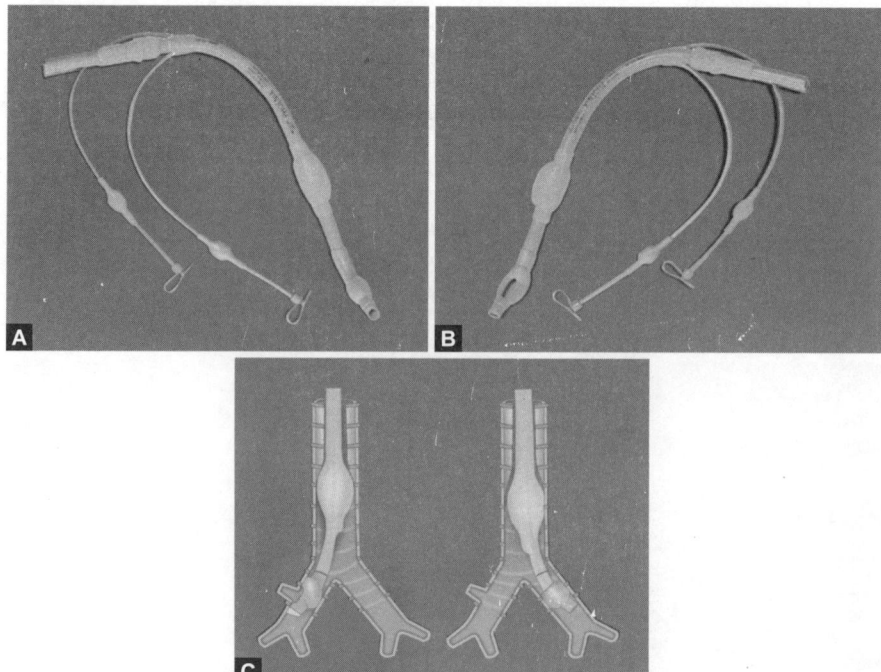

Figs 9.22A to C: Robert shaw double lumen tube for one lung anesthesia. • The two cuffs (bronchial and tracheal) have different colored pilot balloons. The bronchial cuff and pilot balloon are blue colored and the tracheal cuff and pilot balloon are red colored. (A) Left-sided version; (B) Right-sided version—which has a opening in the bronchial cuff for ventilating right upper lobe; (C) The position of the tubes in trachea and bronchus

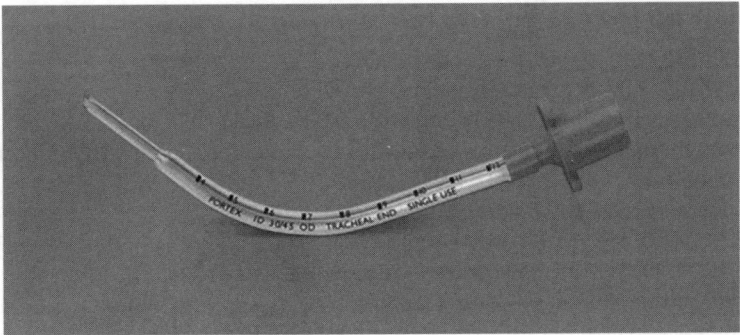

Fig. 9.23: Cole's tube

Laryngectomy Tube

- If the tumor is not obstructing the airway, general anesthesia with oral intubation is managed for the major part of the surgery. When the trachea is severed, surgeon inserts a sterile tube into the trachea and secures it.
- When there is any doubt regarding the maintenance of airway, ideally tracheostomy is done under local infiltration anesthesia and a laryngectomy tube which has performed 'J' shaped curvature is inserted for safe anesthetic management **(Fig. 9.24)**
- Laryngectomy tubes are cuffed tubes available in red rubber as well as reinforced plastic tubes.
- The armoured plastic tubes have a short square cuff.

Endotracheal Connectors

- Different connectors are used to connect the endotracheal tube to the anesthetic breathing system or a resuscitator bag.
- Modern equipment use only the "Universal 15 mm connectors" available in all sizes starting from 2.2 mm tube meant for a premature neonate.
- These connectors fit in almost all adapters used in equipment for anesthesia as well as resuscitation.

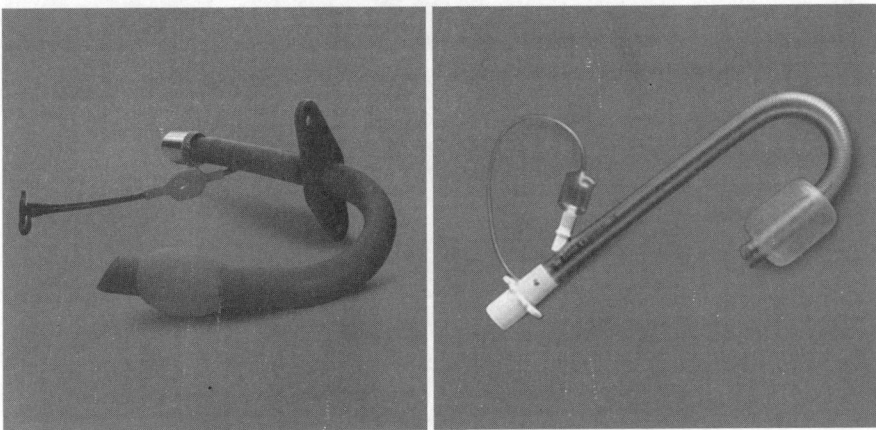

Fig. 9.24: Laryngectomy tube

Magill's Connectors

- In 1930 Sir Ivan Magill designed these curved metal connectors to be used with Magill's red rubber endotracheal tube he invented.
- *Smooth curved* connectors–16 connectors **(Fig. 9.25)**
- Funnel shaped proximal end (flanged) and corrugations on the tip for tight fit to the tube.
- 8 oral connectors and 8 nasal connectors
- 1, 2, 3, 4, 5, 6, 6A and 6B: *Oral*—angle of curvature: obtuse and smooth curve
- 7, 8, 9, 10, 11, 12, 12A, 12B: *Nasal*—very acute curve and nearly right angle
- *Oral*: Less than 90°; nasal—more than 90°.
- Turbulence in flow of gases and increase in resistance with nasal connectors.
- A catheter mount is necessary for using these connectors.
- In both these relatively good laminar flow is maintained, because these are curved connectors.

Rowbotham Connector

- Metal connector
- Right angled with a tapering end with horizontal or transverse ribs for better hold **(9.26)**.

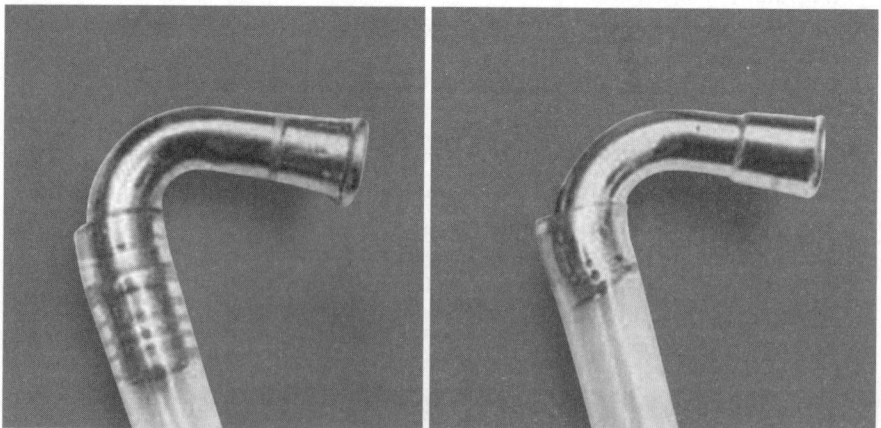

Fig. 9.25: Magill's endotracheal tube connectors—oral and nasal

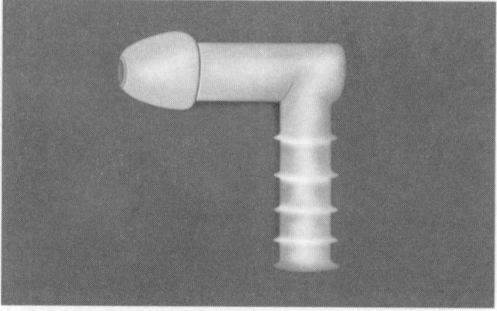

Fig. 9.26: Rowbotham's connector

- *Advantages*: Same connector can be used for a few sizes of ETT, maintains good grip.
- *Disadvantage:* Enormous turbulence and resistance because it is right angled.
- Resistance during inspiration cause more problems in spontaneous breathing. But in controlled ventilation, it is not dangerous.
- Expiratory resistance is dangerous because CO_2 elimination is affected.

Noseworthy Connector

- Curved connector made of chromium plated brass metal.
- Has three pieces of very wide bore **(Fig. 9.27)**.
- Maintains good laminar flow.

Cobb's Suction Union

- Right angle connector, with an extension of a suction port at the angle covered with a metal stopper **(Fig. 9.28A)**
- Metal stopper linked by a chain to the angle.
- These connectors are used for anesthetizing patients with suppurative long diseases posted for lobectomy where purulent secretions from the affected lobe may flow into the proximal bronchial tree during handling necessitating frequent suctioning.

Magill's Suction Union

- Similar to the Cobb's suction union but, the suction port is wide and funnel shaped to facilitate the introduction of catheter easily **(Fig. 9.28B)**.
- Suction port is covered with a metal cap or rubber cap, which fits the outside of suction port.
- These two suction unions are commonly used for *wet lung cases*, which facilitates *frequent suctioning during surgery*.

15 mm Universal Endotracheal Tube Adapter

A set of connectors from 2.5 mm size to 12 mm size are available with a swivel mount adapter **(Fig. 9.29)**.

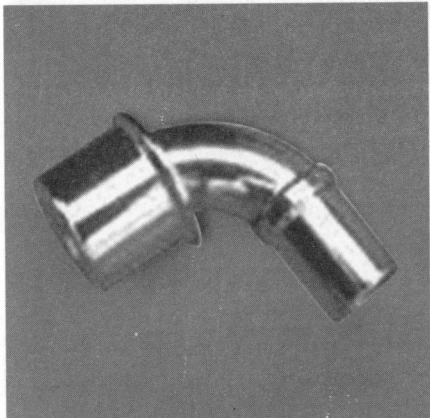
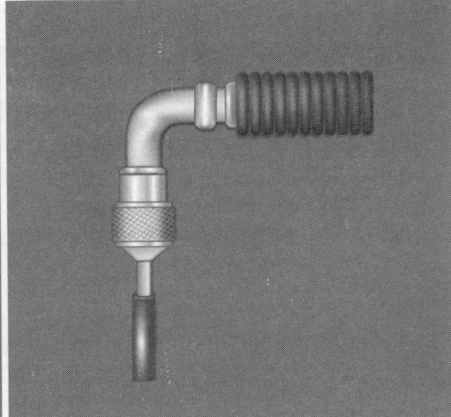

Fig. 9.27: Noseworthy's connector

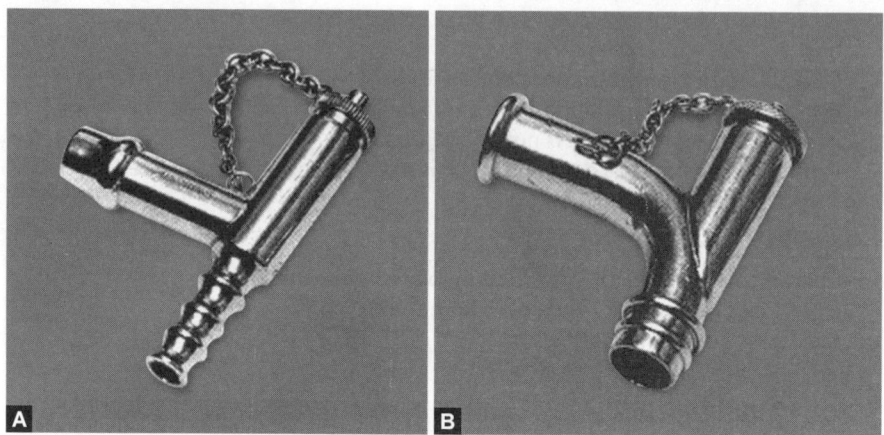

Figs 9.28A and B: Cobb's suction Union and Magills suction Union

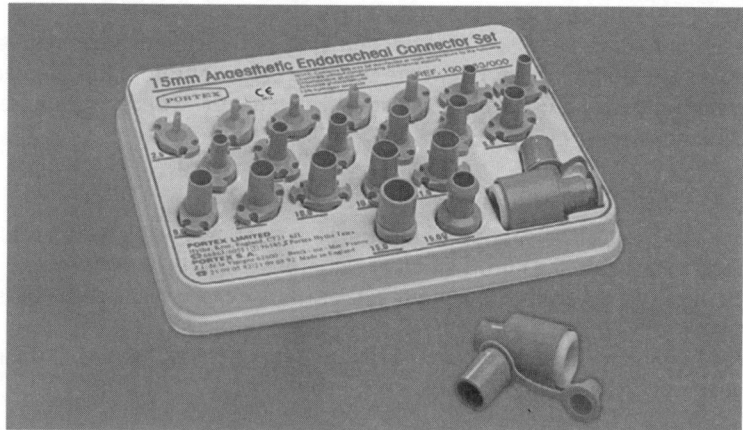

Fig. 9.29: Set of 15 mm Universal connectors with a swivel mount

Swivel Mount with Suction Port

- Permits 360° movement of catheter mount without causing leak
- This is for use with 15 mm universal connectors
- *One way* swivel mount permits 360° movement around the connector
- *Two ways* swivel mount—*axial swivel* and *circular swivel mount* combined. I can be rotated 360° in its axis without leak. Similarly it can be rotated 360° at right angle to the axis. So, no drag on the endotracheal tube is caused during positioning **(Fig. 9.30)**.
- It is provided with a suction port covered with a rubber stopper that helps suctioning without disconnecting the tube.

Stylet

- An endotracheal tube *stylet*, useful in facilitating orotracheal *intubation*.
- An intubating *stylet* is a malleable metal (copper or brass) wire with the tip is rounded up like a globe to prevent injury to any soft structure **(Fig. 9.31A)**.
- Stylets made of aluminium metal covered with PVC are also available **(Fig. 9.31B)**.

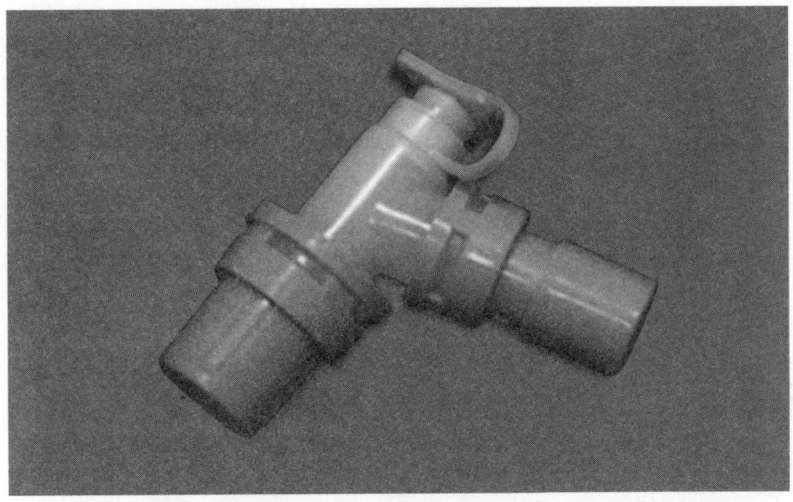

Fig. 9.30: Two way swivel mount for endotracheal connectors

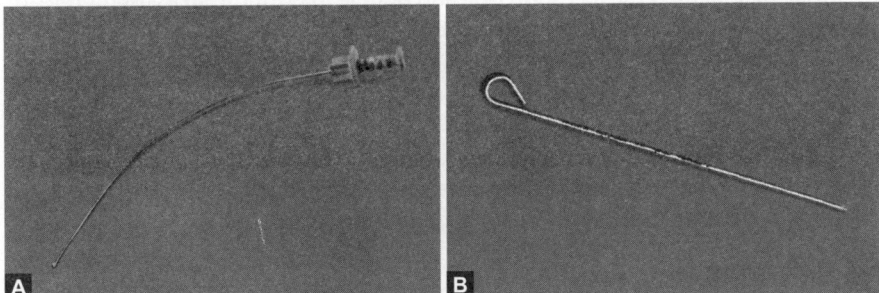

Figs 9.31A and B: Two types of stylet

- Designed to be inserted into the endotracheal tube to make the tube conform better to the upper airway anatomy of the particular individual.
- It is placed into the tube prior to laryngoscopy.
- Then the tube with the stylet in it is bent to resemble a hockey stick.
- It can be used for difficult intubation when the tip of the tube is not reaching the glottic opening when the glottis is very anteriorly placed.
- After insertion of the tube into the trachea, the stylet is removed.

Bougie (Gum elastic Bougie)

- The bougie is also known as 'Endotracheal tube introducer' or 'Intubation Catheter'.
- The bougie is a straight, semi-rigid stylet-like device with a bent tip that can be used when intubation is (or is predicted to be) difficult **(Fig. 9. 32)**.
- It is important to have "the epiglottis only view" during laryngoscopy in the first attempt for using a bougie.
- As an aid to in difficult intubation, Bougie is considered superior to a 'Stylet' especially with limited mouth opening, anteriorly placed glottis.
- During laryngoscopy, the bougie is carefully advanced into the larynx and through the vocal cords until the tip enters a main bronchus.

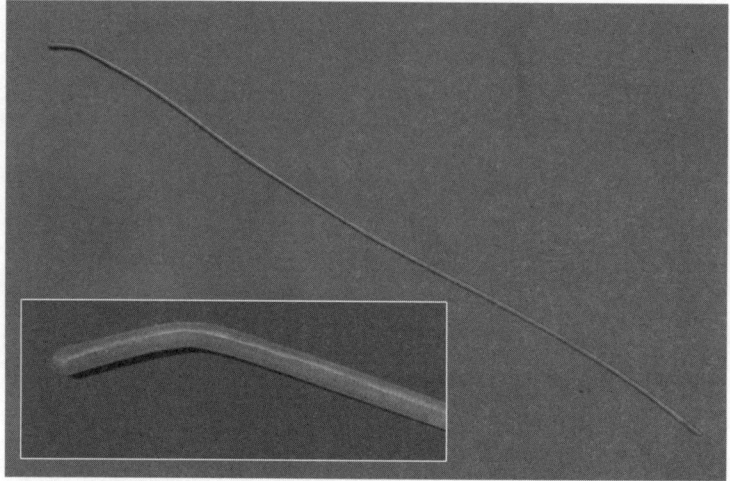

Fig. 9.32: Bougie used for aiding difficult intubation

- While maintaining the laryngoscope and bougie in position, an assistant threads an ETT over the end of the bougie, into the larynx. Once the ETT is in place, the bougie is removed.

Other Uses
- For exchanging ETT. Insert a Bougie through the existing tube. The existing tube is then removed and a new tube is inserted over the bougie.
- It can be used to direct an LMA or for changing an existing LMA.

Magill's Intubating Forceps
- It was introduced by Sir Ivan Magill in 1920.
- The instrument is to guide the tip of endotracheal tube to be introduced into the glottis particularly in nasotracheal intubation.
- Specially designed handle makes it possible to use it without obstructing the view of the operator **(Fig. 9.33)**.
- This instrument is essential for nasotracheal intubation.
- Three sizes are available; small, medium and large.
- Small size for children and medium for normal adults. The large size is for large adults with long neck.
- It has a uniquely designed tip that can hold the tip of endotracheal tube firmly for introducing into the trachea even in the presence of slippery secretions.
- This can be used for packing the throat around the endotracheal tube for preventing aspiration of blood during oral surgery and occasionally for removing a foreign body in oral cavity.

Artificial Airways
Artificial airway is a device that aims to maintain oral or nasal air passages patent. It is to be remembered that the term *'Artificial airway'* includes:
- *Simple supraglottic airway:* Oropharyngeal airway, nasopharyngeal airway
- *Augmented supraglottic airaway:* Laryngeal mask airway
- *Infraglottic airway:* Endotracheal tube, tracheostomy tube

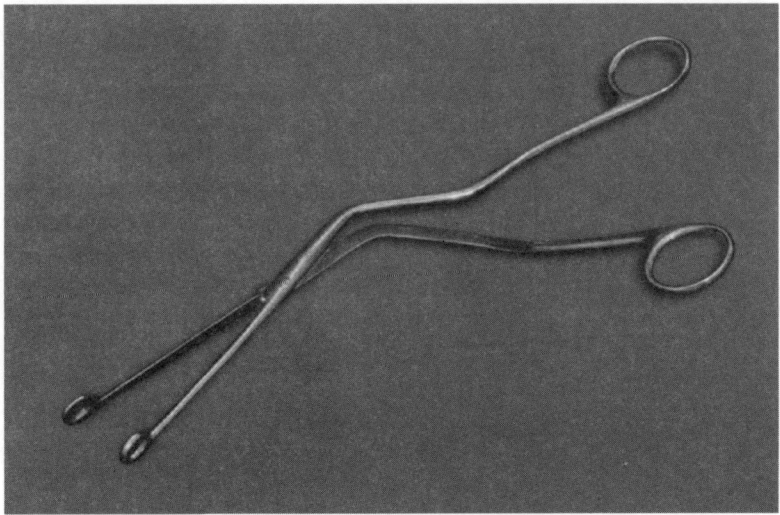

Fig. 9.33: Magill's intubating forceps

Conventionally the term 'Airway' is used to mention about oropharyngeal airways and nasopharyngeal airways.

These are devices that could be used to maintain the patency of the patient's air passage when there is a need.

Airway Obstruction

- In an unconscious patient the muscles that support the mandible are relaxed.
- The *mandible sags behind and the base of the tongue and epiglottis fall backwards and press on the posterior pharyngeal wall causing airway obstruction* **(Fig. 9.34A)**
- The maneuver of lifting the mandible (Jaw thrust), extending the head and supporting the chin is shown in Figure 9.34B
- At this point, an artificial airway when properly placed displaces the base of the tongue and epiglottis from the posterior pharyngeal wall. The lumen of the device maintains a patent airway.

Types of Airways

There are two types of airways:
1. Oropharyngeal airways.
2. Nasopharyngeal airways.

Oropharyngeal Airways

- These are designed in a shape that fits well in the contour of mouth and pharynx.
- It extends from lips to pharynx fitting in the oropharynx between tongue and posterior pharyngeal wall.
- Introducing this airway will keep the tongue away from posterior pharyngeal wall.
- The lumen in the airway is so good that the patency is well-maintained without much resistance.

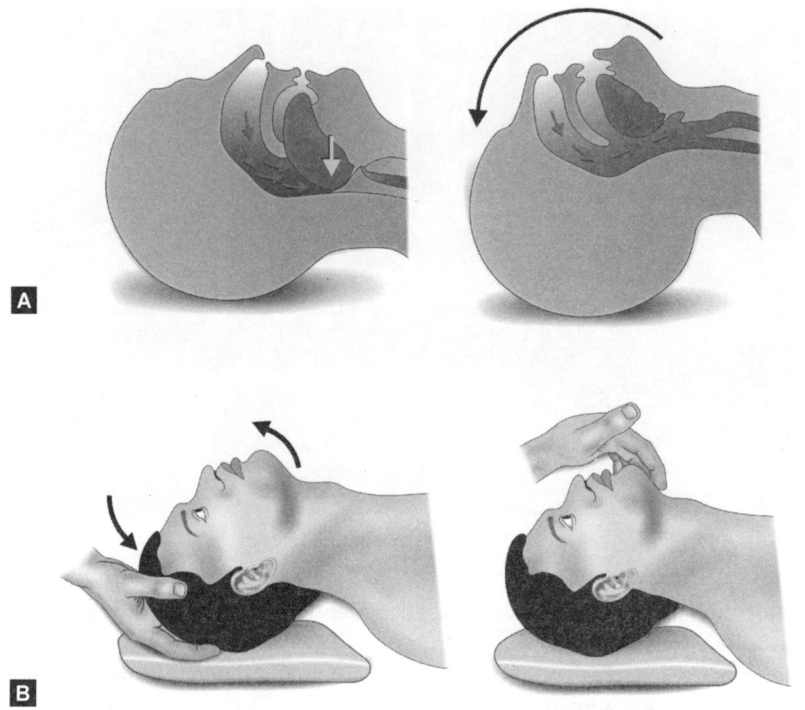

Figs 9.34A and B: (A) Mechanism of airway obstruction in an unconscious patient. • Falling back of tongue causes airway obstruction; • 'Jaw thrust' and extension of the head relieves the obstruction. (B) The maneuver of Jaw thrust, extension of head and supporting the jaw.

- When the patient is unconscious and pharyngeal reflexes are absent, these airways can be tolerated well to maintain a good patency.
- If the patient is conscious, has pharyngeal reflexes, this may induce gagging and vomiting and cannot be tolerated by the patient.
- There are different types of oropharyngeal airways (*See* **Fig. 9.35A to D**).

They are:
- *Water's airway*: 1930 (Metal airway)—Ralph M Waters (1883–1980)
- *Guedel's airway*: 1933—Arthur Ernest Guedel (1883–1956)
- *Phillips airway*: 1920
- *Hewitt's airway*: Sir Frederic William Hewitt (1856–1916)
- *Berman's airway*: Dr Robert A Berman (1914–1999).

Among these, Guedel's airway and Berman's airway are in common use. Parts of the oropharyngeal airway are; *Flange, Bite block* and *Body* **(Fig. 9.36)**.

Flange: It is at the proximal end that prevents the airway slipping deep into hypopharynx.

Bite block: This is the short straight portion of the airway that lies between the incisor teeth. This part is reinforced with a metal insert (sleeve) or hard plastic to prevent the lumen getting blocked if patient bites the airway.

Body: This is the curved portion of the airway that lies in the oropharynx behind the tongue to reach just above the glottis. Usually, it corresponds to the anatomical curvature of the tongue and palate.

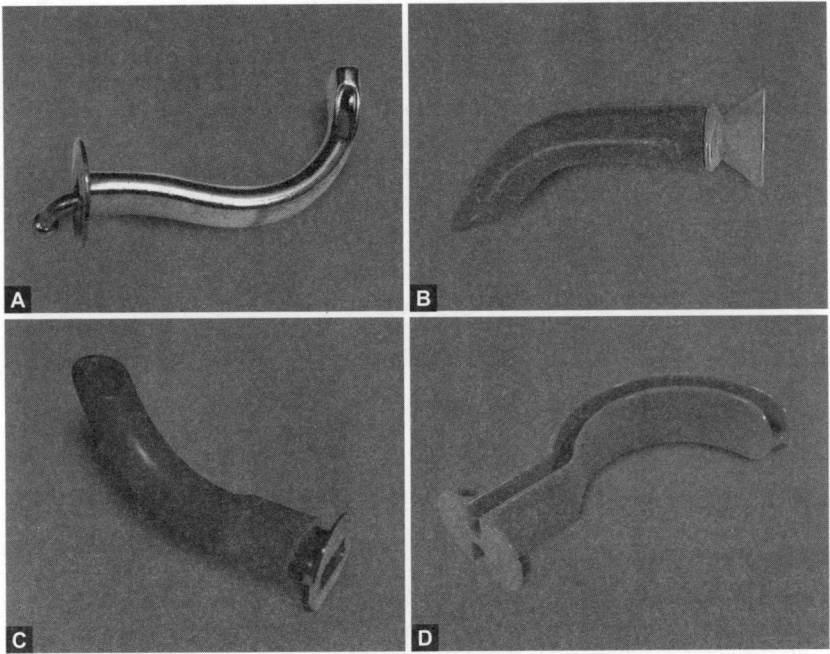

Figs 9.35A to D: Different oral airways; Water's, Hewitt's, Phillips and Berman's

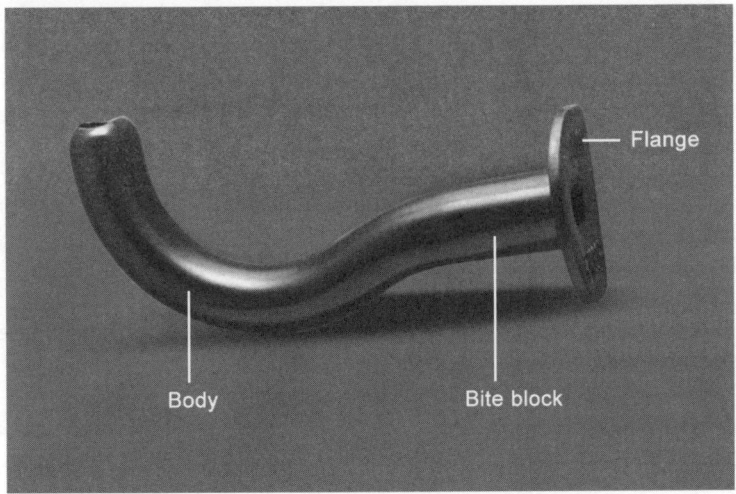

Fig. 9.36: Parts of an airway shown in Guedel's airway

Guedel's Airway

- The most commonly used airway more anatomically shaped, body more deeply curved to accommodate the bulge of the base of tongue **(Fig. 9.36)**.
- Less traumatic introduce
- The flange and the bite black are the same as Water's airway
- Be sure not to push the 'airway' forcefully over the tongue. This may push and move the tongue backward and cause airway obstruction rather than clearing airway obstruction.

- An anatomically curved pharyngeal section and an oval flange at the proximal end prevent over insertion.
- The flattened cross-section made it easy to insert the airway between partially clenched teeth, sometimes an important feature during inhalational anesthesia induction in those times.
- Now Guedel's airways are available in silicon rubber and plastic also (**Fig. 9.37A**).
- The bite block is reinforced with hard plastic which is color coded.
- This prevents the airway-collapsing if the patient bites it.
- The flange prevents the airway slipping into the mouth.
- Available in sizes from 000,00,0,1, 2, 3, 4. Size 000 being the smallest for a neonate.

Types of Guedel's Airway Available
- Black rubber (natural rubber) airway reusable.
- Silicon rubber transparent airway with different color bite blocks to identify the size. It can be sterilized by autoclaving.
- Plastic airways with different color bite blocks to identify the size (disposable).

Technique of Introduction
- When the tongue falls back against the posterior pharynx in anesthetized or unconscious patients obstructing the flow of air, it is inserted over the tongue that creates an air passage between the mouth and the posterior pharyngeal wall.
- The correct size of the airway must be used otherwise it may be blocked.
- The size of the airway to be used is assessed by keeping it on the side of the face. *It must extend from the lips to the angle of mandible* (**Fig. 9.37B**).
- The preferred technique is to use a tongue blade to depress the tongue and then insert the airway posterior to the blade.
- A laryngoscope blade also can be used.
- An alternate technique is to insert the oral airway upside down until the soft palate is reached.
- Then the device is rotated 180° and allowed to slip over the tongue (**Figs 9.38A and B**).
- Be sure not to use the airway to push the tongue backward and block, rather than clear, the airway.

Sizes of Airways
As per American National Standards' specifications 8 sizes of airway are available.

Size	Color	Length
000	Violet	3.5 cm
00	Blue	4.5 cm
0	Black	5.5 cm
1	White	6.5 cm
2	Green	7.5 cm
3	Orange	8.5 cm
4	Red	9.5 cm
5	Yellow	10.5 cm

Laryngoscopes Endotracheal Tubes and Airways 249

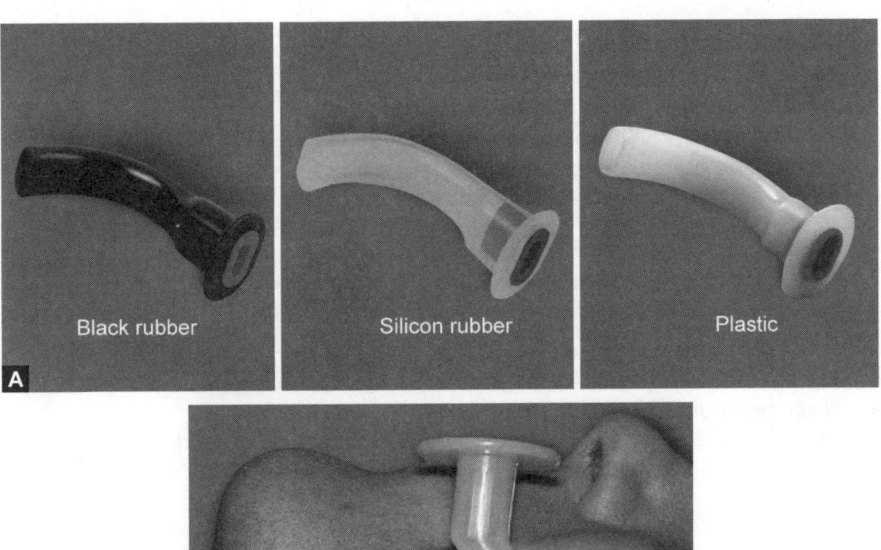

Figs 9.37A and B: (A) Guedel's oropharyngeal airways; (B) The method of assessing the correct size for a patient

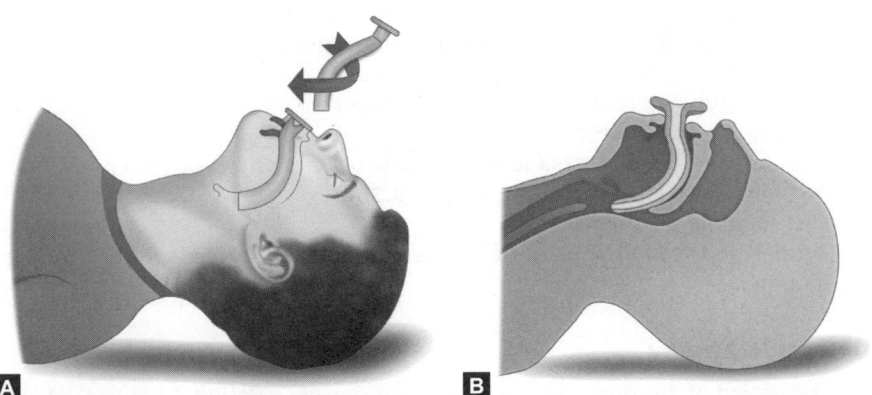

Figs 9.38A and B: The correct technique of inserting the airway (A) It is passed with the tip facing upwards and then gently rotated 180° to make it occupy the normal curvature of tongue. (B) Properly positioned airway maintains the patency

Water's Airway

- Dr Ralph Milton Waters (1883–1980) introduced this *metal oral airway* in 1930.
- It has three parts, *flange, bite piece* and *body*.
- It has a side port or "nipple" to which a tube can be attached to deliver air or oxygen. Its metal construction prevents patients accidentally biting on the airway and blocking the patency of the airway **(Fig. 9.35A)**.
- This airway has flattened cross section and opens at the tip.
- Near the tip there are three alternate pathways for air. Two on either side or one on the posterior aspect. If the tip gets blocked, air will pass through the alternate passages.
- However, metal airways including the Water's airway are prone to cause cut or bruises of lips and dental damage.
- It can be sterilized by autoclaving.
- Three years later, his friend and fellow-inventor, Dr Arthur Guedel, introduced an airway of similar shape but made of rubber with a metal insert at the level of the teeth.

Hewitt's Airway

- A straight and relatively short beveled rubber oropharyngeal airway with a metal mouthpiece **(Fig. 9.35B)**.
- The body is made of red rubber tube with distal curved portion and bevel.
- This is not very anatomically designed airway.
- The metal mouth piece (bite block) has a grove that fits in-between the incisor teeth has a round opening that facilitates suctioning.
- The lumen is round throughout and provides wider airway.
- May stimulate posterior pharyngeal wall and induce vomiting.
- Widest air channel and relatively straight tube which facilitates easy suctioning.
- This airway device was the forerunner of many oropharyngeal airway designs.
- Not commonly used.

Phillips Airway

- The Phillips airway was developed by George Ramsay Phillips. There is no known original description of the airway and the earliest known reference to it is from 1919.
- The airway with its modifications is known now.
- It is a red rubber oropharyngeal airway with a shaped pharyngeal curve section and a metal mouthpiece.
- Bite piece and flange are made of metal. Bite piece has holes on either side which accommodates an oxygen catheter **(Fig. 9.35C)**.
- Less anatomically shaped.
- Further modification of this by *Hirsch* has an additional side feed tube on the metal mouthpiece.

Berman's Airway

- The design of this 'dual-channel' airway was one of Dr Robert A Berman's (1914–1999) earliest innovations.
- The open channel on each side, with a central support, was very different from previous oral airways, which had central tubes **(Fig. 9.35D)**.

- Oral airways with a central tube may contain mucous or other matter that is not easily visible.
- Dr Berman viewed this as a safety concern and designed this airway to prevent unseen occlusion.
- The shape is similar to that of Guedel's airway and fits well in the anatomical space.
- Advantage is airway block by secretions is less and it is easy to clean it.

Nasopharyngeal Airways
- A nasopharyngeal airway is a soft tube designed to be inserted into the nasal passage to secure an open airway.
- Made of mineralized red rubber, silicon rubber or plastic. Various sizes are available.
- When the patient is not tolerating an oral airway, nasopharyngeal airway can be used and is tolerated.
- This airway helps in maintaining the patency of airway in a semiconscious or conscious patient with *active oropharyngeal reflexes* where an oral airway will not be tolerated.
- It is introduced through the *widest patent nostril* and when the tip is just near the glottis opening, it is fixed in that position by *the adjustable flange*.
- If an adjustable flange is not provided it can be fixed by passing a safety pin across the tube that prevents the tube moving further into the nose.
- Position is confirmed by listening to the breath sound through proximal end of airway.
- It extends from nose to pharynx; the pharyngeal end must be below the base of tongue but above epiglottis **(Figs 9.40C and D)**.
- The size noted is the inner diameter of the tube.
- The size required for a particular patient is the same size of a nasal tracheal tube; 0.5 to 1 mm smaller than oral tube.

Two types of nasopharyngeal airways are available.

Airway with an Adjustable Flange
- The adjustable flange is to keep it in position without slipping in or out.
- After passing the tube to the suitable distance, the flange is adjusted to maintain that position.
- Red rubber nasopharyngeal airway with adjustable flange. It is reusable **(Fig. 9.39A)**.
- Silicon rubber nasopharyngeal airway with adjustable flange.
- It causes less irritation to nasal mucosa.
- It is available in different colors. It can be autoclaved **(Fig. 9.39B)**.

Airway with a Widely Flared End
- This is also known as a 'nasal trumpet' because of its flared end and shape.
- Silicon rubber nasopharyngeal airway with a flared end.
- The flared end prevents the airway slipping into the nose **(Fig. 9.39C)**.

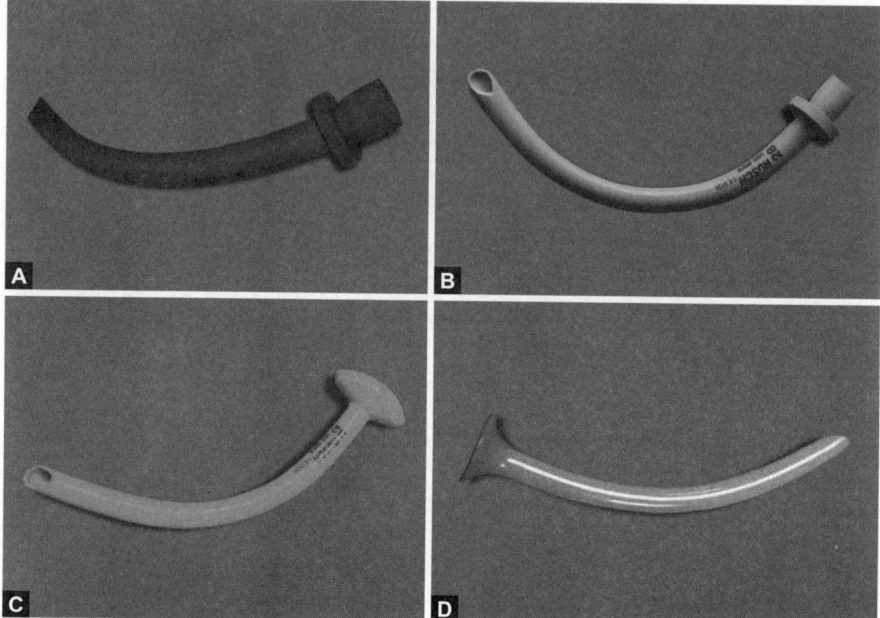

Figs 9.39A to D: Different types of nasopharyngeal airways. (A) Red rubber airway with adjustable flange; (B) Silicon rubber airway with adjustable flange; (C) Silicon rubber airway with flared end; (D) PVC airway with flared end

- A safety pin is used instead of flange to fix the airway in position (passed across the airway)
- It can be autoclaved.
- PVC nasopharyngeal airway with flared end is disposable **(Fig. 9.39D)**.

Choosing the size and inserting the airway:
- The correct size (length) airway is chosen by measuring the device on the patient.
- The device should reach from the patient's nostril to the earlobe or the angle of the jaw is usually 2–4 cm longer than the oral airway **(Fig. 9.40A)**.

Insertion

- Use a nostril that is unobstructed. The widest nasal cavity is identified by feeling the air throw from individual nostril.
- The outside of the tube is lubricated thoroughly with a water-based lubricant jelly along its entire length so that it enters the nose more easily.
- The airway is advanced at an angle perpendicular to the face with the bevel facing the septum **(Fig. 9.40B)**
- The airway is advanced carefully listening to the breath sound and when it is maximally heard, the airway is fixed with the adjustable flange.
- For airways with flared end, a big safety pin is passed through the tube at the appropriate level to fix the tube from slipping into the nose.
- *Remember:* The floor of the nose is the roof of the mouth, and it is the widest portion of nasal cavity.

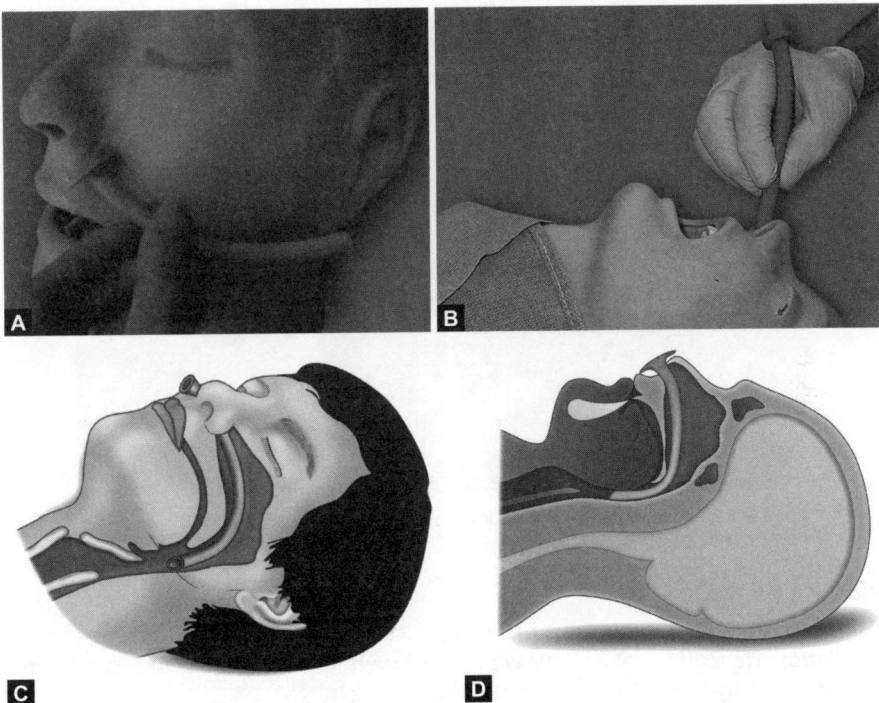

Figs 9.40A to D: Assessing the size and insertion of an nasopharyngeal airway. (A) The size that extends from the nose to the ear lobe is correct; (B) Inserted perpendicular to the face near the floor of the nose and gently advanced posteriorly; (C) The position of the tip is just proximal to epiglottis; (D) The position of the tip just beyond the base of tongue and above epiglottis

Complications

- Epistaxis
- Ulceration and necrosis of nasal mucosa
- Laryngospasm and cough if epiglottis is irritated
- Aspiration or swallowing of part or entire airway
- Latex allergy a rubber airway is used.

London Hospital Mouth Prop

- Though it is not in use now, it has historical importance and was a very useful device during the ether era.
- It is made of aluminum metal and has the shape of a bobbin with one end wider and the other end narrower.
- Assorted sizes linked with a chain to a ring **(Fig. 9.41)**.
- Appropriate size is chosen and passed over the endotracheal tube and kept at the level of incisor teeth. In light plane of anesthesia if the patient clinches the teeth this protects the tube from getting blocked.
- This can be used as a mouth prop in unconscious patient which maintains the patency of airway as well as facilitates suctioning through the wide funnel shaped proximal portion.

254 Anesthetic Equipment Made Easy

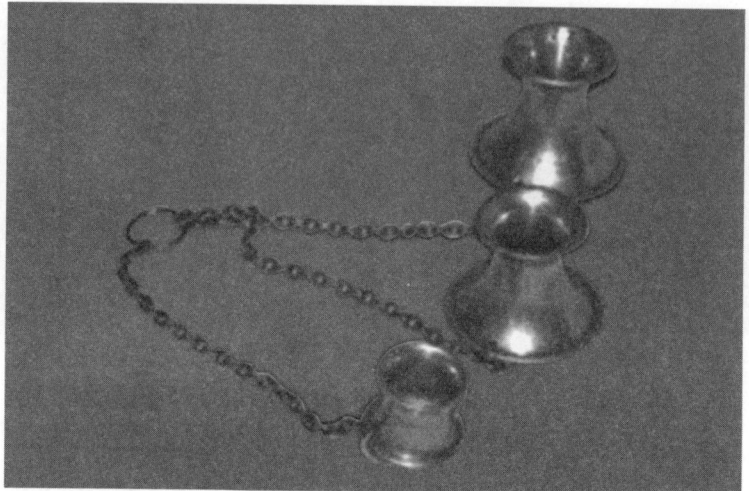

Fig. 9.41: London hospital mouth props

Special Airways Used in CPR

Using an oropharyngeal airway is aesthetically not ideal for mouth-to-mouth ventilation. Hence special airways were developed for the purpose of resuscitation that are more hygienically and esthetically acceptable.

Expired Air Ventilation

Expired air ventilation could be done in the following methods:
- Mouth-to-mouth
- Mouth to nose
- Mouth to airway—using
  - Guedel's airway
  - Resusci airway
  - Safar's airway
  - Brook's airway
  - Mouth to rescue mask.

Resusci Airway

- Simply fixing two Guedel's airways at their flanges with their curvatures facing opposite direction **(Fig. 9.42A)**.
- One is small child size and the other is adult size.
- Used for expired air ventilation during cardiopulmonary resuscitation.

Safar's Airway (Designed by Peter Safar)

- In 1957, *Peter Safar* (Baltimore, Maryland, USA) designed this oropharyngeal airway for mouth-to-mouth ventilation and popularized this device for resuscitation **(Fig. 9.42B)**
- It is a combination of two Guedel's airways fixed together at the flanges, but in the reverse direction, so that it forms an 'S' shaped double airway.

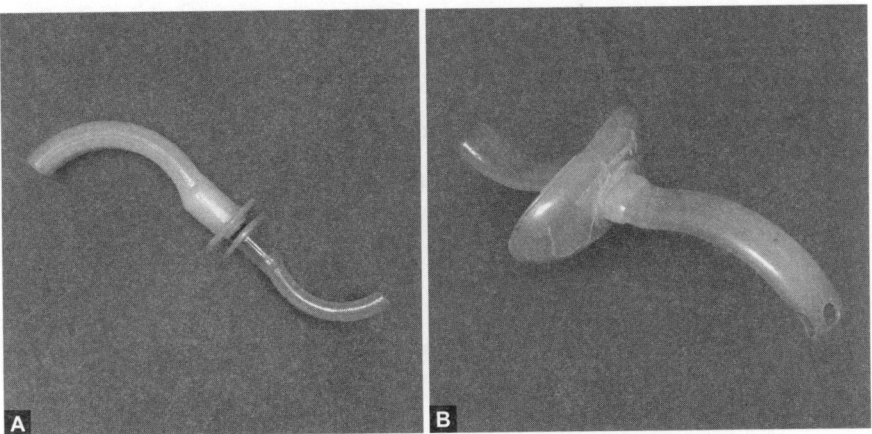

Figs 9.42A and B: (A) Resuci airway; (B) Safar's airway

- One airway is small size for children. The other one large for the adults, which can be used according to the necessity.
- This has a *reversible lip guard* which covers the lip and prevents the leak of air when mouth to airway resuscitation is done.

Brook's Airway

- It is similar to Safar's airway with lip guard.
- But, it has only one airway with a corrugated flexible neck connected to a mouthpiece through which the resuscitator blows into the patient's lung.
- In between the mouthpiece and corrugated tube there is a *unidirectional valve* which diverts the exhaled gases from the victim to the atmosphere without bouncing on the rescuer's face **(Fig. 9.43)**.
- More aesthetically designed and hygienic to use.

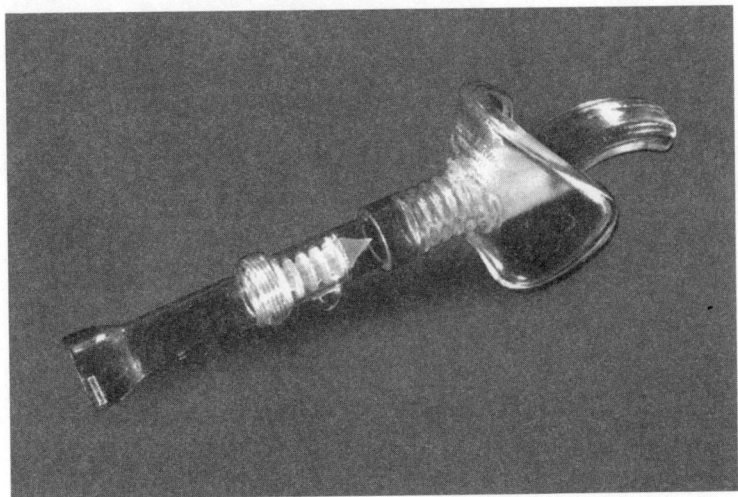

Fig. 9.43: Brook's airway

FURTHER READING

1. Dorsch JA, Dorsch SE. Understanding Anaesthesia Equipment, 5th edn. London: Lippincott Williams and Wilkins, 2008.
2. Dorsch JA, Dorsch SE. Understanding Anaesthesia Equipment. 4th edn. London: Lippincott Williams and Wilkins, 1999.
3. Gardiner AS. The Gordon-Green tube Clinical report. Anaesthesia January. 1963:(18)1.
4. Moyle JTB, Davey A. Ward's Anaesthetic Equipment, 4th edn. London: WB Saunders Company Limited, 1998.
5. Al-Shaikh Baha, Stacey S. Essentials of Anaesthetic Equipment, 1st edn. London: Churchill Livingstone, 1995.
6. Ward CS. Anaesthetic Equipment, 2nd edn. London: Balliere. 1985.
7. Lee's Synopsis of Anaesthesia, 11th edn, London: Butterworth-Heinemann Ltd., 1993.

Laryngeal Mask Airway

chapter 10

- Designed and invented by *Dr AIJ Brain* (Archie Ian Jeremy Brain) in 1981.
- After 6 years of extensive work in cadaver larynx, he made prototype and introduced in clinical use in 1983.
- In 1983, the commercial version had come.
- The laryngeal mask airway (LMA) is a cuff device that provides sufficient seal around larynx to allow positive pressure ventilation to be delivered.
- It is particularly useful in maintaining an airway in anesthetized patients when endotracheal intubation is not desired.
- During emergencies in which mask ventilation is not possible or intubation or ventilation fails, LMA is very useful.

"The laryngeal mask airway is designed to secure the airway by establishing an end-to-end circumferential seal around the laryngeal inlet with an inflatable cuff". It is a useful advancement in airway management, filling a niche between the 'face mask' and 'tracheal tube' in terms of both anatomical position and the degree of invasiveness.

STANDARD LARYNGEAL MASK AIRWAY (LMA CLASSIC)

It is a supraglottic, noninvasive airway management device comprising of three main components; *airway tube, mask* and *inflation line*. It is designed to conform the contour of the hypopharynx with its lumen facing the laryngeal opening.

Description

- It is a *spoon shaped* special device which has a *shallow mask* at the distal end that *resembles somewhat a face mask*, with an inflatable brim or cuff **(Fig.10.1)**.

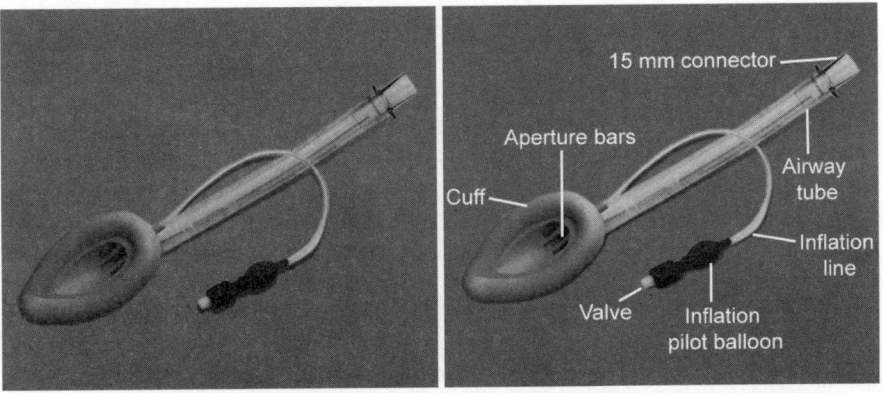

Fig. 10.1: Laryngeal mask airway classic and the parts

- Proximal end of mask is connected to *a wide bore tube* (Silicon plastic) at an angle of 30°.
- The junction between the tube and mask is called as *mask aperture*.
- This aperture has *two vertical bands*, which will prevent the epiglottis folding onto the mask aperture and occluding it. These are known as aperture bars.
- *The 30° angle* is specially chosen to maintain the *curvature of the tube in the pharyngeal cavity*, and if necessary passing an endotracheal tube (ETT) through the mask can be easily done.
- An inflation tube and self-sealing pilot balloon are attached to the proximal wider end of the mask.
- The pilot balloon has a nonmetallic self-sealing valve made of polypropylene for use in MRI.
- The mask is made from medical grade silicon rubber that stands repeated autoclaving for 40 times.
- Before autoclaving, the LMA should be deflated to prevent damage to the cuff.
- A black line running longitudinally along the posterior aspect of the tube helps to orient it after placement.
- When inflated, the elliptical cuff forms a low pressure seal around the entrance of the larynx.
- When the cuff is correctly deflated, it should form a "Wafer-thin" leading edge falling away from the mask aperture.
- Proximal end is connected to a *standard 15 mm connecting tube* and is made of polysulfone.
- In reinforced version, the tube has lesser diameter and more length that permits the use of throat pack.
- It can be used for spontaneous respiration or controlled ventilation.
- It does not guarantee against regurgitation and aspiration of gastric contents.
- Sizes available: 1, 1.5, 2, 2.5, 3, 4, 5 and 6 (8 sizes).

Different LMA Sizes

- The LMA comes in a variety of pediatric and adult sizes and successful insertion requires appropriate size selection.
- The LMA is available in 8 sizes.
- More than one size should always be available because the correct size cannot always be predicted accurately.
- When there is a doubt, a larger rather than a smaller size should be chosen for the first attempt.

Method of Using Laryngeal Mask Airway

- Deflate the cuff to form a smooth "spoon shape" without any wrinkles **(Fig. 10.2B)**.
- A completely flat and smooth leading edge facilitates insertion, avoids contact with epiglottis, and is important to assure success when positioning the device.
- The correct shape can be achieved by pressing the mask with its hollow side down on a sterile flat surface. Use the fingers to guide the cuff into shape **(Fig. 10.2A)**.
- Alternatively, the LMA "cuff-deflator" (available from the distributor) may be used.
- Just before inserting lubricate the posterior surface of the mask with water-soluble lubricant (e.g. K-Y Jelly).

Laryngeal Mask Airway

- Preoxygenate the patient and achieve an appropriate depth of anesthesia.
- In general, the depth of anesthesia needed is slightly more than that required for insertion of a Guedel type airway.
- It is recommended that the less experienced user choose a deeper level of anesthesia.
- In emergency, ensure the absence of protective reflexes.
- Position the patient in the "sniffing position" with the neck flexed and the head extended.
- Hold the LMA like a pen, with the index finger placed at the junction of the cuff and the tube **(Fig. 10.2C)**.
- Under direct vision, press the tip of the cuff upward against the hard plate and flatten the cuff against it. The black line on the airway tube should be oriented toward the upper lip **(Fig. 10.2D)**.
- Use the index finger to guide the LMA pressing upwards and backwards toward the ears in one smooth movement **(Fig. 10.2E)**.
- Advance the LMA into the hypopharynx until definite resistance is felt **(Fig. 10.2F)**.
- Before removing the index finger, gently press down on the tube with the other hand to prevent the LMA from being pulled out of place **(Fig. 10.2G)**.
- Without holding the tube, inflate the cuff with just enough air to obtain a seal.
- Never overinflate the cuff.
- Avoid prolonged intra-cuff pressure greater than 60 cm H_2O.
- Connect the LMA to the anesthetic circuit and employ manual ventilation to airway pressures of less than 20 cm H_2O.
- Check adequate gas exchange with auscultation and capnography.
- Insert a bite block and secure it and secure the LMA by taping to the patient's face
- Ensure that the airway tube is taped downwards against the chin not to the mandible **(Fig. 10.2H)**.

Directions for Removal
- Keep the bite block in place until the LMA is removed.
- Leave the patient undisturbed until reflexes are restored, except to administer oxygen and perform monitoring procedures.
- Watch for signs of swallowing.
- Remove adhesive tape when swallowing begins.
- Only when the patient can open the mouth on command, deflate the cuff and simultaneously remove the LMA and bite block.
- Verify airway patency and respiratory depth.
- Oral suctioning may now be performed, if required.

Indication and Use
- The LMA is indicated for use as an alternative to the facemask for achieving and maintaining control of the airway during routine and emergency anesthetic procedures in fasted patients.
- It is also indicated for securing the immediate airway in known or unexpected difficult airway situations.
- During cardiopulmonary resuscitation (CPR) in the profoundly unconscious patient with absent glossopharyngeal and laryngeal reflexes requiring artificial ventilation. It may be used to establish an immediate and clear airway.

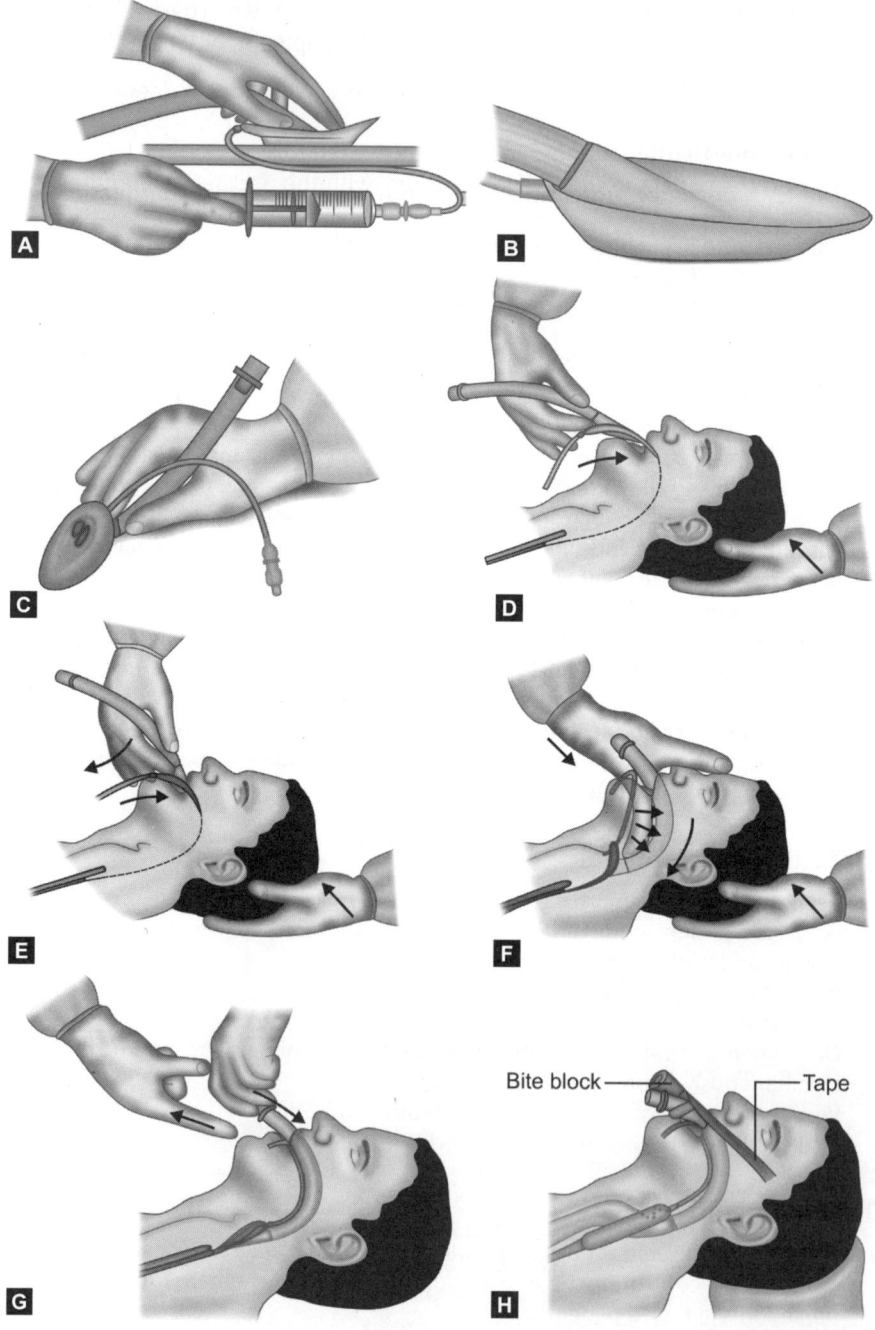

Figs 10.2A to H: Method of inserting a LMA: (A) Deflating the cuff; (B) Deflated cuff; (C) Holding the LMA like a pen; (D) Under vision, pressing the tip upwards against hard palate; (E) Guiding the LMA upwards and backwards with index finger; (F) Advancing the LMA to hypopharynx with index finger; (G) Pressing down the LMA with left hand and removing the index finger; (H) After inflation of cuff, a bite block is inserted and the LMA is secured with tapes

- The LMA may also be used to secure an immediate airway when tracheal intubation is precluded by lack of available expertise or equipment, or when attempts at tracheal intubation have failed.

Contraindications
- The LMA does not protect the airway from the effects of regurgitation and aspiration.
- It is therefore contraindicated in nonfasted patients, patients suspected of being nonfasted, or patients who may have retained gastric contents (except in "cannot intubate-cannot ventilate" situations in which the user must decide on the risk benefit ratio of using this device).
- Such situations include, but are not limited to:
  - Symptomatic hiatus hernia
  - Morbid obesity
  - Pregnancy past 14 weeks
  - Multiple or massive injury
  - Acute abdominal or thoracic injury
  - Conditions associated with delayed gastric emptying.
  - Use of opiate medication prior to fasting.
- When used in the profoundly unresponsive patient in need of cardiopulmonary cerebral resuscitation (CPCR), the risk of regurgitation and aspiration must be weighed against the potential benefit of establishing an airway.
- In addition, the LMA is contraindicated in patients with fixed decreased pulmonary compliance, e.g. patients with pulmonary fibrosis because it forms a low pressure (approx 20 cm H_2O) seal around the larynx.

Precautions
The user should be familiar with the following precautions when considering or attempting LMA use.
- In order to avoid laryngeal spasm, ensure anesthesia or unconsciousness is sufficient to obtund the reflexes.
- Lubricate only the posterior surface of the mask to avoid blockage of the aperture or aspiration of the lubricant.
- Patients should be monitored at all times during its use.
- To avoid trauma, force should never be used during insertions.
- Over-inflation may cause malposition, loss of seal, or trauma.
- Cuff pressure should be checked periodically.
- If airway problems persist or ventilation is inadequate, the LMA should be removed and reinserted or an airway established by other means.
- The presence of a nasogastric tube does not rule out the possibility of regurgitation and may even make regurgitation more likely because the tube makes the esophageal sphincters incompetent.

Sizes and their Specifications
Table 10.1 shows sizes and their specifications.

Table 10.1: Sizes and their specifications

Size	ID/OD (mm)	Length (cm)	Cuff volume	Patient size
1	5.25/8.2	8	Up to 4 mL	Neonates/Infants up to 5 kg
1.5	6.1/9.6	10	Up to 7 mL	Infants between 5 and 10 kg
2	7/11	11	Up to 10 mL	Infant/Child between 10 and 20 kg
2.5	8.4/13	12.5	Up to 14 mL	Children between 20 and 30 kg
3	10/15	16	Up to 20 mL	Children/Small adults >30 kg
4	10/15	16	Up to 30 mL	Normal adults 50–70 kg
5	11.5/16.5	18	Up to 40 mL	Large adults 80–100 kg
6	11.5/16.5	18	Up to 50 mL	Adults > 100 kg

Adverse Effects

- Throat soreness may be expected of the same order as that which occurs with facemask use.
- Transient dysarthria (difficulty in speaking) has been reported in patients undergoing prolonged procedures, or in whom the cuff has been over inflated.
- The effects on the pharyngeal mucosa from prolonged use are presently unknown.
- Rare cases of hypoglossal, lingual and laryngeal nerve injury and transient tongue numbness have been described in patients following use of the LMA airway.
- However, the relationship of these adverse events to the device has not been established.
- The incidence of aspiration is low (2:10,000) and is comparable to the incidence of aspiration associated with outpatient general anesthesia with the facemask or endotracheal tube.

MODIFIED VERSIONS OF LMA

Apart from the original *Standard LMA* or *LMA Classic*, there are several variants of LMA. These include:
- Flexible LMA or Reinforced LMA
- Short tube LMA
- LMA-Unique or Single-use LMA
- Intubating LMA or LMA-Fastrach
- LMA Pro-Seal
- LMA Supreme.

Flexible LMA

- The flexible (wire-reinforced) LMA differs from the standard version in that it has a flexible, wire-reinforced tube **(Fig. 10.3)**.
- It is available in sizes 2, 2.5, 3, 4 and 5.
- In each size, the tube is longer and has a smaller diameter than the standard LMA.
- The flexible LMA can be bent to any angle allowing it to be positioned away from the surgical field without occluding the lumen or losing the seal against the larynx.

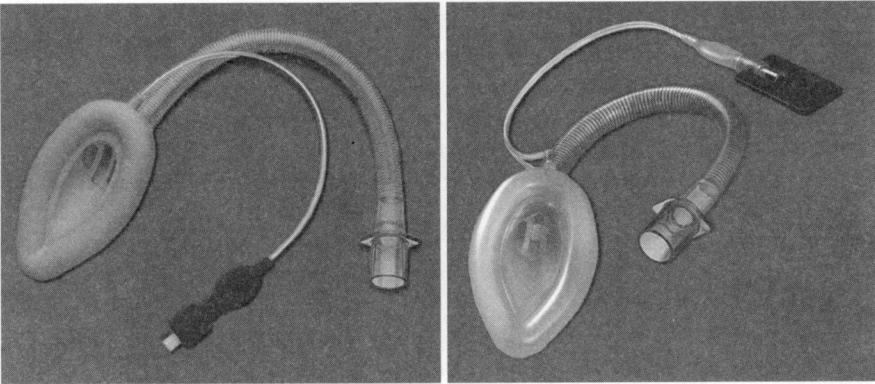

Fig. 10.3: Flexible LMA (Reinforced LMA) reusable and single use

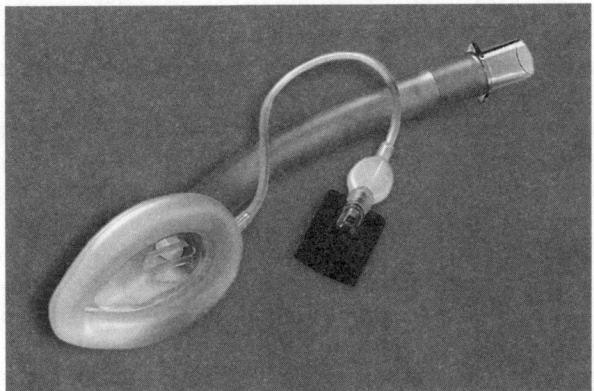

Fig. 10.4: LMA unique

Short Tube LMA

- It has a tube that is 2 cm shorter than the standard LMA.
- It is designed to allow proper positioning of tracheal tube passed through it.
- An endotracheal tube passed into the standard LMA may not reach the level of the mid trachea because of the length of LMA tube.
- The short tube LMA has been designed to circumvent this problem. It is available in size 3.

LMA Unique

- This is a disposable LMA for single use, available in a presterilized pack in sizes 3, 4 and 5 **(Fig. 10.4)**.
- The cuff of this LMA is made from polyvinylchloride (PVC).
- It has been designed for use in emergency airway management, inside and outside the operating room.

Intubating LMA (Fastrach)

- A specially devised LMA that helps in intubating difficult airways.
- Designed to aid endotracheal intubation with an appropriate size tube without any manipulation of the head and neck during placements.
- It consists of a rigid stainless steel 'right angled' airway tube and a metallic handle specially designed for intubation. The metal handle is for holding the mask during insertion.
- The convex radius of the curve of the metal tube is 41.5 mm.
- The tube is curved around a minimum arc of 128° corresponding to the approximate alignment axis.
- This curve avoids the need for head and neck manipulation and permits the ILMA *to be placed with the head in neutral position*.
- The minimum internal diameter of the tube is 13 mm, with a wall thickness of <1 mm. This accepts up to an 8 mm ID cuffed TT.
- Stainless steel is chosen because of its compatibility with silicone, high strength, and malleability, ease of sterilization and cleaning and absence of toxicity.
- The stainless steel tube is covered with a silicone sheath to minimize trauma and facilitate secure bonding with the mask portion, giving an outer diameter of 17.6 mm **(Fig. 10.5A)**.
- There is an integral stainless steel 15 mm connector incorporated into the proximal end of the tube. These permit its use as a standard LMA and avoid risk of accidental disconnection. Once inserted, it can be connected to the breathing system to ventilate the patient.
- In place of the aperture bars of the standard LMA, the LMA has of a single *epiglottis elevating bar* (EEB), attached only at the upper rim of the aperture of the mask, so that its free end can swing out by the advancing TT pushing the epiglottis out of the way as it does so.
- The passage immediately behind the EEB is provided with a 'V' shaped 20° guiding ramp in its floor, which centers the tracheal tube and guides the tube anteriorly to reduce risk of arytenoids trauma and esophageal placement.
- Specially manufactured straight, soft, wire reinforced cuffed silicone endotracheal tubes are used when intubating through the ILMA **(Figs 10.5B and C)**.
- Silicone significantly retains the curvature imposed by passage through the metal airway tube, even when the tubes are warmed to 37°C.
- The endotracheal tube is marked transversely with a depth marker to show the point at which the tip of endotracheal tube is about to lift away the EEB.

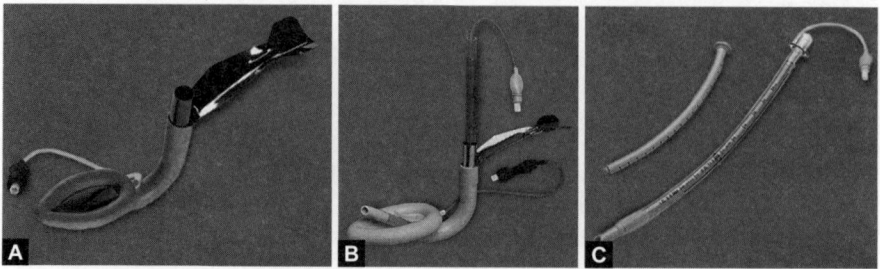

Figs 10.5A to C: Intubating LMA (Fastrach), endotracheal tube and obturator

Laryngeal Mask Airway

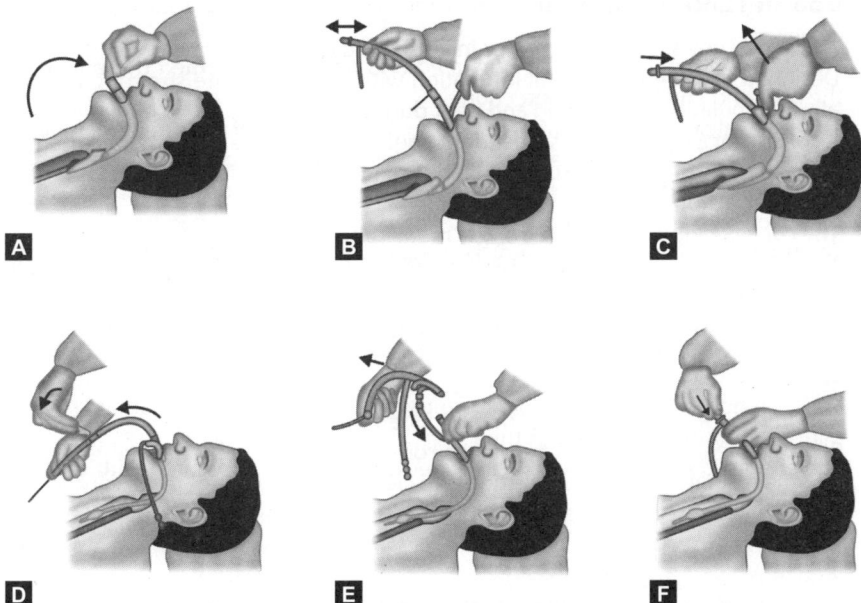

Figs 10.6A to F: The steps and technique of intubating with an intubating LMA

- In addition, a longitudinal line similar to the black line on an LMA tube is provided to serve as a guide to the orientation of the tracheal tube bevel.
- The pilot balloon and valve are small enough to pass easily through the metal tube of the ILMA, and the tracheal tube connector is removable in order that the ILMA could be removed from the patient when intubation has been achieved **(Fig. 10.5C)**.
- Now the intubating LMA can be removed gently simultaneously pushing the ETT and retaining it in its place with the help of an obturator **(Fig. 10.5B)**.
- The steps and the technique of intubation with intubating LMA are shown in **Figures 10.6A to F**.

Technique of using LMA Fastrach for Intubation

- The patient's head and neck must be in the neutral position.
- The cuff must be fully deflated.
- The LMA Fastrach must be lubricated on the posterior aspect for easy sliding.
- The LMA is held in such a way that the metal tube is touching the patient's chin before advancing.
- Mouth is gently opened and the LMA is slowly advanced in a way it is swung into its place. The curved body of the LMA must gently follow the natural curvature of the oropharynx.
- Once fully introduced, the cuff is inflated without holding the tube or handle.
- Now the breathing system is connected and patient is ventilated and adequate seal and effective ventilation is confirmed.
- With the handle of LMA held steady, the special endotracheal tube is inserted up to the 15 cm depth marked on its body.
- The handle of LMA is gently lifted as the tube is advanced.

- If no resistance is encountered, the tube can be advanced until intubation is achieved.
- The cuff of endotracheal tube is inflated and position confirmed by ventilating the lung and end tidal CO_2 detection.
- The removal of LMA is done after removing the connector of endotracheal tube, so that the tube is not dislodged in the process. Now the cuff of LMA is deflated and the LMA is slowly withdrawn into the oral cavity. During this time counter pressure is applied with the other hand.
- The rubber stabilizer or 'Obturator' is attached to the endotracheal tube.
- The LMA is gently pulled over the endotracheal tube and stabilizer rod until is cleared of the oral cavity.
- Stabilizer rod is then removed and the endotracheal tube is secured in position at the level of incisors.
- LMA can now be removed taking care to gently unthread the inflation line and pilot balloon through the LMA tube.
- The endotracheal connector is reattached and the tube is secured with strips of adhesive plasters

Uses

- If there is difficulty in intubation, there is difficulty in laryngoscopy, it can be used.
- To intubate a patient with cervical spine injury.
- If opening the mouth is possible, intubation can be done in neutral position.

LMA ProSeal

(LMA with an integral gastric access and venting port)
- It is an advanced form of LMA that may be used for the same indications as the original LMA.
- It has been specifically designed for use with positive pressure ventilation with and without muscle relaxant at higher airway pressures.
- It does not however protect the airway from the effects of regurgitation and aspiration.
- The LMA ProSeal has *four main components*;
  1. Cuff
  2. Inflation line with pilot balloon
  3. Airway tube
  4. Drain tube.
- The cuff is made of a softer material than the standard LMA.
- The mask has *a main cuff that seals around the laryngeal opening* and *rear cuff that acts to increase the seal* **(Fig. 10.7C)**.
- Attached to the mask is an inflation line terminating in a pilot balloon, which inflates and deflates the mask via a valve.
- Within the mask, a drain tube provides a conduit that communicates with the upper esophageal sphincter.
- The *airway tube is wire reinforced* which resists kinking and terminates with a standard 15 mm airway connector.

- The position of the drain tube inside the cuff is designed to prevent the epiglottis from occluding the airway tube. This eliminates the need for aperture bars **(Figs 10.7A and B)**.
- The revised cuff arrangement allows a higher seal than the standard LMA for a given intra-cuff pressure.
- The drain tube communicates with the upper esophageal sphincter and permits venting of the stomach and blind insertion of standard gastric tubes in any patient position without the need to use Magill's forceps.

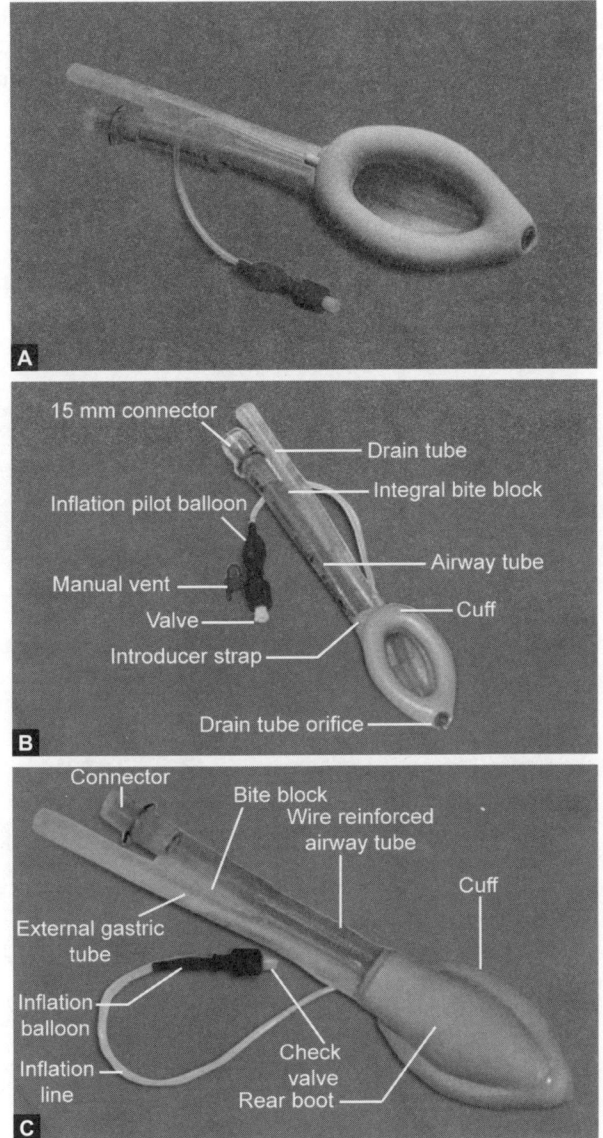

Figs 10.7A to C: LMA ProSeal and its parts

- The double tube arrangement reduces the likelihood of device rotation; the revised cuff profile, together with the two tubes, results in the device being more securely anchored in place.
- The LMA ProSeal can be introduced with the help of the introducer or using the thumb and forefinger in the same manner as that used for standard LMA.
- The position of LMA ProSeal in a patient and its anatomical relations are shown in **Figure 10.8**.

Accessories to the LMA ProSeal include:
- A removable introducer to aid insertion of the LMA ProSeal without the need to place fingers in the mouth.
- A dedicated deflation device to help obtain complete deflation of the LMA ProSeal for successful sterilization, optimum insertion and positioning within the patient. **(Fig. 10.9)**.

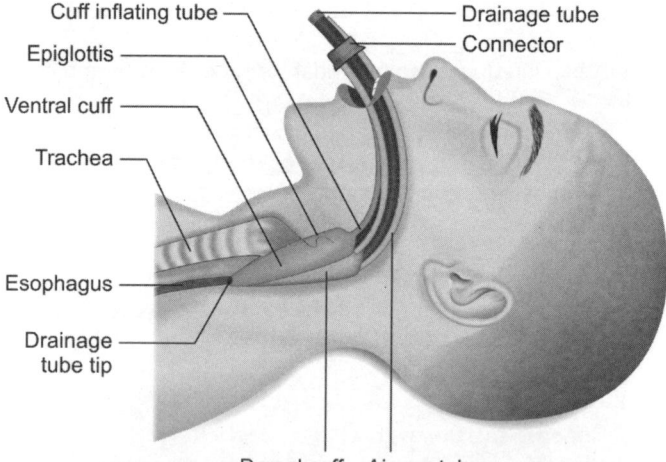

Fig. 10.8: LMA ProSeal and its anatomical relations

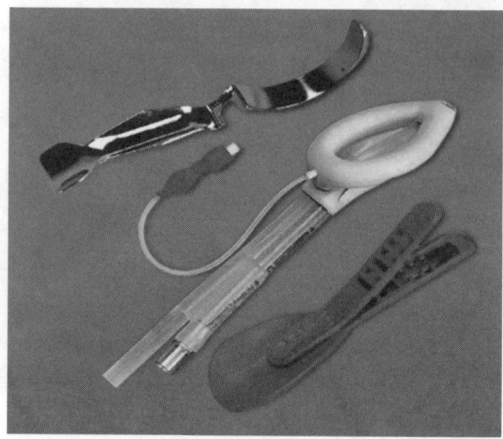

Fig. 10.9: LMA ProSeal with introducer and deflator

LMA Supreme

- It is similar to LMA ProSeal with a built-in curvature and additional features.
- The LMA Supreme provides access to airway at the same time functional separation of the respiratory and digestive tracts. The anatomically-shaped airway tube is elliptical in cross section and ends distally at the laryngeal mask.
- The inflatable cuff is designed to conform to the contours of the hypopharynx, with the bowl and the mask facing the laryngeal opening.
- It has a drain tube which emerges as a separate port proximally and continues distally along the anterior surface of the cuff bowl, passing through the distal end of the cuff to communicate distally with the upper esophageal sphincter.
- The drain tube may be used for the passage of a well lubricated gastric tube to the stomach, offering easy access for evacuation of gastric contents.
- It provides easy insertion without the need for digital or introducer tool guidance and enough flexibility to permit the device to remain in place if the patient's head is moved in any direction.
- The two lateral grooves in the airway tube are designed to prevent the airway tube kinking when flexed.
- A built-in bite-block reduces the potential for tube damage and obstruction by patient biting.
- It has a new fixation system (Fixation tab) which prevents proximal displacement. If correctly used, this enhance the seal of the distal end around the upper esophageal sphincter thereby isolating the respiratory tract from the digestive tract, so reducing the danger of accidental aspiration.
- It is supplied after ethylene oxide sterilization and is for single use only.
- It is made of medical grade PVC.
- The LMA Supreme airway combines the best features of previous LMA airways to provide superior safety and ease of use.
- This LMA specially designed to permit easy insertion and provide higher seal pressure with a gastric access.
- The cuff is designed in such a way that it provides better seal in the airway and also at the esophagus level (sometimes it is mentioned as First seal and Second seal).
- The gastric access is designed to channel fluids away from the airway in the event of active or passive regurgitation of gastric contents and eliminates the chances of aspiration **(Fig. 10.10)**.
- It can be used to decompress the stomach by passing a Ryle's tube and suctioning.
- Both for a routine procedure or to manage a higher risk patient, the higher seal pressure and gastric access provide a higher degree of safety.

First Seal (Laryngeal)

- Provides adequacy of ventilation and gas exchange
- Advantageous for patients with decreased thoracic compliance, heavy patients, and certain procedures requiring mechanical ventilation with higher pressures.

Second Seal (Esophageal)

- Reduce the risk of insufflating the gases into the stomach during ventilation
- Provide a passive conduit for unexpected regurgitation
- Provide a conduit for active suctioning of the stomach
- Enhance the effectiveness of the first seal (oropharyngeal seal)

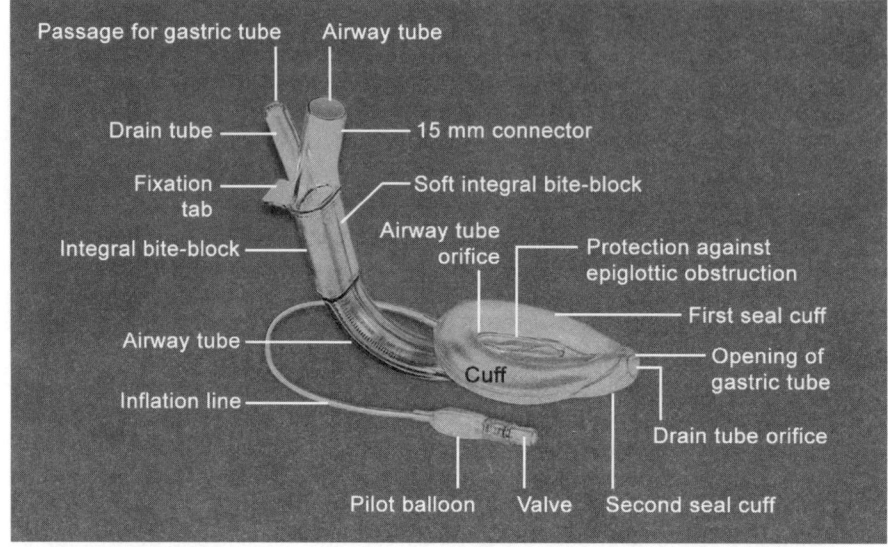

Fig. 10.10: LMA Supreme

Method of Using

The correct size of LMA for the particular patient can be assessed by keeping the LMA Supreme on the side of the face. With the bite block positioned at the level of palate, the distal end of the mask must be at the level of cricoids cartilage **(Fig. 10.11)**.

- Deflate the cuff
  Fully deflate the mask by attaching a syringe. Compress the tip of the mask with thumb and index finger. Apply suction on the inflation line to remove all air until a vacuum is felt. Remove the syringe.
- Lubricate posterior side of the mask
- Generously lubricate the posterior surface of the cuff and airway tube.
- Keep the patient in neutral position
  Place the patient's head in a neutral or slight "sniffing" position. Hold the LMA Supreme at the proximal end with the connector pointing downward to the chest and the tip of mask pointing toward the palate.
- Hold the mask by fixation tab
- Press the tip of the cuff against the hard palate
- Maintaining the pressure, rotate the mask inwards with a circular motion following the curvature of palate.
- Advance the airway in to the hypopharynx until resistance is felt. Now airway is fully inserted and the distal end of the mask will be in contact with upper esophageal sphincter.
- Maintaining inward pressure, using adhesive tape secure the mask in position across the fixation tab from cheek to cheek. This should be done prior to inflation.
- Inflate the mask with half the volume recommended and continue to increase till seal is achieved. The recommended cuff pressure should not exceed 60 cm H_2O.
- After fixation, the taping tab should be seen 1–2.5 cm from the upper lip. If the taping tab is more than 2.5 cm from the upper lip, this suggests the LMA is

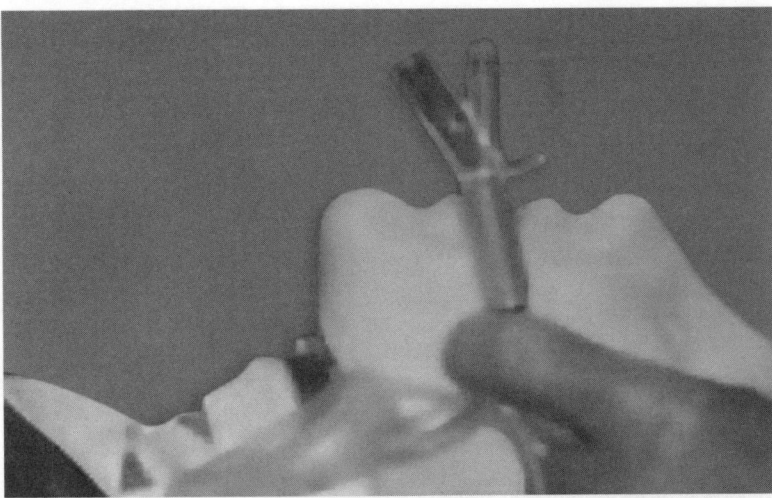

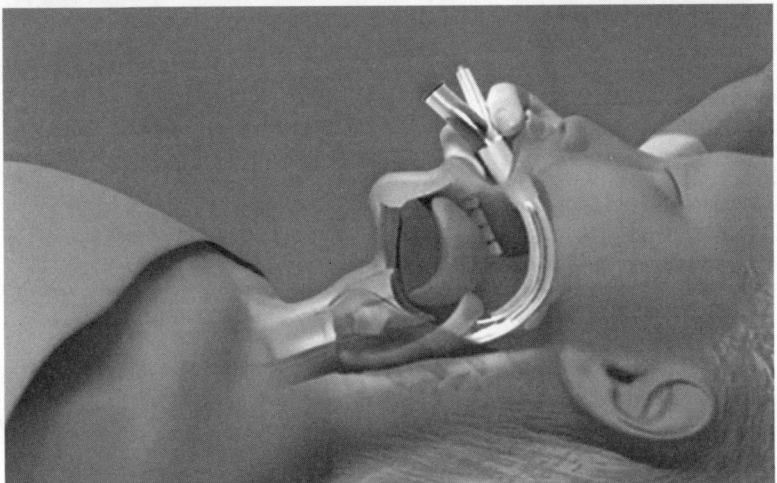

Fig. 10.11: Assessing the correct size and properly positioned LMA Supreme

too big. If the taping tab is less than 1 cm from the lip, the LMA is too small. At no time should the taping tab be in contact with the upper lip.
- Replace a mask that appears too big or small.
- Connect the bag to ventilate.
- Lubricate the gastric tube and insert it to decompress the stomach by suction (14 size for 3 size airway and 16 size for 4 and 5 size airway) **(Table 10.2)**.

Indications
- Used in emergency procedures in which tracheal intubation has failed.
- As a rescue airway device in known or unexpected difficult airway situations.
- To establish an immediate clear airway during resuscitation in profoundly unconscious patient with absent glossopharyngeal and laryngeal reflexes who may need artificial ventilation.

Table 10.2: Sizes available and specifications

Size	Cuff volume	Patient size	Size of Ryle's tube
1	5 mL	Neonate/Infant (Up to 5 kg)	6 French
1.5	8 mL	Infants (5–10 kg)	6 French
2	12 mL	Infants (10–20 kg)	10 French
2.5	20 mL	Children (20–30 kg)	10 French
3	30 mL	Children (30–50 kg)	14 French
4	45 mL	Adult (50–70 kg)	14 French
5	45 mL	Adults (70–100 kg)	14 French

FURTHER READING

1. Al-Shaikh Baha, Stacey S. Essentials of Anaesthetic Equipment, 1st edn. London: Churchill Livingstone, 1995.
2. Cook TM. et al. Anaesthesia. 2009;64:555-62.
3. Dorsch JA, Dorsch SE. Understanding Anaesthesia Equipment, 4th edn. London: Lippincott Williams and Wilkins, 1999.
4. Dorsch JA, Dorsch SE. Understanding Anaesthesia Equipment, 5th edn. London: Lippincott Williams and Wilkins, 2008.
5. Lee's Synopsis of Anaesthesia, 11th edn. London: Butterworth-Heinemann Ltd., 1993.
6. Moyle JTB, Davey A. Ward's Anaesthetic Equipment, 4th edn. London: WB Saunders Company Limited, 1998.
7. Sharma V. et al. BJA. 2010;105(2):228-32.
8. The LMA-Supreme TM. Instruction Manual. Maidenhead: Intavent Orthofix Ltd, 2007.
9. Van Zundert A, Brimacombe J. Anaesthesia. 2008;63:202-13.
10. Verghese, Ramaswamy B. LMA-Supreme—a new single-use LMA with gastric access: a report on its clinical efficacy. Br J Anaesth. 2008;101:405-10.

Monitors

chapter 11

Universally accepted basic minimum mandatory monitoring during anesthesia are:
- Noninvasive blood pressure (BP)
- Pulse oximetry
- Capnography
- ECG.

There are multiparameter monitors available that incorporate ECG, pulse oximeter, capnography, respiration, noninvasive BP and invasive BP. But individual parameter monitors are available for selected use.

PULSE OXIMETER

- Pulse oximeter was first introduced in Japan by Nelcor in 1983.
- It is a noninvasive monitor for the cardiorespiratory system.
- This is one of the most important and versatile inventions in electronics in the field of noninvasive monitoring that had saved many lives in the past three decades.
- It is mandatory that every patient on the operating table is monitored with a 'Pulse Oximeter' **(Figs 11.1A and B)**.

It can show:
- O_2 saturation in hemoglobin
- Pulse rate
- Pulse waveform.

It cannot show:
- O_2 content of blood
- Amount of O_2 dissolved in blood

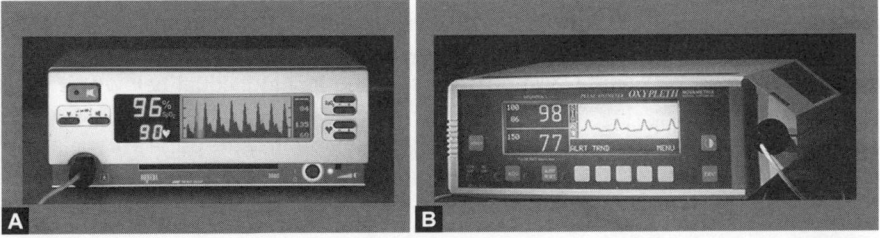

Figs 11.1A and B: Pulse oximeters; (A) The display of saturation and pulse rate are in bigger digits (about 1 cm height); • The alarm setting is displayed for each parameter; • The pulse waveform clearly shows the dicrotic notch; (B) A sophisticated pulse oximeter having all the required features; • The most important feature is the perfusion indicator (signal bar) that shows the degree of perfusion to the limb; • Has facilities for analyzing the previous data by using the trends; • For record purposes, 'printouts' can be taken by connecting to a printer

- Respiratory rate and tidal volume (adequacy of ventilation)
- Cardiac output and BP.

Working Principle

It works on the following principle:
- Absorption spectra of oxyhemoglobin and that of reduced hemoglobin are different.
- By calculating the values of each in the arterial blood (arteriole) the percentage of O_2 saturation can be deducted.
- During a pulsatile flow in the systolic phase there will be a slight increase in oxyhemoglobin levels than in the diastolic phase.
- This small difference is sensed by the sensors and processed.
- So the venous blood which is not pulsatile is ignored. So also the light absorbed by other tissues is ignored.
- The probes are commonly applied on the fingertips. Reusable probes as well as disposable probes are available **(Fig. 11.2A)**.
- There are two light emitting diodes (LED) in the probe which emit light with wavelengths of 660 nm (Red) and 940 nm (Infrared) on one side.
- Reduced hemoglobin absorbs more light in the red band (660 nm) and oxyhemoglobin absorbs more light in infra red band (940 nm)
- The average requirement is 811 nm.
- The two LEDs alternatively emit light many hundred times per second which passes through the tissues in the fingertips.
- The light which comes out on the other side of the finger after being absorbed by various tissues will fall on a photo sensor called the *Photodiode*.
- The light passing through the pulsatile structures (arterioles) have a minimal difference between the systolic and diastolic phase which will be picked up by the sensor converted into electrical signals and sent for processing.
- The nonpulsatile structures like tissues, bones, tendons and nails also absorb light but as there are no differences they are ignored and are not processed.
- So, depending on the wavelengths of the light absorbed by the oxyhemoglobin and reduced hemoglobin, the microprocessor calculates the percent saturation and displays it digitally on the screen.
- The heart rate is also displayed as the number of pulses is counted.
- So, it cannot sense the saturation in nonpulsatile flow as in extracorporeal circulation (heart-lung machine).
- The response time varies from 5 to 20 seconds with various models.
- Any value less than 70% carries little meaning as the calibration is done with healthy volunteers and it is impossible to bring any individual below this level safely.
- Some monitors have a plethysmographic representation of the pulse in a waveform which will give an idea about the arterial pulse and its waves.
- The absorption spectrums of adult Hb A (Adult) and Hb F (Fetal) are almost the same.
- So in a neonate, where the percent of Hb F is considerably higher, the adult probe can be used.
- One molecule of hemoglobin carries four molecules of O_2.
- There are miniature fingertip pulse oximeters available **(Fig. 11.2B)**.
- Two laws of light absorption are used in the pulse oximeter.

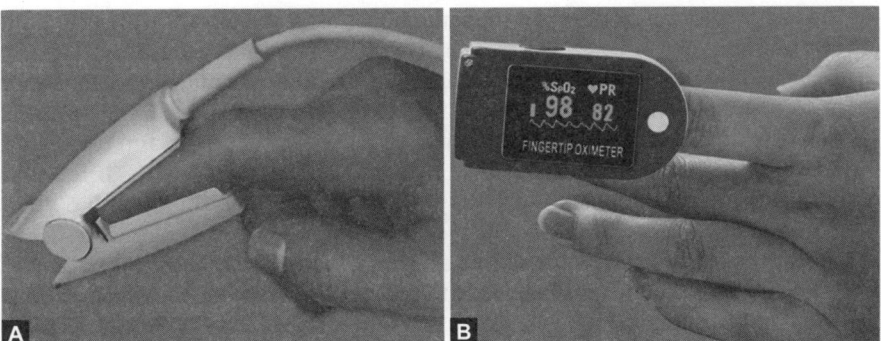

Figs 11.2A and B: Finger probe of pulse oximeter and finger pulse oximeter

Beer's law: Amount of light absorbed is proportional to the concentration of the light absorbing substance

Lambert's law: Amount of light absorbed is proportional to the length of the path that the light has to travel in the absorbing substance.

These laws cannot be simply applied as the tissues (finger or ear lobe) vary in its size and contents in different patients, complicated calculations in the microprocessor are needed.

A good pulse oximeter must be able to provide the 'functional saturation' (SaO_2) not 'fractional saturation'.

Fractional saturation (HbO_2) is the ratio of the oxyhemoglobin to the sum of all the hemoglobin present whether available for reversible binding with oxygen or not.

Functional saturation represents the amount of oxyhemoglobin as a percentage of hemoglobin that can transport oxygen. Dysfunctional hemoglobins such as carboxyhemoglobin (COHb) or methemoglobin (METHb) are not included in the measurement of functional saturation.

$$\text{Functional saturation} = HbO_2/100 - (COHb + METHb)$$

Functional saturation displayed in a pulse oximeter is referred to as SpO_2.

Features

- Basically, it is meant for knowing the functional oxygen saturation of hemoglobin.
- This equipment uses *pulsatile blood flow in the arterioles* for assessing the saturation.
- Incidentally, it counts the pulse rate also.
- Any basic models of pulse oximeter will show *oxygen saturation* and *pulse rate* on display.
- Most of the instruments provide audible beep of pulse with variable pulse tone; the pitch increase with increasing saturation and vice versa.
- The display shows oxygen saturation and pulse rate against a background light so that it is visible in dark environment.
- The size of the numbers is ideally minimum 1 cm high for viewing from a distance of 10 feet.
- Alarm settings for both *oxygen saturation* as well as *pulse rate* are displayed.

- The alarm is set to sound when the saturation crosses the higher or lower limit of the setting.
- Usually, it is set as 100% (upper limit) and 90% (lower limit) or it can be set according to the need of the individual patient.
- Similarly for pulse rate the alarm limits can be set so that the alarm will sound when the limits are crossed.
- In healthy adult patient it is usually set as 120/min (upper limit) and 60/min (lower limit).
- Ideally the *alarm setting* must also be seen in the form of *display on the screen*.
- When an alarm sounds the display of the particular parameter for which alarm is triggered must blink.
- In sophisticated machines, there will be display in words which also blinks.
- For example, the words 'Pulse High' will blink indicating that the pulses rate is higher than that set in the alarm.
- Beyond this there will be *a visual alarm* of a *red light blinking*, to attract the attention of the anesthesiologist in case the audible alarm is not noted.
- Many pulse oximeters have provision for interface for printers for getting printouts.

Functioning of pulse oximeter is modified by:
- Very bright ambient light
- Movements of the limb and thereby the movement of the probe
- Shivering
- Vasoconstriction or low perfusion
- Diathermy
- Nail-polish
- Dyes in the blood, e.g. methylene blue.

Pulse Waveform (Plethysmograph)

- Further sophistication is the presence of a *pulse waveform* meant for pulse monitoring.
- This is known as pulse plethysmography **(Figs 11.3A and B)**.
- Pulse plethysmography is based upon the measurement of *the increase in the volume of an extremity, usually a finger or an ear lobe, during or shortly after systole.*
- All pulse oximeters use a special technique known as *photoplethysmography* for producing the pulse waveform.
- A low level of electromagnetic energy (infrared light) is passed through the extremity.
- The pulsatile flow of blood absorbs the light and the remaining light that passes through the nonpulsatile tissue is detected by a semiconductor sensor or photo-detector.
- An increase in volume of the part is then detected as an increase in absorption of the incident light during systole.
- The signal from the photodetector is then amplified and may be displayed on the screen.
- This technique is so sensitive that the dicrotic notch of the pulse wave is easily visible. If the pulsatility of the signals decreases below a critical level, the alarm is initiated.
- No pulse oximeter should be used unless a plethysmograph trace is displayed.

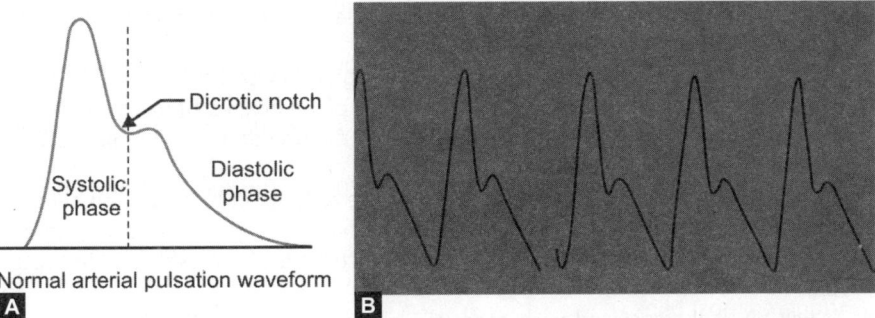

Figs 11.3A and B: (A) Arterial pulse waveform; (B) Waveform of pulse oximeter

- Some of the monitors have *a perfusion indicator* (Signal Bar) which indicates the degree of perfusion in the finger (periphery) *(See* **Fig. 11.1B)**.
- The signal bar reflects the pulsatile strength as detected by the SpO_2 sensor. Strong signals produce a tall bar; weak signals produce a short bar. Typical signals are 25–75% of the signal bar height. A good signal bar is seen in Oxypeth 520A model of Novametrix *(See* **Fig. 11.1B)**.

Interpretation of Waveform and Perfusion Indicator

The waveform and the perfusion indicator can be very useful during anesthesia for assessing two aspects.
- The depth of anesthesia
- The volume status of the patient.

Depth of Anesthesia

- When the right plane of anesthesia is maintained with respect to the triad of anesthesia for the particular step of surgery, then there will be very little sympathetic stimulation and vascular tone is reduced with good peripheral perfusion. In deeper plane, there may be even depression of sympathetic tone with increase in perfusion.
- This status will be indicated by a normal pulse rate, normal or a little lower BP, and a very good peripheral vasodilatation seen as good venous filling.
- As it is earlier discussed, the *perfusion indicator* which is otherwise known as *signal bar* is a special feature not found in all pulse oximeters *(See* **Fig. 11.1B)**.
- It will indicate the degree of perfusion in the periphery; the finger tip.
- It is a vertical tube like column which gets filled up from the bottom towards the top and maintains a level that fluctuate minimally according to the sympathetic tone.
- In fact this works by the increase in the volume of the part during or immediately after systole and indicates the amount flow through the arterioles.
- Usually, it is found at the left side of the screen at the starting point of the waveform.
- When the oximeter probe is clipped to the finger of a normal person the column gets filled up to a level of anything from 25–75% depending upon the sympathetic tone of the individual.
- In a well-relaxed individual it may be more than 75%.

- Depending upon the level seen we may assess the degree of perfusion in the peripheral level.
- When the volume of flow is high, the level is high and vice versa.
- During anesthesia if everything is fine with the plane of anesthesia the perfusion indicator must fill at least a little more than 50% provided the volume status is normal.
- *If the plane of anesthesia is inadequate* and the reflexes induced by the surgical procedure are not adequately suppressed, then there may be *severe sympathetic stimulation* resulting in the fall of level in the column of the perfusion indicator bar.
- It will be well correlated with other signs of sympathetic stimulation such as sweating, elevation of BP, tachycardia poor peripheral venous filling, etc.
  Thus, it is a very good indicator for assessing the level of anesthesia and for modulating it.

Volume Status of the Patient

- If everything is fine with the plane of anesthesia, and the volume status of the patient is good, the column must fill almost fully indicating that both anesthesia as well as circulating volume is good.
- This is clinically correlated by a normal pulse rate and volume, normal or a little reduced BP, and adequate filling of peripheral veins.
- In case of circulating volume deficit, which has not been corrected, there will be fall in the level of this column.
- This hypovolemic state can be clinically correlated with a low volume pulse, lower BP, and poor filling or totally contracted peripheral veins.
- If an anesthetized patient has a pulse rate of 70/min, a BP of 110/70 mm Hg, well filled up peripheral veins, and the signal bar fully filled to the top has good level of anesthesia with good volume status and excellent vascular relaxation with good tissue perfusion.

Advantages

- Accurate even in the presence of arrhythmia. Error is less than 3%
- Any value less than 70% is incorrect as the calibration is done with healthy human volunteers and it is unsafe to take anyone below that level.
- Noninvasive, continuous monitoring of oxygen saturation, pulse rate and blood flow.
- Response time is small—about 5 seconds.

Other Uses

- Cardiorespiratory status assessment
- To assess the vascularity of the limb by plethysmography.

Some Important Information about Pulse Oximeter

A good pulse oximeter must have the following minimum features.
- It must display the O_2 saturation value on the screen.
- It must have the display of pulse rate on the screen.

- Alarm settings for both pulse rate as well as oxygen saturation must be displayed on the screen.
- *Perfusion indicator* or *signal bar* must be available that indicates the degree of perfusion to the peripheral tissues. (It is not the pulse indicator or pulse ladder).
- There must be a pulse waveform (plethysmograph) available for analyzing various components.
- All the display on the screen must be LCD (liquid crystal display) display and not LED (light-emitting diode).
- Display with a Backlit screen of either blue or green color with letters and numbers in white color.
- The numbers indicating the saturation and pulse rate (main display) must be at least 1 cm high with round corners to be read clearly from a distance of 10 feet (3 mts).
- There must be variation in the pitch of sound to indicate the fall or rise of saturation or pulse rate.
- The alarm must be both audible alarm as well as visual alarm. The parameter for which the alarm sounds must blink and there must be a display in words blinking, e.g. pulse high.

When choosing a pulse oximeter the above-said features must be emphasized:
- The backlit blue screen with white letters will be very comfortable to read even in less illuminated areas like radiology department.
- The LCD display will give normal contour to the numbers and letters that cannot be mistaken from distance particularly the main display. At least 1 cm high.
- Alarm settings must be seen on the screen so that the user knows the setting at a glance.
- Moreover when the alarm sounds, the setting must blink and ideally a written display comes on the screen indicating the parameter that has caused the alarm.

The perfusion indicator or signal bar gives idea about two things:
1. The degree of perfusion to the periphery.
2. The relative volume status of the patient at that moment.

The Purpose of Perfusion Bar

- This is a vertical rectangular bar (column) looking like a tubular jar on the side of the screen usually on the left side of the screen.
- This box or column, when the probe is not connected to the patient is empty. When applied to the patient's finger there will be filling from the bottom and a level will be seen.
- The normal level of filling seen is anything from 25–75%. This indicates the degree of filling of the arterioles.
- When the arterioles are well relaxed as in deep anesthesia where there is no undue sympathetic activity, the column will be filled more than 75% fully indicating that the peripheral perfusion is very good or excellent.
- When the arterioles are constricted, either due to sympathetic stimulation during light plane of anesthesia or in hypovolemia the level in the column falls. This indicates that peripheral perfusion is reduced. Anything from 25% to 75% of the column filled is considered normal depending upon the clinical condition.

- With normal heart rate, if good venous filling is also seen in the dorsum of the hand, it indicates that the volume status is good.
- When the volume status is good, assessed by other clinical parameters or by central venous pressure monitoring and still there is a gross reduction in the level of the column, poor plane of anesthesia with inadequate reflex suppression is indicated. This patient may need either supplementation of analgesia or muscle relaxant as the case may be.

Thus the perfusion indicator helps the anesthesiologist to modulate the plane of anesthesia according to the requirement of surgical procedure (reflex stimulation).

In other words, it indicates the degree of vascular relaxation available and also the intravascular volume.

When a patient shows tachycardia, very poor level in perfusion indicator and no cutaneous venous filling, it may indicate two things.

1. The plane of anesthesia is poor that has stimulated the sympathetic response with tachycardia and vasoconstriction explaining the necessity for deepening the plane of anesthesia to relax the vasculature.
2. It may indicate hypovolemia. These two have to be clinically differentiated by other signs or if a central venous line is thereby the central venous pressure (CVP).

CAPNOGRAPHY

The capnogram is a direct monitor of the inhaled and exhaled concentration or partial pressure of CO_2 and an indirect monitor of CO_2 in arterial blood.

Principle

Infrared Absorption Spectrometry

Capnographs usually work on the principle that CO_2 absorbs infrared light rays. A beam of infrared light is passed across the gas sample to fall on a sensor. The presence of CO_2 in the gas sample leads to a reduction in the amount of light falling on the sensor. The change of voltage caused by this in a circuit is used to measure. The analysis is rapid and accurate, but the presence of N_2O in the gas mixture changes the infrared absorption by a phenomenon known as 'collision broadening'. This is corrected by measuring its infrared absorptive power.

Infrared Analyzer

- Gases with molecules that contain at least two dissimilar atoms absorb radiation in the infrared region of the spectrum.
- Using this property CO_2 concentration can be measured directly and continuously throughout the respiratory cycle.

Components

- The sample chamber—either in the main stream or in the side stream
- A photo detector measures light reaching it from a light source at the correct infrared wavelength after passing through two chambers.
- One chamber acts as *a reference chamber*, where as the other is *sampling chamber*.

Capnography (End-tidal CO_2 Monitoring)

- End-tidal carbon dioxide monitoring ($EtCO_2$) is the noninvasive measurement of alveolar CO_2 at the end of expiration when the CO_2 concentration is at its peak. The normal range is 35 to 37 mm Hg. The amount of CO_2 in exhaled gases is determined by three factors.
  1. Metabolic rate
  2. *Perfusion status* (to remove the gas from the tissues and bring it to the lungs).
  3. Alveolar ventilation
- Therefore, the measurement of concentration of CO_2 at the end of tidal breath provides a reflection of the alveolar CO_2 ($PACO_2$) which in turn reflects the arterial CO_2 ($PaCO_2$).
- At the beginning of expiration, the gas from the anatomical dead space that is free from CO_2 is exhaled.
- CO_2 elimination rapidly rises, reaching a plateau as the alveolar gases are exhaled.
- Therefore, the concentration of CO_2 in the expired gases is maximum or at the peak at the end of expiration (end-tidal).
- It can be measured near the proximal end of endotracheal tube.
- The measurement of CO_2 concentration at the end of expiration is called *capnography*.
- Noninvasive measurement of CO_2 concentration and giving in numerical display is called *capnometry* and the equipment is *capnometer*.
- The numerical and graphic display of CO_2 in respired gases in a waveform is known as *capnography* and the equipment is *capnograph*. The display of actual waveform pattern is called as capnogram. *It is a real time waveform record of the concentration of carbon dioxide in the respiratory gases* **(Figs 11.4A and B)**.
- The main purpose of capnography is to monitor the patient's ventilatory status ($PaCO_2$), as the maintenance of normal $PaCO_2$ depends upon adequacy of alveolar ventilation.
- The method of analyzing CO_2 in the expired gases is *infrared absorption spectrometry*.

Uses

- Warns of errors in airway, intubation and ventilation, i.e. esophageal intubation. Control of CO_2 level during surgery.
- Efficiency of closed system in CO_2 absorption can be monitored continuously.

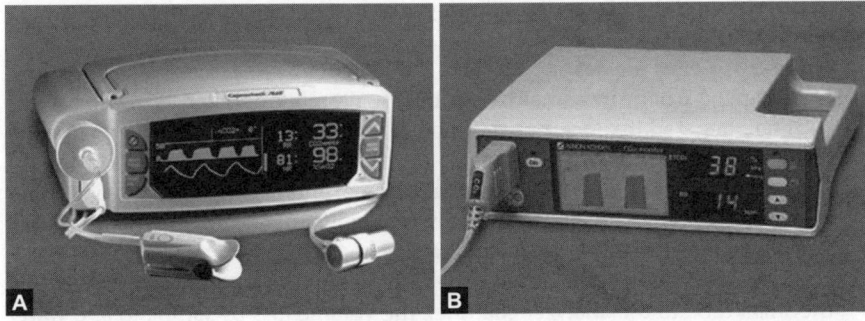

Figs 11.4A and B: Capnographs. (A) Capnograph and pulse oximeter combined with a side stream sampling adapter; (B) Capnograph alone

Infrared Absorption Spectrometry or Infrared CO_2 Analyzer
- This equipment is less expensive, portable, and most commonly used.
- It works on the principle of infrared light absorption by CO_2 in the mixture of gases.
- An IR analyzer simply has a source of IR radiation, an analysis chamber, a reference chamber, and a detection cell.
- The light absorption by CO_2 in the analyzing chamber is compared to that reference chamber which has no CO_2.
- It provides continuous monitoring of the patient.
- There are two systems of sampling available based on which there are two types of monitors available; one is *mainstream analyzer* and the other is *sidestream analyzer*.
- Actual deference between these two is not in the technology but is in the site of analysing the gas. Both the modules can be made available in the same machine.

Mainstream CO_2 Analyzer
- In this type of analyzer, the sensors are placed directly on the breathing system.
- It incorporates, the analyzer cell with IR source, detector, and the associated electronics into a especially designed airway adopter which is interposed into the breathing system **(Figs 11.5A and C)**.
- There is no volume loss of respiratory gases and the system offers a very fast response.
- The highest content of the CO_2 is found at the end of expiration and that is called as end tidal CO_2.
- The possibility of condensation of water vapor is prevented by heating the measuring chamber to about 40°C.
- The possibility of contamination with secretions that absorbs IR light may give an erroneously high value of CO_2 is a disadvantage.
- The added apparatus dead space is disadvantageous in children.
- There can be a drag on the endotracheal tube because of the weight.

Sidestream CO_2 Analyzer
- It consists of an adapter that can be fixed near the endotracheal tube from which sample of gases is drawn through a long slender tube to a measuring chamber at a distance. After processing the value is displayed **(Fig. 11.5B)**.
- A continuous sample of respired gases is withdrawn from as near to the trachea as possible and the CO_2 content displayed as percentage on a continuous record **(Fig. 11.5B)**.
- A pump aspirates the gas sample from the patient's airway.
- The sampling is done by a small bore tube (usually made of Teflon as PVC may react with halogenated hydrocarbons) of about two meters length to the measuring chamber.
- The end of sampling tube is kept at the proximal end of endotracheal tube using a T-piece assembly. The sampling rate is in the order of 50–200 mL/min.
- The advantage is that there is no addition of apparatus dead space.
- The disadvantages include delay in the response, as the gas has to travel through the small tube to the analyzer chamber, the volume loss by sampling and water condensation in the sampling tube.

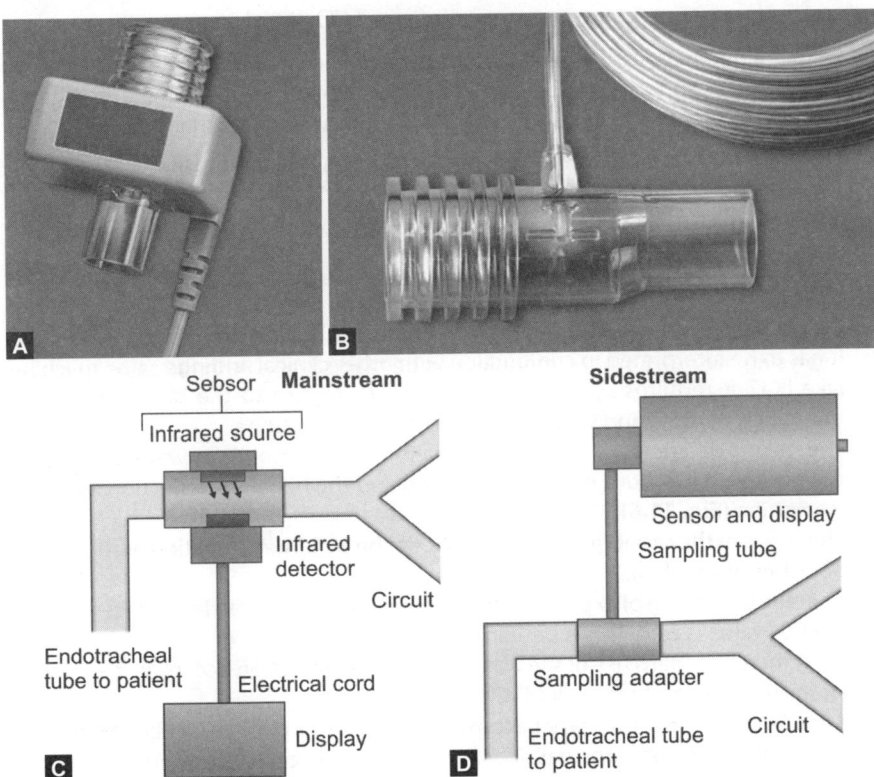

Figs 11.5A to D: (A) Mainstream analyzer adapter; (B) Side stream analyzer adapter with sampling tube; (C) Schematic diagram of mainstream analyzer; (D) Schematic diagram of side stream analyzer.

- In patients without intubation, 'nasal prongs' are used for sampling of expired gases. The values are unlikely to be correct as there is continuous mixing of atmospheric air at the level of nose.

The schematic representation of the two types of analyzers is shown in **Figs 11.5C and D**.

Interpretation of Values

- The normal value is usually 2–5 mm Hg lesser than the $PaCO_2$.
- For example, if the $PaCO_2$ is 39 mm Hg and the $EtCO_2$ is 35 mm Hg, it is normal.
- Certain factors may modify the $EtCO_2$ value (raised or lowered).

Factors that Increase $EtCO_2$

- *Ventilation:* Hypoventilation due to any reason.
- *Perfusion:* Increased transport of CO_2 to lungs as in postcardiac arrest state.
- *Metabolism:* Increased CO_2 production due to any reason, most commonly pyrexia, trauma, shivering, or malignant hyperthermia, etc.
- *Equipment:* Rebreathing due to any reason, partially obstructed airway, or leak in the breathing circuit delivering low volume, etc.

Factors that Decrease EtCO$_2$

- Hyperventilation
- Reduced pulmonary perfusion as in decreased cardiac output, pulmonary embolus, etc.
- Decreased CO$_2$ production as in hypothermia, heavy sedation, etc.
- Obstruction or kink in endotracheal tube
- Ventilator disconnection.

Normal Capnogram

- Capnogram is not a measurement of respiratory function only.
- It has to be interpreted in conjunction with other clinical findings.
- Like ECG, it requires systematic analysis with regard to the baseline, height, frequency, rhythm, and shape to get the best information.
- The striking difference of capnogram waveform other respiratory waveforms is that the positive deflections indicate expiration and the negative deflection indicates inspiration **(Fig. 11.6)**.
- The shape of the capnogram is diagnostic of abnormal lung function or suggestive of technical problem.
- As at the beginning of expiration, the air from the anatomical dead space escapes, the CO$_2$ value is zero. This is baseline (A–B).
- Then there is a sharp rise of the wave when CO$_2$ elimination occurs as the alveolar air mixes with dead space air (B–C).
- After this sharp rise, the wave becomes a plateau. This plateau is called as *alveolar plateau* where most of the gas flow from the alveoli occurs. The plateau gradually ascends and reaches a peak (C–D).
- This point at the end of plateau is the end of expiration and the PCO$_2$ at this point is the end tidal CO$_2$.
- Therefore, the EtCO$_2$ is the highest concentration of CO$_2$ exhaled.
- The curve then takes a sharp downstroke as the fresh gas free from CO$_2$ is inhaled.
- Individual capnogram wave can be analyzed for studying each characteristic.
- A trend of capnogram over a period of time can be analyzed to know the changes that have occurred during that period **(Fig. 11.7)**.

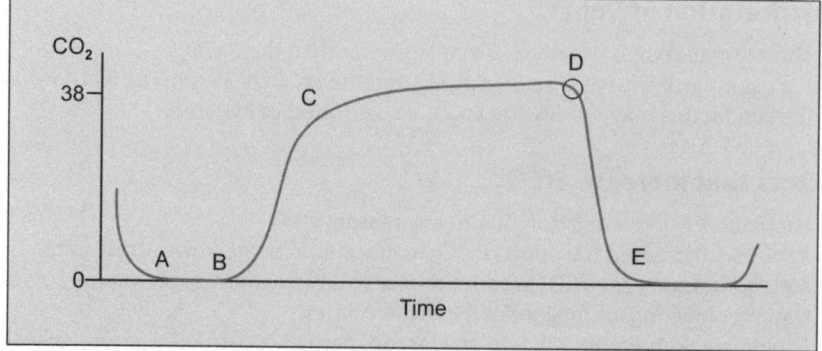

Fig. 11.6: Normal capnogram; • Inspiratory baseline: A–B Just before expiration; • Expiratory upstroke: B–C Active expiration; • Expiratory plateau: C–D Expiration of alveolar air; • Inspiratory down stroke: D–E Inspiration

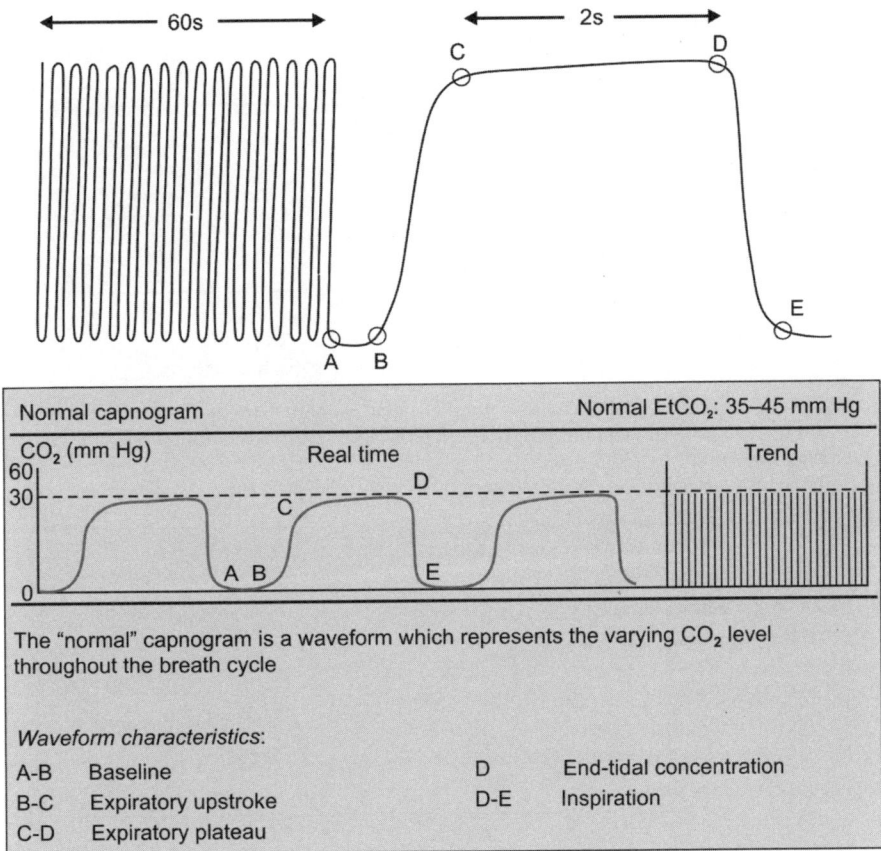

Fig. 11.7: Normal capnogram, the trend for 60 seconds and a single waveform

The square graph thus generated has the following parts.
1. Inspiratory baseline
2. Expiratory upstroke
3. Expiratory plateau
4. Inspiratory downstroke.

Some abnormal capnogram patterns and the possible causes are discussed below:
- Elevated EtCO$_2$ with good alveolar plateau **(Fig. 11.8)**.
- Progressively increasing EtCO$_2$ with normal alveolar plateau **(Fig. 11.9)**.
- A rise in baseline and increasing EtCO$_2$ **(Fig. 11.10)**.
- Alveolar plateau showing a cleft on the top (alveolar cleft) **(Fig. 11.11)**.
- Oblique expiratory upstroke **(Fig. 11.12)**.
- Progressively decreasing end-tidal CO$_2$ **(Fig. 11.13)**.

ELECTROCARDIOGRAM MONITOR
- ECG monitors are available as independent units or along with other modules like pulse oximeter, capnography, noninvasive BP, etc. (Multiparameter monitors).
- Valuable information concerning cardiac rhythm may be obtained by monitoring the electrocardiogram.

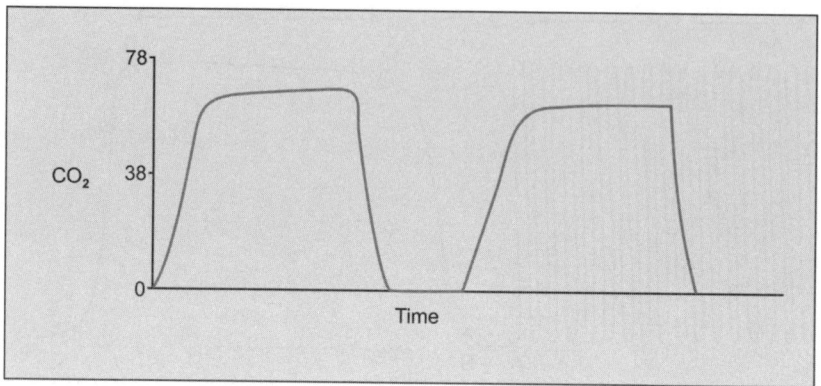

Fig. 11.8: Elevated end-tidal CO_2 with a good alveolar plateau; • Inadequate minute volume (VE) with tidal volume sufficient to empty the alveolar gas; • Increased metabolic rate such as fever, pain, shivering

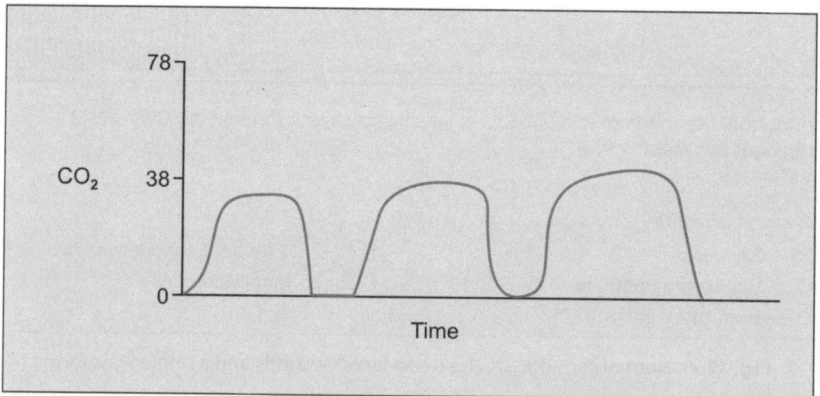

Fig. 11.9: Gradually increasing end-tidal CO_2 with normal alveolar plateau; • Hypoventilation; • Malignant hyperthermia; • Factors that raise the body temperature

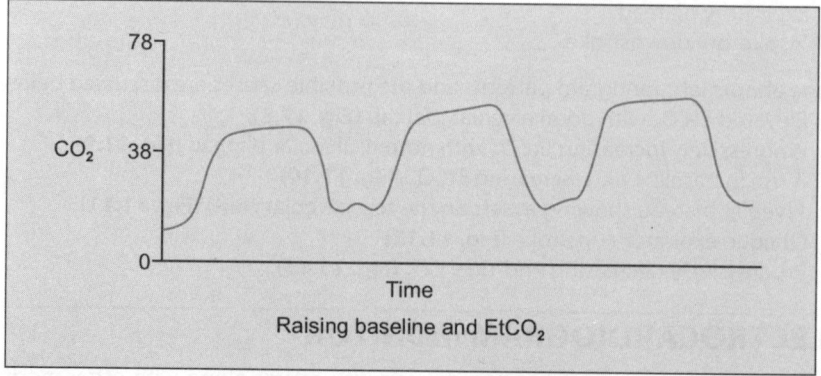

Raising baseline and $EtCO_2$

Fig. 11.10: Increase in end-tidal CO_2 and elevated inspiratory baseline; • Rebreathing of exhaled CO_2; • Increased apparatus dead space; • Exhausted sodalime in anesthesia; • Defective expiratory valve

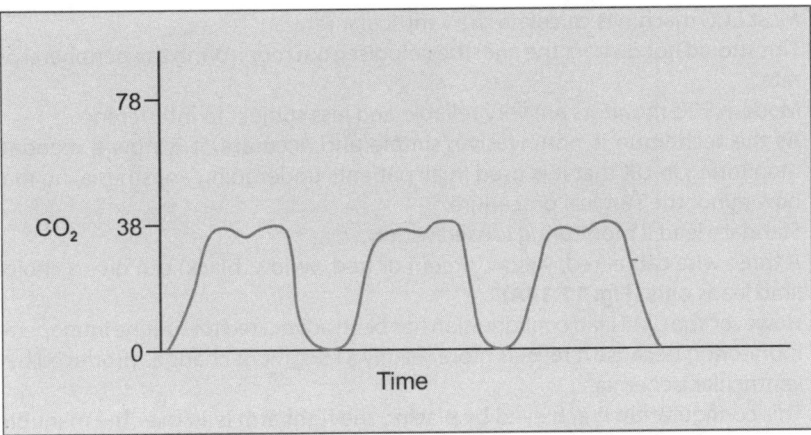

Fig. 11.11: Normal capnogram with "alveolar cleft"; • Inadequate neuromuscular blockade or neuromuscular block wearing off; • The patient's inspiratory attempts are seen as a depression on the top of the alveolar plateau, known as "Alveolar cleft".

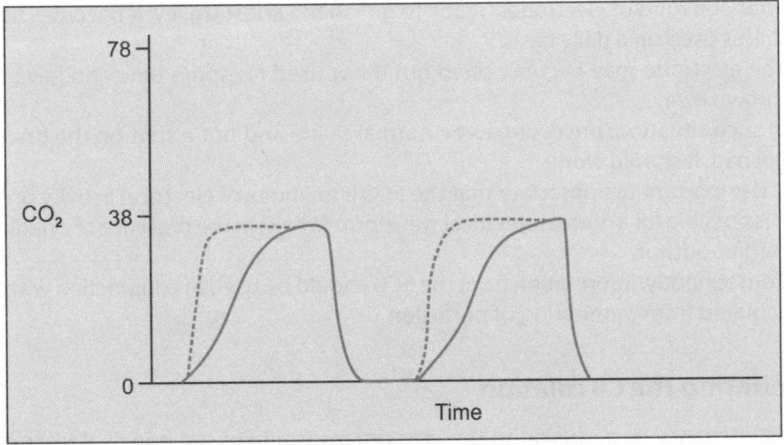

Fig. 11.12: Sloping alveolar plateau; • Expiratory obstruction as in bronchospasm; • The airway obstruction causes a delay in alveolar air and CO_2 to be expelled, so, the upstroke is not sharp and merges with the plateau. The dotted line indicates the normal upstroke and plateau.

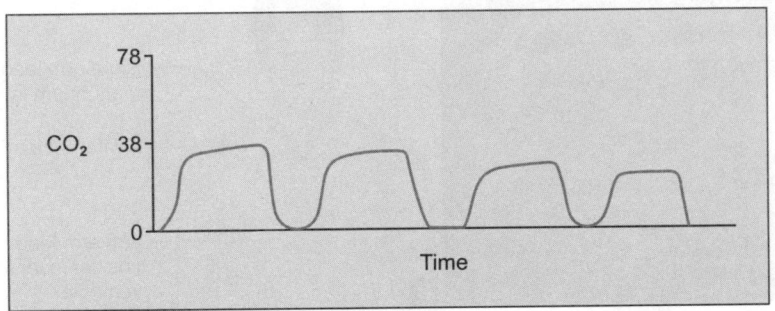

Fig. 11.13: Progressively decreasing end-tidal CO_2; • Reduction in blood flow to the lung.; • Severe hypotension or pulmonary embolus

- Most ECG machines calculate the ventricular rate.
- This should not distract the anesthesiologist from monitoring the peripheral pulse rate.
- Modern ECG monitors are very reliable and less subject to interference.
- As the technique is noninvasive, simple and accurate, it is now a mandatory monitoring in UK that it is used in all patients undergoing anesthesia, no matter how minor the surgical procedure.
- Standard lead II monitoring is used widely.
- A three wire cable (red, yellow, green) or (red, yellow, black) can give a choice of limb leads only **(Fig. 11.14A)**.
- However, the CM5 lead configuration has been advocated for routine intraoperative monitoring because it reveals more readily ST segment changes produced by left ventricular ischemia.
- This configuration is achieved by placing the right arm lead over the manubrium sterni, the left arm lead on the V5 position over the left ventricle, and the indifferent lead over the shoulder. Red-Right arm, Yellow-Left arm, Green-Left leg (indifferent lead placed on left shoulder) **(Fig. 11.4B)**.
- It is not correct to leave electrodes attached to the patient cable, or put neatly arranged rows of electrodes "ready to go" on the arrest trolley. It becomes useless unless used on a daily basis.
- The electrode may become dried out if not used for some time and have to be thrown away.
- In such situation, break out some normal saline and put a spot on the dried out gel pad, it should work.
- It is important to appreciate that the ECG is an index of electrical activity only.
- It is possible for a normal electrical waveform to exist in the presence of a negligible cardiac output.
- Consequently, information from the ECG should be used in conjunction with data acquired from monitoring of perfusion.

Monitoring the Circulation

- Maintenance of perfusion to the vital organs is one of the principal tasks of the anesthesiologist during surgery.

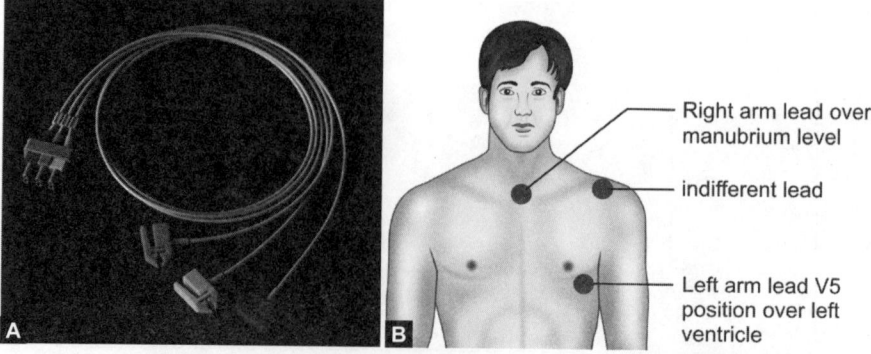

Figs 11.14A and B: CM5 lead configuration for ECG monitoring and the cable; Red—*Right arm* and Yellow—*Left arm*

- Adequate perfusion is dependent on adequate venous return to the heart, cardiac performance and arterial pressure.
- Direct measurement of cardiac output requires invasive procedures.
- However, adequacy of cardiac output and circulating blood volume may be inferred from observation of the following variables:
  - Arterial pressure
  - Peripheral pulse
  - Arterial oxygen saturation
  - Peripheral perfusion
  - Urine production

Arterial Pressure

- Perfusion of vital organs (brain, heart and kidney) requires an adequate systemic blood pressure.
- Anesthesia, surgery, the patient's underlying condition, and adverse events that occur during surgery may all affect blood pressure. So, it must be monitored in all patients.
- In most patients, intermittent noninvasive readings are sufficient.
- Continuous direct (Invasive) measurement of blood pressure requires an arterial cannula, but it is invaluable for some patients and procedures.
- Noninvasive technique usually produce good estimate of systolic pressure but less accurate diastolic and mean arterial pressures.
- For general purposes, either a sphygmomanometer or automated noninvasive BP monitor is quite reliable.
- It is advised that BP is checked every 5 to 10 minutes initially and once things are stable, the interval may be made every 15 minutes.

Peripheral Pulse

- Regular palpation of peripheral pulse (Radial pulse) is one of the simplest and most useful methods of monitoring during anesthesia.
- Valuable information may be obtained by monitoring the rate, volume and rhythm.
- It is mandatory even in the most minor surgery.

Pulse Plethysmography

- Automated devices are available for monitoring peripheral pulsation.
- Usually, it is available with sophisticated models of pulse oximeters.
- Pulse monitors provide a guide to the pulse pressure.
- Thus, an increase in signal may be seen in peripheral vasodilatation or increased cardiac output.
- Low pulse pressure is seen during vasoconstriction or low cardiac output states. It has been discussed in detail in pulse oximeter.

Arterial Oxygen Saturation

Pulse oximeters measure the arterial oxygen saturation and pulses rate accurately within 2% variation.

Peripheral Perfusion

- Pink skin indicates adequate peripheral perfusion; cold white peripheries indicate the reverse.
- This is particularly true in children, in whom cold peripheries indicates a degree of hypovolemia.
- The core-peripheral temperature gradient is a useful index of adequacy of peripheral perfusion.
- One probe is placed in nasopharynx and the other on the great toe. Temperature gradient increases with vasoconstriction and low cardiac output.

Urine Output

- Adequacy of renal perfusion may be inferred from the volume of urine produced. Kidney is the only organ whose function may be monitored directly in this way.
- A urine production of 0.5 mL/kg/hour is considered adequate.
- Adequate production of urine implies that perfusion of other vital organs is likely to be adequate.

Defibrillator

It is not uncommon to meet with a catastrophic situation of cardiac arrest during anesthesia due to either surgical or anesthetic causes. As most of the time an ECG monitor is always there attached to the patient, it is easy to assess the status of heart whether it is in aystole or ventricular fibrillation. If it is in ventricular fibrillation, electrical defibrillation, if available is the choice of management. Defibrillator is the equipment used for that. It is worth discussing it with ECG monitor.

- Defibrillation consists of delivering a therapeutic dose of electrical current to the heart with a device called a *defibrillator*. This depolarizes a critical mass of the heart muscle, terminates the dysrhythmia and allows normal sinus rhythm to be re-established by the body's natural pacemaker, in the sino-atrial node of the heart.
- Defibrillators are available as independent units or available in combination with ECG monitor and ECG recorder **(Fig. 11.15)**.
- Defibrillators may be external, or internal.
- Same unit usually provides the paddles for external and internal use.
- Commonly external paddles are used. But during cardiac surgeries when the thoracic cage is open and the surgeon has the access to the heart, sterile internal pads are used.
- Only the cardiac arrest rhythms ventricular fibrillation and pulseless ventricular tachycardia are normally defibrillated. This is because the whole point of the exercise is to shock the patient *into* asystole and then let their heart start back beating normally.
- A patient who is already in asystole cannot be helped by electrical means, and usually needs urgent CPR and intravenous medication.
- There are also several heart rhythms that can be "shocked" when the patient is not in cardiac arrest, such as supraventricular tachycardia and ventricular tachycardia that produces a pulse; this more-complicated procedure is known as cardioversion, not defibrillation.

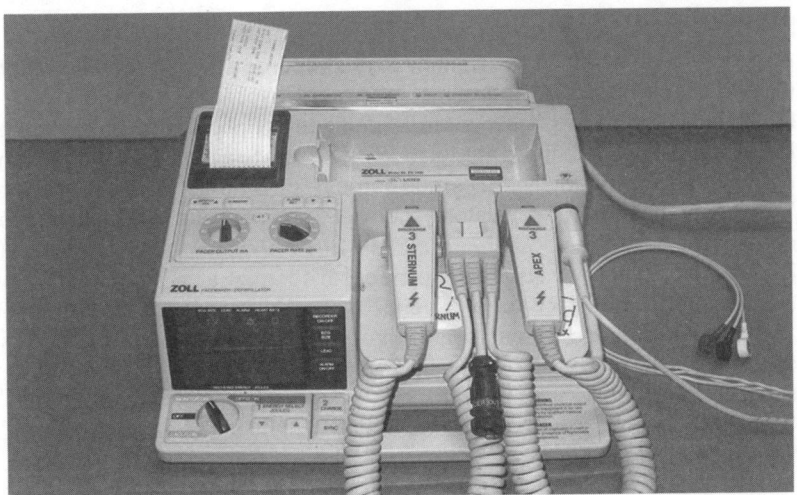

Fig. 11.15: A defibrillator unit with ECG monitor and recorder

Treatment of Ventricular Fibrillation

- Adrenaline 0.5 to 1 mg IV given to convert slow fibrillation to fast fibrillation.
- Acidosis is corrected by sodium bicarbonate as acidosis inactivates adrenaline.
- Calcium chloride 1 gm as 10% solution IV converts slow fibrillation to faster fibrillation and improves the tone before electrical defibrillation.
- Now electrical defibrillation could be done effectively.

Defibrillation

What is Defibrillation?

- Fibrillation is ineffective fascicular incoordinate contraction of bundles of ventricular muscles.
- Therefore, effective contraction of ventricle does not occur and blood is not pumped out of ventricles.
- So, the fibrillation of myocardium is converted into normal effective ejectile contraction of ventricles in normal rhythm.
- It is done by passing calculated dose of electrical current through the ventricles for a very short time.
- This is called as electrical cardioversion or defibrillation.

The Principle of Defibrillation

- Electrical current is passed through the heart causes all the fibers to go into their refractory period simultaneously.
- At this moment, the normal sinus rhythm takes over. If not, normal beat can be stimulated by a manual compression.

DC Defibrillation

- AC defibrillation which was in use early days is not used now as its duration is longer (0.25 to 1 sec—60 Hz 6 A) and so results in more myocardial damage.
- DC defibrillation causes less myocardial damage as the duration is very short.
- In this, a capacitor is charged at a relatively slow rate to a high DC voltage from the AC mains and then rapidly discharged at the desired time.
- The energy stored in the capacitor is then delivered at a relatively rapid rate to the chest of the patient.
- The amount of energy discharged by the capacitor may range from 2 to 400 joules (watt seconds) with peak value of current 20 A. The duration is less 3 to 10 mseconds.
- Two paddles one near the apex and the other near the base of the heart with conductive jelly on the bare skin **(Fig. 11.16A)**.
- *Dose 100 to 400 joules (watt seconds).*
- Usually, the heart responds to 100 joules.
- If the response is not good in two attempts, it can be increased to 200 joules.

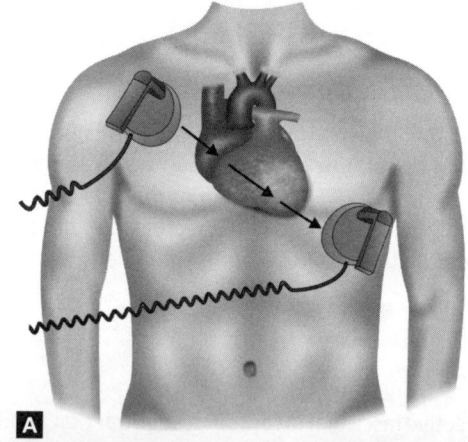

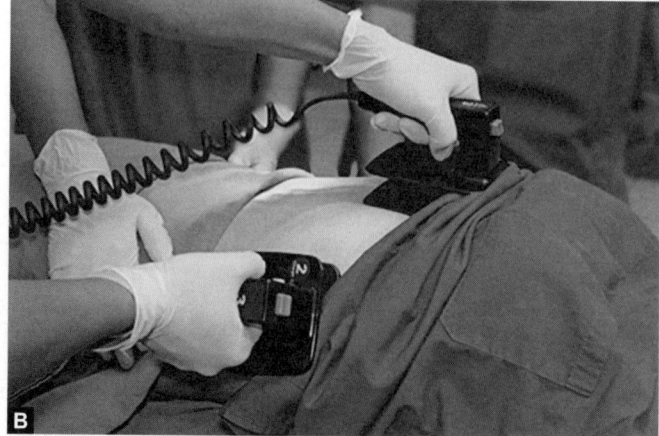

Fig. 11.16A and B: (A) The position of defibrillator paddles on the chest wall; (B) The way of applying the external paddles

- Defibrillation (shock success) is defined as termination of VF for at least 5 seconds following the shock.
- VF frequently recurs after successful shock, but this recurrence should not be equated to shock failure.

Placement of Paddles
- The anterior electrode is placed on the right, below the clavicle.
- The apex electrode is applied to the left side of the patient, just below and to the left of the pectoral muscle **(Fig. 11.16B)**.
- This works well for defibrillation and cardioversion.
- *Paddle size:* Adult 10 to 13 cm diameter, Children >10 kg 8 cm, Infants <10 kg 4.5 cm.
- Smaller paddles concentrate current and may cause burns. Larger paddles reduce the current density.
- Conducting jelly is used on the paddles (ECG jelly).
- Pressure applied is 25 pounds. In children about 10 pound.
- Deflated lungs reduce the distance of path of current.

MONITORING NEUROMUSCULAR BLOCK

History
In 1958, Christie and Churchill Davidson described the use of a nerve stimulator to monitor neuromuscular block.

However, until 1970 it was not in popular use. Only when the TOF pattern of stimulation was described and handy equipment was made available, it came into routine clinical use.

As there is no clinical method of assessing the neuromuscular blockade a tool is needed, that is the peripheral nerve stimulator.
- It provides a means of application of a current up to 50 mA (milliamperes) for a fraction of a millisecond (0.2 ms) to a peripheral motor nerve and to assess the response evoked in the muscle innervated by the nerve. The voltage necessary may be up to 300 volts.
- A nerve which is easily accessible such as ulnar, facial or lateral popliteal is chosen. Most commonly ulnar nerve is used for convenience.
- As the skin resistance vary, the stimulator that automatically adjusts the output to discharge a constant direct current is needed.
- The skin where the electrodes are applied is cleaned with alcohol that removes the oil and thus reduces the resistance.
- When the nerve is stimulated with sufficient current all the fibers contract and that is called *maximal current*.
- An intensity of current a little more than maximal (*supramaximal*) is used to ensure contraction. Usually it is 30 mA.
- In awake patients *a submaximal* (15 mA) current is used to reduce the discomfort to the patient.
- In common practice it is assessed by visual or tactile means.
- Two electrodes are placed along the course of nerve and current is passed. Generally surface electrodes with adhesive periphery and central jelly for electrical conductivity are used. Metal electrodes and needle electrodes are available, but less commonly used.

- Usually the peripheral nerve stimulator is set to deliver the stimulus at specific intervals to evaluate the degree of neuromuscular block.
- Mini stimulator with two electrodes with globular ends to be applied directly on the skin **(Fig. 11.17)** and also with wires to be connected to the skin electrodes **(Fig. 11.18)** are available.
- The current delivered is direct current and has a red positive and a black negative electrode. Preferably the positive electrode is placed where the nerve is superficial and the negative along the course of the nerve **(Fig. 11.19)**.

Peripheral Nerve Stimulator

The objective assessment of the status of neuromuscular block during anesthesia is an absolute necessity and that is the purpose of this equipment.

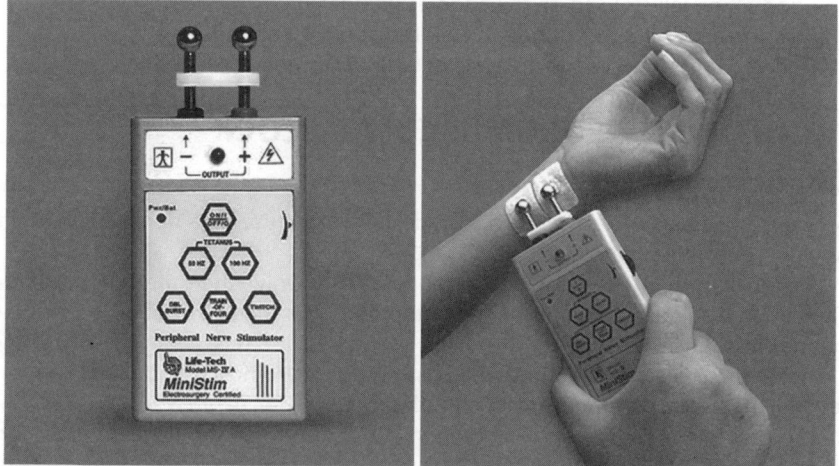

Fig. 11.17: Small peripheral nerve stimulator with metal ball electrodes

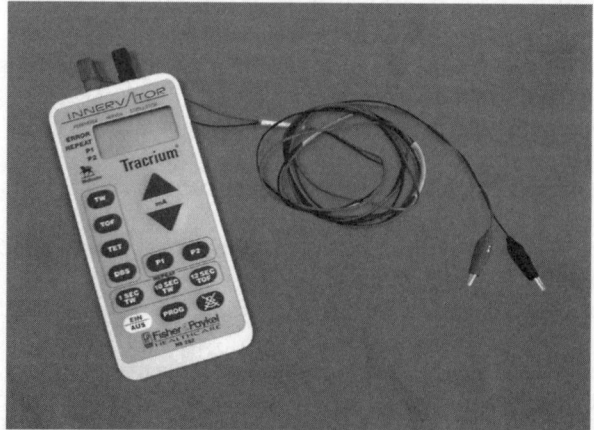

Fig. 11.18: Peripheral nerve stimulator with wires to reach electrodes

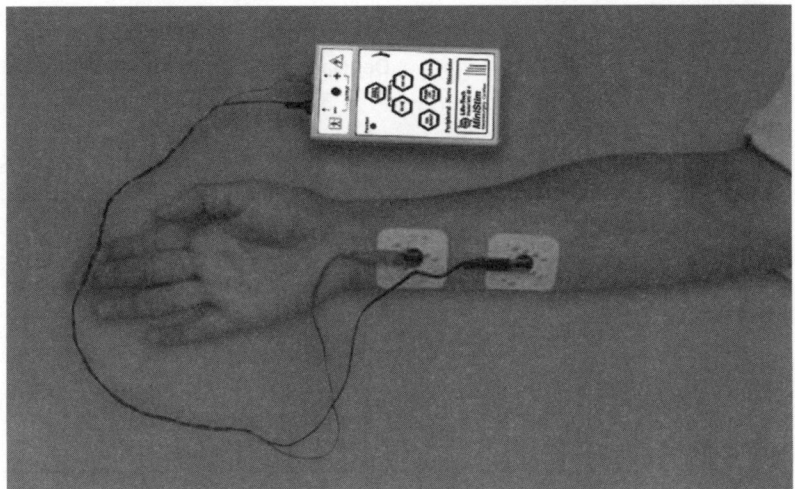

Fig. 11.19: Application of electrodes of peripheral nerve stimulator

Frequency
- Frequency of stimulus applied is expressed in Hz.
- One Hz is one cycle/second.
- 0.1 Hz means one stimulus every 10 seconds

Duration
- The duration of stimulus must be 0.2 ms (milliseconds).
- If the duration is more than 0.5 ms, then a second action potential may be triggered.

Three types of electrical stimulations were in vogue for a long time.
1. Single twitch
2. Train of four (TOF)
3. Tetanic stimulation

Later two newer modes have been added.
1. Post-tetanic count (PTC)
2. Double burst stimulation (DBS).

The five commonly used types of electrical stimulations namely; **Single twitch, Train of four, Tetanic stimulation with post-tetanic twitch** and **Double burst stimulation** are shown in **Fig. 11.20**.
- In clinical anesthesia, there are two types of neuromuscular blockade possible namely—depolarizing block and non-depolarizing block.
- Depolarizing block is caused by the drug succinylcholine (Suxamethonium chloride), the only drug available in this group. Though it is still in use worldwide, many developed countries have stopped using it.
- Non-depolarizing drugs are in common use. The first one used in the world was D-Tubocurarine derived from a plant *Chondrodendron tomentosum* was introduced clinical anesthesia by Griffith and Johnson in 1942. Now it has been replaced by numerous synthetic drugs having very desirable properties.

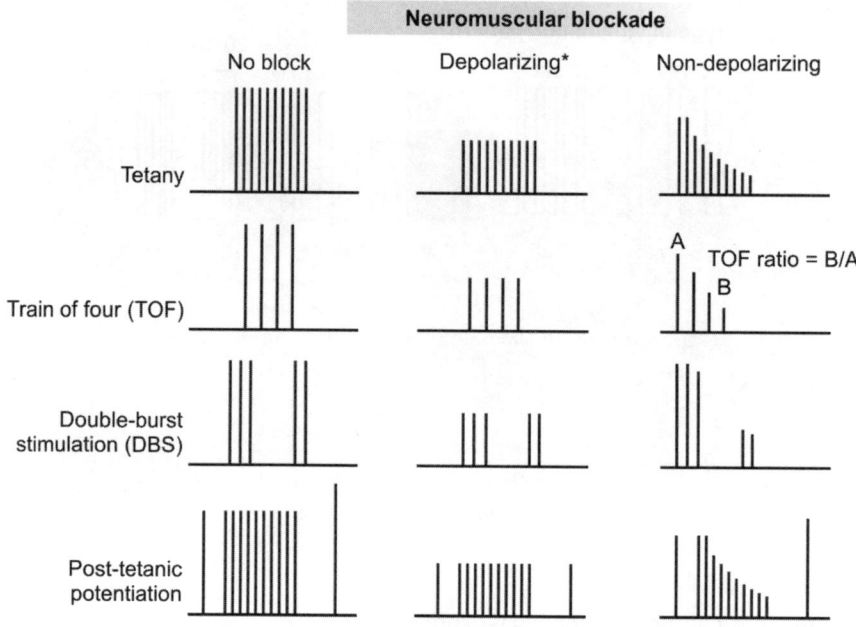

Fig. 11.20: Comparing normal response with that of depolarising and non-depolarising blocks

- It is essential to compare the normal response of contraction for the stimulus from a peripheral nerve stimulator and difference in the pattern of depolarizing block and non-depolarizing block **(Fig. 11.20)**.

Train of Four

- Application of four twitch stimuli each of 2 Hz (2 seconds) with 10–12 seconds intervals between trains **(Fig. 11.21)**.
- The ratio of the 4th twitch (T4) to the 1st twitch (T1), that is TOF ratio is measured.
- The clinical response of contraction and the percentage of block is shown in **Figures 11.22 and 23**.

Single Twitch

- Electrical stimulation for short duration (0.2 ms) usually to ulnar nerve at every second (1.0 Hz) or every 10 seconds (0.1 Hz) and observe muscle contraction **(Fig. 11.21)**.
- Not a very sensitive test.
- About 75% of postsynaptic junctions have to be blocked before any depression in twitching.
- About 90% of depression in twitch response is required for ideal operating conditions **(Fig. 11.21)**.

Response
Depolarizing block : Reduction in all the four twitches
Nondepolarizing block : 4th twitch reduced in relation to 3rd, 2nd and 1st (decrement)

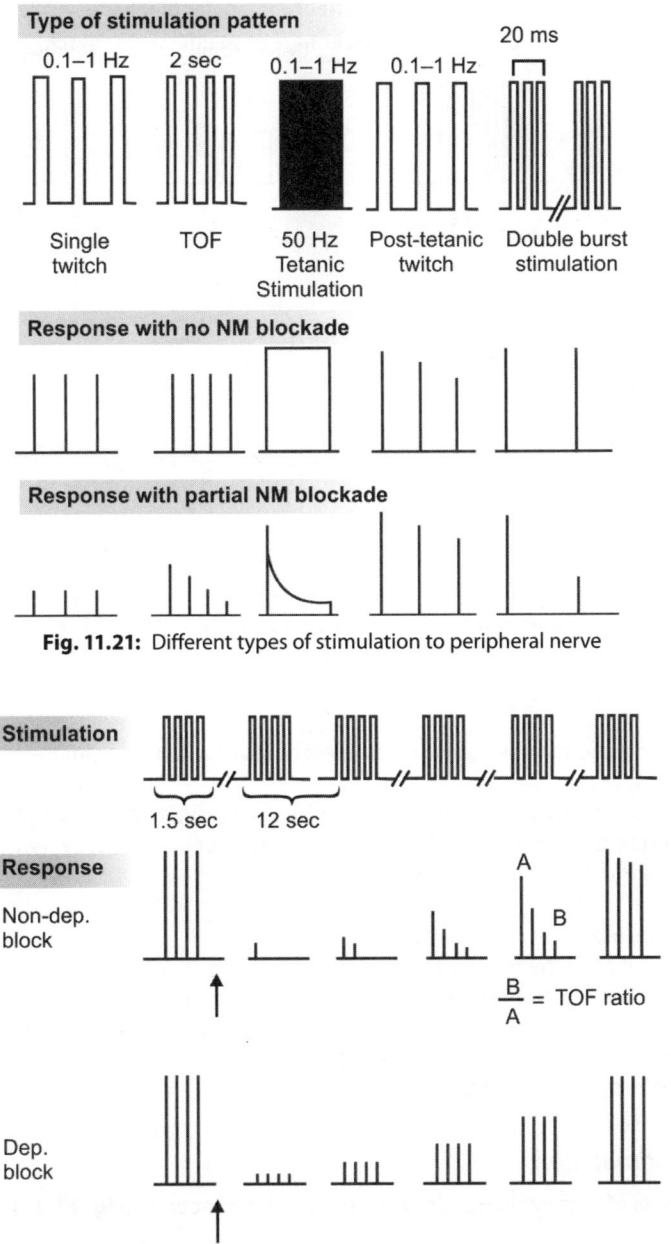

Fig. 11.21: Different types of stimulation to peripheral nerve

Fig. 11.22: Train-of-four response in non-depolarizing block and depolarizing block

Interpretation
T4 Disappears at 75%—depression of T1.
T3 Disappears at 80–85%—depression of T1.
T2 Disappears at 90%—depression of T1.

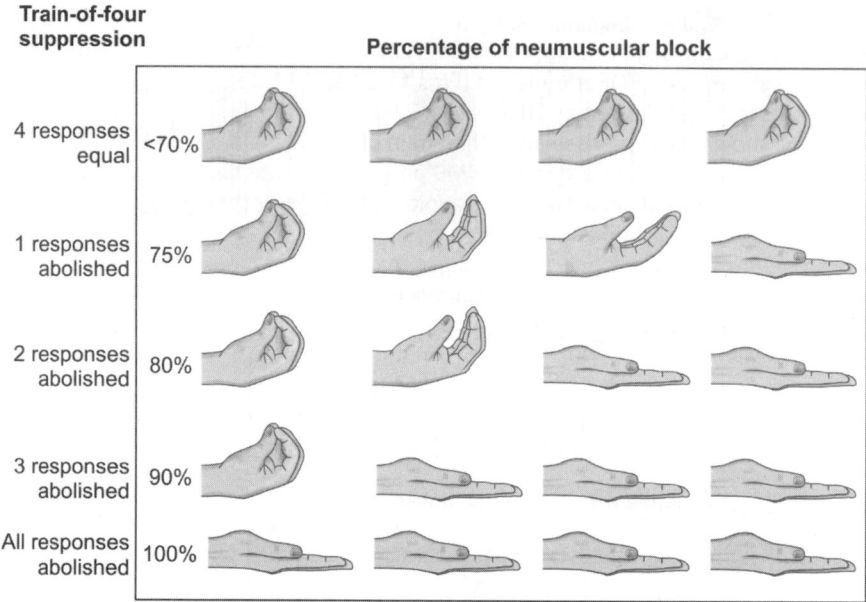

Fig. 11.23: The percentage of block judged by clinical observation of contraction. The response of twitch is equated to the corresponding percentage of block.

- Counting the number of twitches present gives a rough estimate of the extent of block.
- Anticholinesterase should be given only after the appearance of T2 and the subsequent recovery of T4 70% is considered a very good recovery clinically and considered safe for extubation.

Depolarizing Block
- Recovery of all the four twitches of TOF should be at similar rate.
- The TOF nerve stimulation has become "Gold Standard" for nerve stimulation because, it allows easy quantification of the degree of block, even though the preoperative values may be lacking.
- This is less painful than the Tetanic stimulation.

Tetanic Stimulation

- Consists of at least 50 Hz stimulation given for 5 seconds **(Fig. 11.21)**.

Depolarizing block
- Stimulation is sustained.

Nondepolarizing block
- The response will not be sustained and fade occurs.
- Post-tetanic facilitation is encountered in nondepolarizing block.
- In Phase II block also these two features are seen.
- But it is painful, if applied on conscious patients.

Post-tetanic Count

- To evaluate the degree of block during very intense block, when there is no response to single twitch or TOF stimulation **(Figs 11.21 and 11.24)**.
- It is 5 s tetanus followed by 20 pulses of 2 Hz.
- It will show fade response earlier than train of four.
- It helps to assess the degree of NMB and to eliminate sudden movements as necessary in ophthalmic surgery or avoiding bucking or coughing in response to tracheobronchial stimulation.
- Sometimes, the block may be so intense that PTC cannot be evoked.
- During recovery from neuromuscular blockade (NMB), the degree of residual block is determined by this response.
- This evaluation is by visual or tactile method without any recording equipment and may pose difficulty in estimation even in clinically significant NMB.
- "TOFGUARD" is the equipment available to visualize the graphical representation of block with recording facilities **(Fig. 11.23)**.

Double Burst Stimulation

- Provides three 0.2 ms bursts of 50 Hz tetanus each separated by 20 ms and repeated after 750 ms **(Figs 11.21 and 11.25)**.
- It is similar to TOF, but tactile evaluation is more sensitive because the fade of the two resultant contractions is more marked.
- Absence of tactile fade response to DBS means that severe residual NMB does not exists, but it does not exclude clinically significant residual block.

In Clinical Practice

Useful Hints to Assess Adequate Reversal of NMB

- TOF ratio minimum 0.9, 0.8
- Sustained head raising for 5 seconds
- Sustained handgrip for 5 seconds
- Minimum inspiratory pressure—50 cm of H_2O—will enable a vital capacity of 15 mL/kg.
- Infants hip flexion for more than 90°—equals with a maximum inspiratory force of 30 cm of H_2O which is adequate for spontaneous respiration.
- About 80% of the postoperative deaths occur in the first postoperative hour. In that, nearly 80% of the patients die because of recurarization caused by the residual effect of NM blocking drugs and resultant hypoventilation or respiratory arrest.

Post-tetanic count
- 5 s tetanus followed by 20 pulses at 2 Hz
- Shows fade response earlier than train of four
- Used under deep paralysis to estimate time to recovery

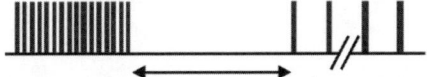

Tetanus 5 s Recovery 3 s 20 single twitches
1 s spart

Fig. 11.24: Post-tetanic count in relation to TOF response

Double burst stimulation
- Two bursts 0.5 s apart
- Either 3 pulses followed by 2 pulses (3:2) or 2 followed by 3 (3:3)
- Used under light paralysis where train of four ratio is difficult to distinguish

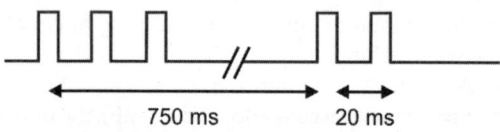

Fig. 11.25: Double burst stimulation

FURTHER READING

1. Aitkenhead AR, Smith G. Textbook of Anaesthesia, 3rd edn. Edinburgh: Churchill Livingston, 1996.
2. Al-Shaikh Baha, Stacey S. Essentials of Anaesthetic Equipment, 1st edn. London: Churchill Livingstone, 1995.
3. Dorsch JA, Dorsch SE. Understanding Anaesthesia Equipment, 4th edn. London: Lippincott Williams and Wilkins, 1999.
4. Dorsch JA, Dorsch SE. Understanding Anaesthesia Equipment, 5th edn. London: Lippincott Williams and Wilkins, 2008.
5. Lee's Synopsis of Anaesthesia, 11th edn. London: Butterworth-Heinemann Ltd., 1993.
6. Moyle JTB, Davey A. Ward's Anaesthetic Equipment, 4th edn. London: WB Saunders Company Limited, 1998.
7. Ward CS. Anaesthetic Equipment, 2nd edn. London: Balliere, S;1985.

Equipment for Spinal and Epidural Anesthesia

chapter 12

TECHNIQUES OF REGIONAL ANESTHESIA
- *Spinal*: Subarachnoid block (Intrathecal block)
- *Epidural*: Extradural
  - Sacral epidural (Caudal)
  - Lumbar epidural
  - Thoracic epidural.
- *Epispinal* (combined spinal and epidural)
  Spinal, epidural and epispinal anesthesia are commonly known as *Central Neural Block*
- *Nerve block:* Digital nerve block
- *Plexus block:* Brachial plexus block
- *Field block:* A few nerves are specifically blocked. For example, for inguinal herniorrhaphy.
  - Ilioinguinal nerve
  - Iliohypogastric nerve
  - Femoral branch of genitofemoral nerve
  - *Drug*: Xylocaine 0.5 to 1%
- *Infiltration block:* Infiltrating subcutaneous tissue with 0.25–0.5% Xylocaine and block cutaneous nerves crossing there.
- *Topical analgesia:* Intact mucous membranes—nose, mouth, larynx, etc.
  - Xylocaine 4% (spray or packing)
- *Intravenous regional analgesia:* After exsanguination of the limb, tourniquet is applied to the limb. Then through an indwelling cannula, required quantity of (30–40 mL) 0.25 to 0.5% of xylocaine is injected into the vein.
  - Peripheral nerve endings are blocked and through the vasa nervorum nerves are also blocked.
  - This technique is useful for limbs particularly for upper limbs.
- *Eutectic mixture of local analgesics (EMLA):* Fixed proportions of Xylocaine 2.5% and Prilocaine 2.5% can penetrate intact skin and cause local anesthesia when applied as a cream and an occlusive dressing is given for 1 hour—useful for taking skin grafts and for doing venepuncture in children.

SPINAL ANESTHESIA

History
- The first spinal analgesia was administered in 1885 by *James Leonard Corning* (1855–1923), a neurologist in New York. When experimenting with cocaine on

the spinal *nerves* of a dog, he accidentally pierced the dura, and it became a subarachnoid block.
- The first planned spinal anesthesia for surgery in man was administered by *August Bier* (1861–1949) on 16 August 1898, in Kiel, when he injected 3 mL of 0.5% cocaine solution into a 34-year-old laborer. After using it on 6 patients, he and his assistant each injected cocaine into the other's spine. They recommended it for surgeries of legs, but gave it up due to the toxicity of cocaine.

Other Names

- Spinal analgesia
- Subarachnoid block
- Subarachnoid central neural block

Anatomy

- The spinal cord ends at the level of lower border of L1
- The dural sac ends at the level of lower border of S2
- The dural sac below the level of L1 is filled with CSF
- The dural sac below L1 contains CSF, cauda equina and filum terminale interna (**Fig. 12.1**).

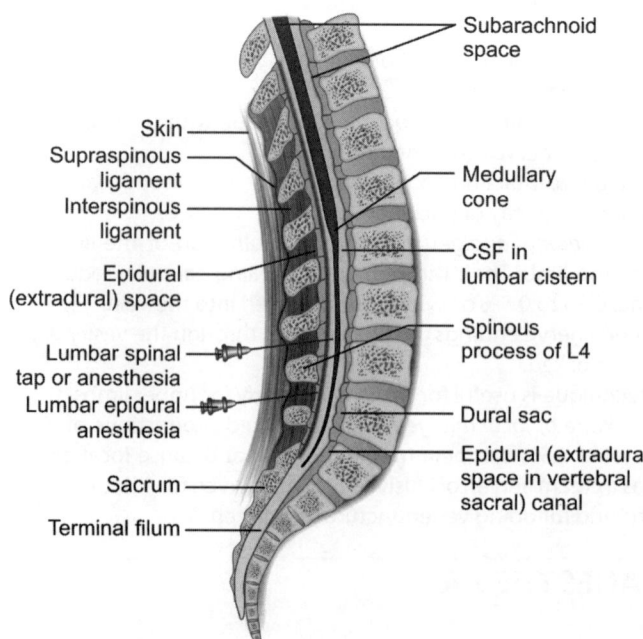

Fig. 12.1: Anatomy of lower end of spinal column–sagittal section; • The spinal cord ends at the lower border of L1; • Cauda equina and filum terminale interna in CSF; • Needle are shown to indicate the position of needle tip for spinal and epidural

LUMBAR PUNCTURE

- It is the procedure of passing a fine long needle through an interspinous space in lumbar region below the level of L2 to reach the subarachnoid space of the dural sac so that CSF can be drained or drugs may be deposited inside the sac.
- Lumbar puncture can be performed in any interspinous space between L2 and L4, when the patient is kept in right lateral position with well-flexed spinal column **(Fig. 12.2)**.
- Right lateral position is the most common position used.
- Lumbar puncture can be done when the patient is in sitting posture with the back bent forwards **(Fig. 12.3)**.

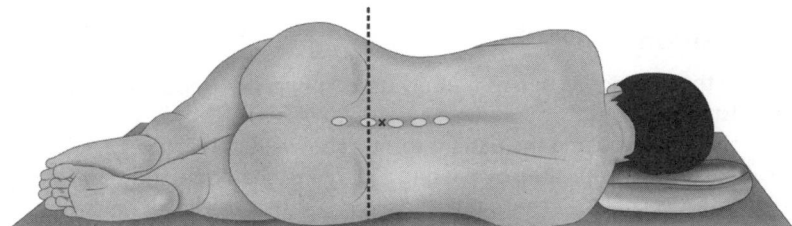

Fig. 12.2: Position of the patient for lumbar puncture. The table top is horizontal; should not be head-up or head-down. A pillow of comfortable size supports the head. Back is bent forward in a smooth curve. The lumbar spines are marked. Highest point of the iliac crest is marked corresponds to L4. The marked point is the space between L3 and L4

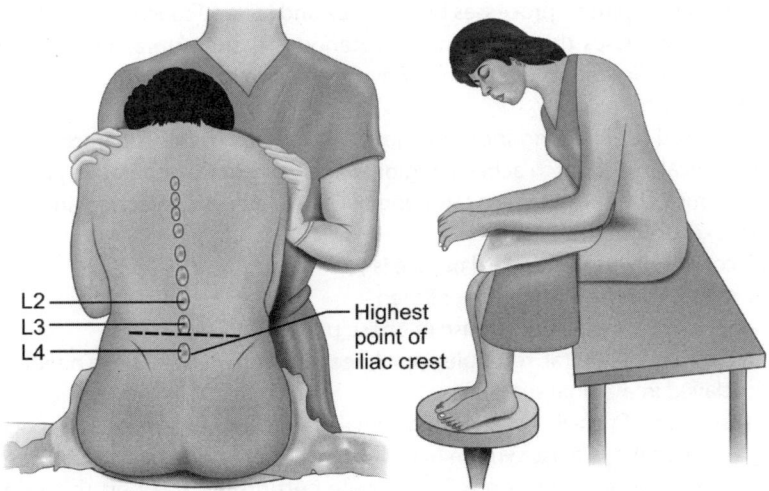

Fig. 12.3: Ideal sitting position for spinal anesthesia. • The anesthesia technician is supporting the patient by holding the shoulder and allowing the head to rest on his chest; • The levels of the spine are shown as seen from behind; • The feet must be supported by an adjustable stool; • The landmarks are being marked on the skin; • The spinous processes of L2, L3, and L4 are marked; • A line connecting the highest point of iliac crests pass through L3–L4 interspace or a little lower

POSITIONING FOR GIVING SPINAL ANESTHESIA

Right Lateral Position
- The lumbar puncture is done usually by keeping the patient in right lateral position with a good flexion of spine on a horizontal table
- The line connecting the highest point of iliac crests, pass through the L3–L4 interspace
- Lumbar dural puncture (spinal tap) is done by passing the spinal needle at this level and the 'Heavy Spinal' solution is injected slowly into the subarachnoid space.
- When the patient is turned supine, the solution being "Heavy" (heavier than CSF), settles in the site of injection backwards (posterior), acts more on the posterior nerve roots and spread to a higher level by rapid diffusion is prevented.

Sitting Position
- Though this position is not commonly used, it may be needed in certain special circumstances.
- The right way of making the patient to sit is shown in *see* **Figure 12.3**.
- Local analgesic is deposited by passing a long fine needle through the interspace below the level of L2. Because the spinal cord ends at the lower border of L1, the needle passed below L2 will not damage the spinal cord (*see* **Fig. 12.1**).

SPINAL NEEDLES
- These are long fine needles which are used to reach the subarachnoid space through the midline of back—usually in the lumbar region in the inter space between the spinous processes between L2 and L5 (any space can be chosen).
- The needle passes through skin, subcutaneous tissue, supraspinous ligament, interspinous ligament, ligamentum flavum and two layers of dura and arachnoid **(Fig. 12.4)**.
- This is used for injecting local analgesics or opioids in the subarachnoid space (Intrathecal injection) to achieve regional analgesia or postoperative pain relief.
- Sometimes, they are used for sampling of CSF for analysis, injecting antibiotics or cytotoxic drugs intrathecally.
- The commonly used standard needle is 9 cm long.
- The shorter ones are for use in children.
- Longer ones are available for use in obese patients.
- In olden days all metal, reusable spinal needles were in use. These needles were autoclaved in a "spinal set".
- The "spinal set" usually consists of a spinal needle (either 20G or 21G) packed in a glass test tube, a glass syringe (usually 2 mL), a xylocaine heavy spinal ampule, a IV needle to load the drug, an ampule cutting file to open the xylocaine ampule.
- All these were packed in especially made thick linen cover, rolled as a pack and tied.
- These packs were loaded in a separate bin and are autoclaved.
- Now, disposable needles are in use and are available easily.

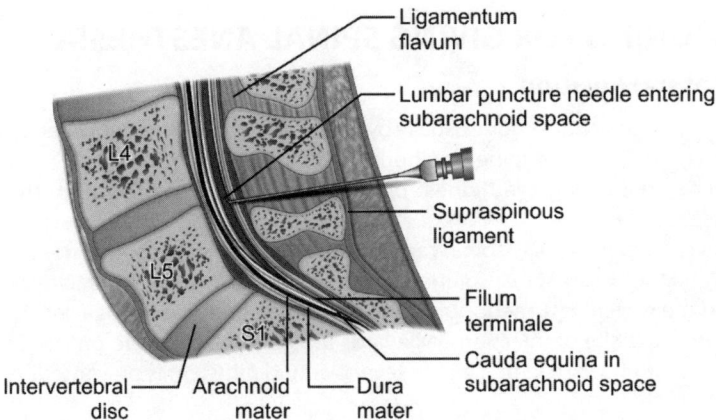

Fig. 12.4: Structures passed through by the spinal needle; • Skin, subcutaneous tissue, supraspinous ligament, interspinous ligament, ligamentum flavum, dura and arachnoid

Parts of Spinal Needle

- The needle has a hub, shaft and a tip (bevel).
- There is a stylet, which fits very snugly from hub to the tip (bevel) to prevent tissues blocking the lumen.
- There is a lock for the stylet on the hub and when placed correctly, the bevel of the needle and the stylet set smoothly at the tip.
- The lock indicates the direction of the bevel.
- It is advantageous to pierce the dura with the bevel facing the side so that the longitudinal fibers of the dura are not cut but separated by the tip of the needle. The hole seals easily and the chance for postdural puncture headache is minimized.
- The needle hub, in disposable needle is made of transparent plastic.
- When the needle tip enters the subarachnoid space, once the stylet is removed, CSF will flow out through the needle.
- The flow of CSF will be very slow and it can be observed through the transparent hub **(Fig. 12.5)**.
- The thickness of the needle may be from 18G to 29G (29G is the finest).
- G indicates the thickness and refers to "standard wire gauge".
- The thinner needles make a smaller hole in the dura—so less chance of postdural puncture headache (PDPHA) or postspinal headache.

The Tip of the Needle

- Commonly used needle has a tip in the form of a bevel cut obliquely. It is called a 'Quinke point'
- To prevent cutting the dural fibers 'pencil tip needles are also available. The tips may be 'Whitacre', 'Sportte' or 'Gertie' tips **(Fig. 12.6)**.
  The local analgesic solution is 'hyperbaric' (heavy). It means the specific gravity of the solution is higher than that of CSF. Hence, the drug settles where it is injected.

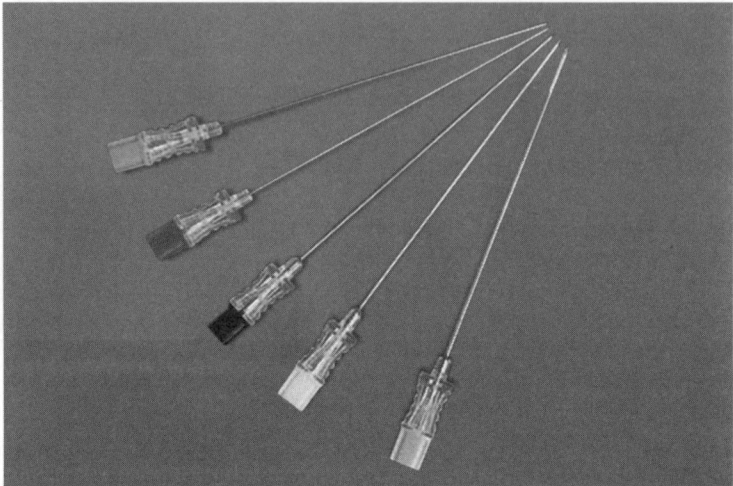

Fig. 12.5: Disposable spinal needle with transparent hub and lock. • The color-coded stylet head indicates the size of the needle; • Through the transparent hub of the needle flow of CSF could be easily visualized

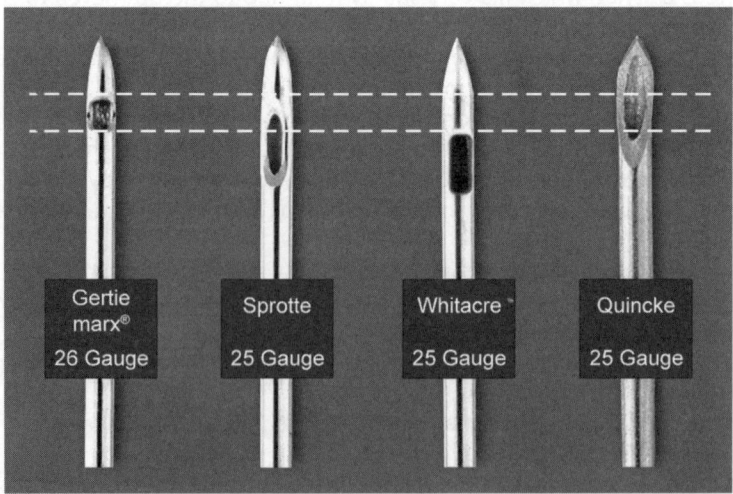

Fig. 12.6: Different types of tip of spinal needles

The CSF containing the local anesthetic baths the spinal nerves passing through the point. High lipophilic nature of the drug causes immediate and rapid absorption of the drug into the nerve fibers and cause conduction block, effectively causing anesthesia of the area supplied by these nerves. This regional anesthesia technique involves—blocking all the modalities of nerve conduction (motor, sensory and autonomic) below one particular spinal segment level.

EPIDURAL ANESTHESIA

History
- In 1921, Spanish military surgeon *Fidel Pagés* (1886–1923) developed the technique of lumbar epidural anesthesia.
- Italian surgery professor *Achille Mario Dogliotti* (1897–1966) popularized this technique in the 1930s.
- Dogliotti described "loss-of-resistance" technique for identifying the epidural space.
- Loss of resistance technique is application of constant pressure to the plunger of a syringe while advancing the Tuohy needle—a technique sometimes referred to as *Dogliotti's technique*.
- In October 1941, Robert Andrew Hingson (1913–1996), Waldo B. Edwards and James L Southworth, working at the United States Marine Hospital at Stapleton Island in New York, developed the technique of continuous caudal anesthesia.
- The first continuous caudal epidural anesthesia was done in a laboring woman January 6, 1942.
- The first continuous lumbar epidural with a catheter was performed by *Pío Manuel María Martínez Curbelo*, Cuban anesthesiologist (1906–1962) on January 13, 1947.

Technique of Epidural Anesthesia
Depositing the local anesthetic solution in appropriate concentration and volume with or without Adrenaline (1 in 200,000) in between the two layers of dura, i.e. the investing layer and the periosteal layer so that the mixed spinal nerve that crosses the epidural space before entering the inter vertebral foramen is acted upon by the local anesthetic to cause a conduction block **(Fig. 12.7)**.
- Sufficient volume of the solution has to be used to block the required number of spinal nerves.
- The mixed spinal nerve drags and takes a cuff of investing layer of dura along with it before entering the inter vertebral foramen.
- So the local anesthetic has to penetrate this dural cuff before acting on the nerve.
- This is the reason for the delay in the onset of action of epidural anesthesia.
- This causes slow onset of sympathetic blockade so that the compensatory mechanisms have adequate time to work, to prevent rapid fall of BP. The differences of this technique from spinal anesthesia are:
  - Low percentage of local anesthetic is needed.
  - Large volume of solution is necessary to cover the required number of spinal segments.
  - Adrenaline can be added to the solution to increase the duration of anesthesia by delaying the absorption by vasoconstriction.

Depending upon the region where the epidural injection is given, it is classified as:
- Lumbar epidural
- Caudal epidural (Sacral epidural)
- Thoracic epidural
- Segmental epidural (only required segments are blocked selectively)

EPIDURAL NEEDLES
- The construction of the needle is almost similar to that of the spinal needle.
- This is a special needle which has a bevel turned to the side instead of facing forward (Huber point) **(Fig. 12.8)**.

308 Anesthetic Equipment Made Easy

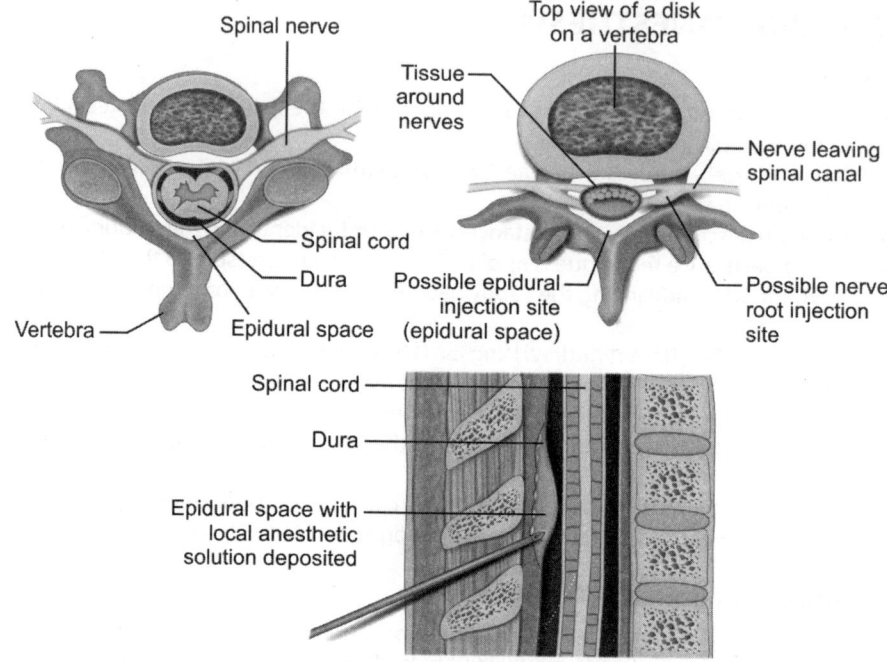

Fig. 12.7: Injection of local anesthetic in between the two layers of dura in epidural space.
• The mixed spinal nerve entering into the intervertebral foramen with a cuff of dura; • Below L2 level, the epidural space is a little wider. Here, sub-arachnoid space contains cauda equina and filum fermin de interna; • The local analgesic deposited penetrates the dural cuff and acts on the mixed spinal nerve

- This Huber point prevents accidental dural puncture and incidentally helps in feeling the variation of resistances offered by the ligaments on the way.
- This has smooth curve corresponding to the stylet lock on the hub, helps in identifying the direction of the bevel and also smooth introduction of the catheter.
- The needle with Huber point is called *Tuohy needle*.
- Huber point/Tuohy needle : 8 cm/Long
- Total length : 9 cm
- Needle length : 8 cm
- Hub and stylet : 1 cm
- Gauge : 16, 17 or 18 SWG (Standard Wire Gauge)
- There will be 1 cm markings from the tip with alternating color to assess the depth of epidural space from the skin **(Fig. 12.8)**.
- The tip is having a slight curvature and the bevel of the needle points to the side fully and is blunt (Huber point).
- Can be used for single dose and continuous epidural anesthesia.

Epidural Catheter

- Continuous epidural is by using a blunt-tipped catheter with two or three side eyes.
- There will be marking from the tip of tube every centimeter and for every 5 cm there will be different markings up to 20 cm **(Fig. 12.9)**.

Equipment for Spinal and Epidural Anesthesia 309

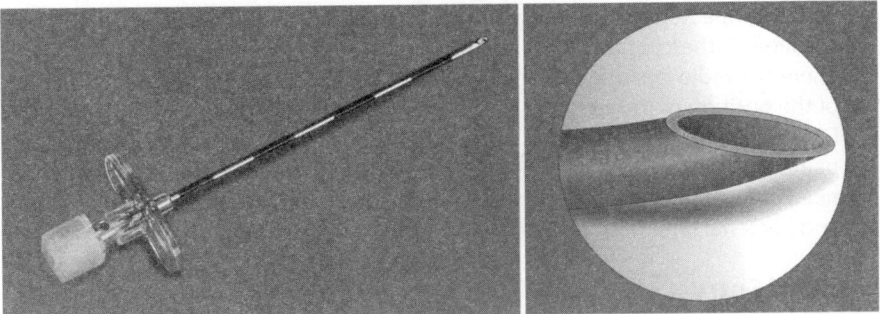

Fig. 12.8: Epidural needle with markings of 1 cm (8 cm); • Huber point is shown

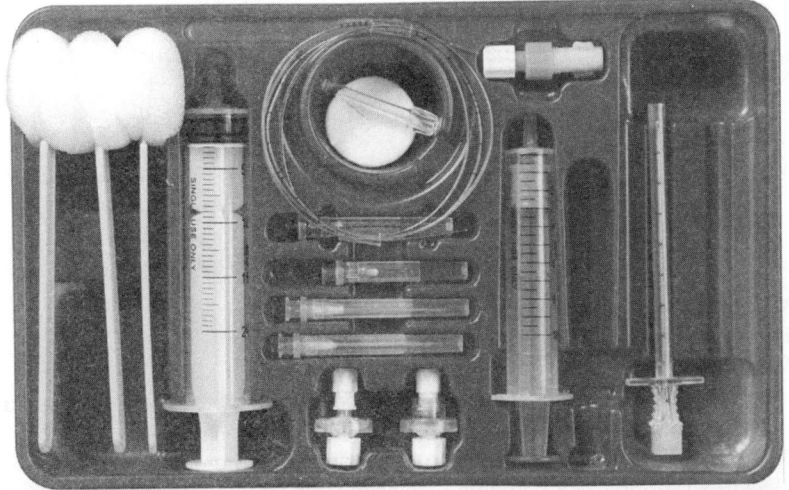

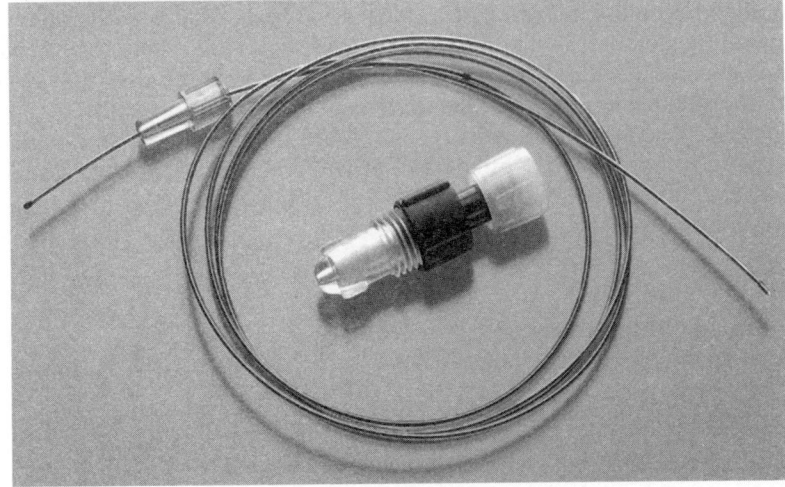

Fig. 12.9: An epidural set in a sterile pack and an epidural catheter

- This is connected to a bacterial filter and analgesic solution is injected through the filter. Catheter with filter is essential.
- There is a radio-opaque, black line on the catheter for radiological confirmation of the position of the catheter.
- Disposable epidural sets in EO sterilized pack is available. This contains swabs for painting, syringes, epidural needles, and epidural catheter with director and hub, needles for loading the syringe and for giving skin infiltration at the site of puncture and bacterial filter **(Fig. 12.9)**.

Route of Entry

- Lumbar
- Thoracic—selective or segmental
- Caudal

Methods for Identifying Epidural Space

- Loss of resistance signs; by passing through ligamentum flavum
- Negative pressure sign; caused by the following:
  - Indentation of the dura by the point of the advancing needle.
  - Flexion of the spine
  - Transmission of negative intrapleural pressure through para-vertebral space to the epidural space.

Some of the Methods Used for Identifying Negative Pressure

- Macintosh needle with spring-loaded stylet
- Brunner and Like's spring-loaded syringe
- Macintosh's indicator—a small balloon with air
- Hanging drop being sucked in when the space is reached—the Gutierrez sign.
- Odom's indicator—movement of air bubble in the capillary tube
- Broolle's indicator—Odom's indicator with an air-filled bulb.
- Macintosh spring-loaded needle—devised by RH salt.
- Modified Broolle's indicator—Dawkins (The indicator is partially filled with colored sterile water so that the capillary tube shows one meniscus). The bulb is momentarily heated with the spirit lamp creating a positive pressure. As epidural space is entered it is shown by the movement of the meniscus.
- When the fluid in room temperature is injected in the epidural space, there is an increase in the rate and depth of respiration. *'Durren's sign',* particularly useful in unconscious patient.

Routinely, loss of resistance technique is used.

Drugs

- Xylocaine 1.5% with adrenaline (1 in 200,000).
- Bupivacaine 0.5% (without adrenaline).

Advantages

- Onset of hypotension is sow and relatively minimal.
- No chance of postspinal headache.
- Continuous epidural can be used.

Continuous Epidural

- A fine-graduated polyvinyl catheter passed through the Tuohy needle into the epidural space. There are 1 cm markings with special marking every 5 cm (*see* **Fig. 12.9**).
- Sterile disposable sets (Gamma ray sterilized) containing the epidural needle, epidural catheter with adapter, and bacterial filter are available (*see* **Fig. 12.9**).
- After placing the catheter in the epidural space correctly, the needle is removed and the catheter is secured in position with sterile dressings (**Fig. 12.10**).
- To the proximal end of the catheter, a hub and microbacterial filter are attached.
- Now this catheter is secured with waterproof plasters along the midline of the back and brought above the shoulder near the patient's neck (**Fig. 12.10**).
- Repeated injections of local analgesic can be made through this catheter to continue the anesthesia.
- Continuous epidural technique may be used for prolonged surgeries where it is possible to continue the anesthesia with repeated doses of local analgesic and also for providing pain relief in postoperative period.
- The patient on continuous epidural analgesia receives stable, consistent pain relief instead of experiencing the peaks and valleys associated with most other pain control methods.

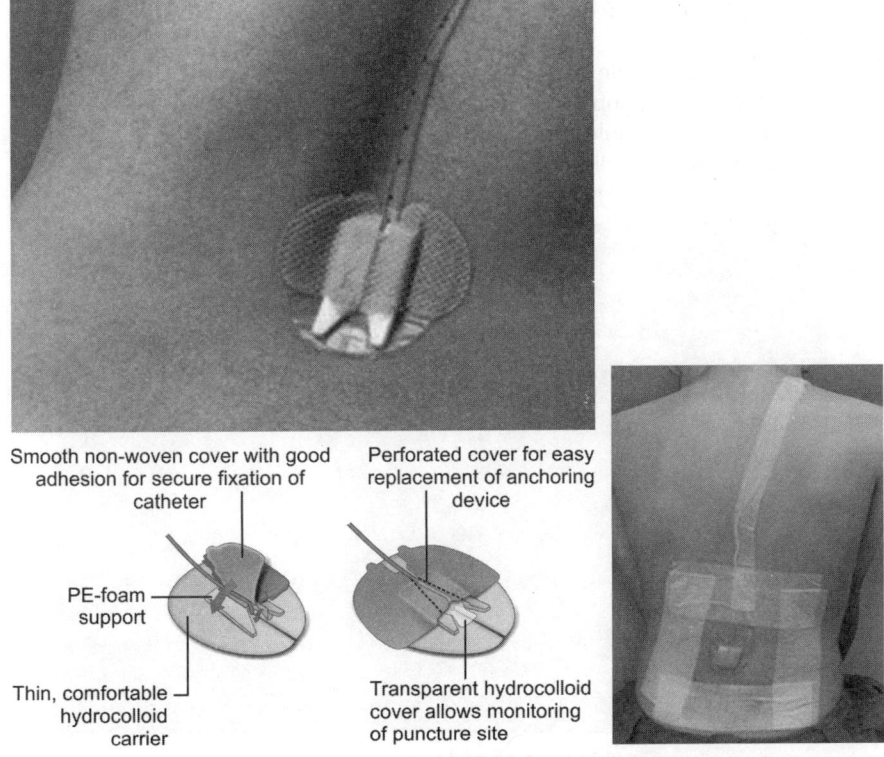

Fig. 12.10: Fixing the epidural catheter with sterile dressings and plaster

Disadvantages and Complications
- Accidental total spinal.
- Likelihood of over dosage and toxicity because of the larger volume used.

Combined Spinal-epidural Anesthesia (CSEA)
- In *1937* Soresi, a surgeon used a fine needle into the epidural space and after injecting the drug in epidural space, pushed the needle further into the subarachnoid space to inject the drug further intrathecally. Procaine was the local anesthetic. He called it "episubdural."
- In *1987* Sprotte et al. in Germany used similar technique.
- In *1979*, Curelaru in Romania inserted an epidural catheter at one inter space and inserted a spinal needle in the adjacent space for giving spinal.
- In *1982*, Coates used an epidural needle being placed in the epidural space; a fine spinal needle is passed through the epidural needle to pierce the dura to inject the drug in subarachnoid space. Then the spinal needle is removed and the epidural catheter is placed in epidural space for continuing the anesthesia. The spinal needle must be sufficiently longer to pierce the dura **(Fig. 12.11)**.
- As the name indicates this central neural block is a combination of the two namely the spinal and epidural.
- First a small dose of local anesthetic is injected into the subarachnoid space for immediate effect and then the epidural injection is given to continue the anesthesia.

There are *four methods* by which this combination of the two techniques can be performed:
1. Single needle single interspace method
2. Double needle double interspace method
3. Double needle single interspace method
4. Needle beside needle single interspace method.

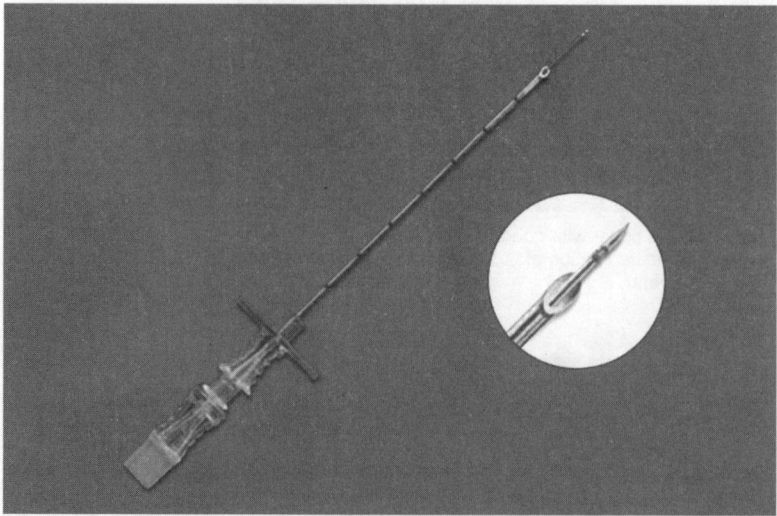

Fig. 12.11: Combined spinal epidural needles

- Now it has been standardized to have a spinal needle protruding for 1.2 cm beyond the tip of epidural needle **(Fig. 12.11)**.
- The anteroposterior diameter of epidural space in lumbar region is about 1.3 to 1.8 cm.
- So the 1.2 cm distance into the subarachnoid space is quite adequate. Too long a needle may reach the epidural space anteriorly.
- In 1988 a special needle was designed in such a way that it is an epidural needle with a spinal needle guide attached to it. It is called as combined spinal epidural needle (CSEN).
- The technique of combined spinal epidural is shown in **Figure 12.12**.

Advantages

- This technique combines the speed of onset, reliability and low toxicity of spinal block with the ability of the epidural catheter to modify or prolong the anesthesia.
- This provides flexibility of technique and flexibility of choice of drugs.
- Opioids and other antinociceptive drugs may be used for postoperative analgesia.

Uses

- Cesarean sections, by adding opioids for excellent postoperative analgesia.
- For relief of labor pain by using quick acting fat soluble opiates such as fentanyl or sufentanil followed, if needed by bolus injection of local anesthetics.

Infusion Pumps for Continuous Epidural

- Infusion pumps are devices, which can be used to infuse the calculated amount of fluid in the given time **(Figs 12.13 and 12.14)**.
- Usually, a roller pump acting on the infusion tube at the set speed does this job.
- This may be simply for delivering fluids or fluids containing medications thereby delivering the calculated doses of the drug in the given specific time.

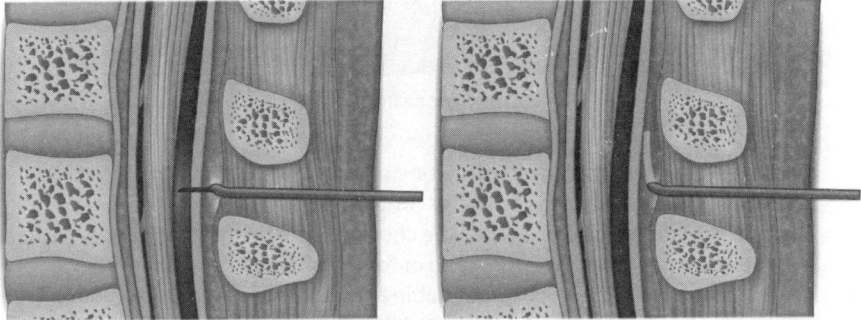

Fig. 12.12: Technique of combined spinal epidural; • Epidural needle is placed in the epidural space; • Dura is punctured with the spinal needle and local anesthetic is injected into the subarachnoid space; • The spinal needle is withdrawn and removed; • Epidural catheter is introduced and placed in the space; • Then epidural needle can be removed, leaving the catheter in position

314 Anesthetic Equipment Made Easy

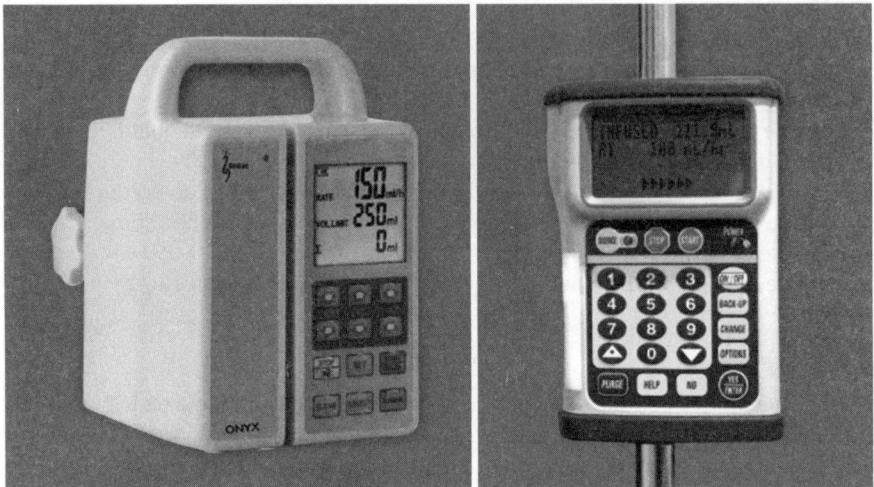

Fig. 12.13: Infusion pumps two different makes for continuous epidural

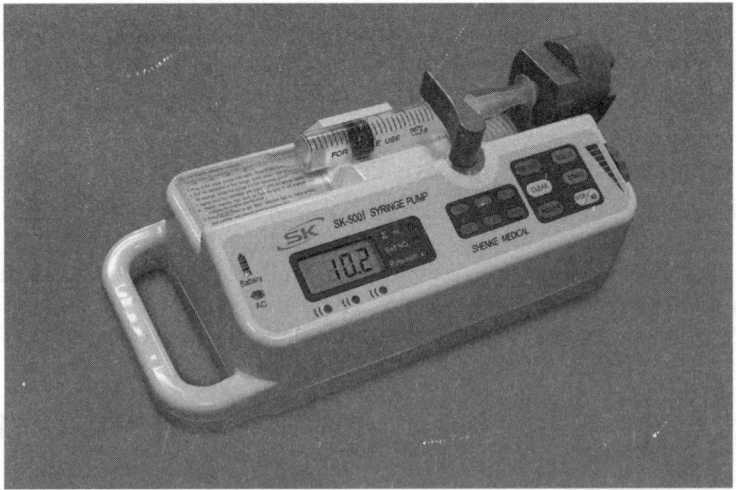

Fig. 12.14: Syringe infusion pump

- Medications either local anesthetic alone or local anesthetic with opioids such as fentanyl or sufentanil premixed in the container.
- The concentration of the drugs may be chosen as per the requirement, whether it is for surgery, postoperative analgesia or for labor analgesia.
- These infusion pumps are programmable and deliver the required volume. There is a constant display on the screen regarding the rate of infusion and the volume infused.
- The volume is calculated as mL/kg/hour and is set on the pump.
- The tubing has to be fixed in the machine and rate of infusion can be fixed.
- The setting and the total fluid infused will be constantly displayed on the screen.

Syringe Infusion Pump

- In this infusion pump, a syringe loaded with the drug in the required concentration and is placed in it. The plunger of the syringe is pushed by a motor **(Fig. 12.14)**.
- The piston of the syringe is moved as per the requirement set in the program. The program is controlled by an embedded computer device.
- These pumps are mainly used for delivering drugs in the IV line or for continuous epidural.
- For continuous epidural, the rate of infusion can be set in the machine.
- For top up doses, the rate and volume to be infused and time interval of delivery can be fixed on the machine.

FURTHER READING

1. Cousins MJ, Bridenbaugh PO, Carr DB, Horlocker TT. Cousins and Bridenbaugh's Neural Blockade in Clinical Anesthesia and Pain Medicine, 4th edn. Lippincott Williams & Wilkins, Philadelphia, 2009.
2. Gurudatt CL. Unintentional dural puncture and postdural puncture headache: can this headache of the patient as well as the anaesthesiologist be prevented? Indian J Anaesth. 2014;58(4):385-7.
3. MacIntosh SRR, Lee JA, Atkinson RS, Livingston C. Sir Robert Macintosh's Lumbar Puncture and Spinal Analgesia: Intradural and Extradural, 1978.

Index

Page numbers followed by *f* indicate figures.

A

Absorber type of 208
Adam's
  pressure 29*f*
  valve 29*f*, 121
Adjustable airway pressure limiting
    valve 33
Adjustable pressure limiting valve 45, 46*f*,
    47, 60, 66
Air
  brake 58
  ventilation, expired 254
Airway
  artificial 244
  Berman's 246, 250
  Brook's 255, 255*f*
  Guedel's 246, 247, 249*f*
  Hewitt's 246, 250
  mechanism of 246*f*
  nasopharyngeal 251
  obstruction 245
  oropharyngeal 245
  parts of 247*f*
  Phillips 246, 250
  pressure release valve 204
  Resuci 254, 255*f*
  Safar's 254
  sizes of 248
  tube 257, 266
  with widely flared end 251
  types of 245
Aladin cassette vaporizer 166, 167
Allen key 43*f*
Aluminium float, made of 127
Alveolar
  cleft 287*f*
  plateau 285
Ambu bag 64
American National Standard
    Institute 33, 61
Anesthesia
  clinical 295
  depth of 277
  exhausted sodalime in 286*f*
  gas machine 27
  machine 27, 28
    checking 63
      equipment 64
      system 63
      gas supply and suction 63
      monitors 64
      power supply 63
      scavenging 64
      two bag test 64
      ventilator 64
    color coding of cylinders in 77*f*
    components of 30
    essential components 33, 34*f*
    history of 28
    modern 29, 32*f*
    modern pressure reducing
        valve of 119
    pressure reducing valve used in 42
    various components of 1
    worktop of 48
  spinal 301
  techniques of regional
      anesthesia 301
  workstation 32*f*, 104
Anesthetic
  breathing system 33, 173, 174
    classification 175
    closed system 176
    criteria for 177
    modern classification 176
    non-rebreathing system 176, 177
    open system 175
    rebreathing system 176
    semi-closed system 176
    semi-open system 175
  gas
    cylinders 77
    mixture of 174
  mixture 48, 57

vapor concentration 61
waste gas scavenging system 58f
Antinociceptive drugs 313
Anti-spill 159, 164, 169
　　funnel filling device 170f
Antistatic
　　black rubber 211
　　rubber
　　　　tyres 34
　　　　wheels 59
Applied physics 1
Arterial
　　blood pressure 61
　　oxygen saturation 289
　　pressure 289
　　pulse waveform 277f
Arteriole 274
Atomic weight 2
Atomizer vaporizer 154
Automatic thermocompensating
　　　　valve 149
Avogadro's
　　constant 3
　　hypothesis 3, 3f
　　hypothesis specific weight 4
Ayre's t-piece system 178, 191, 192, 192f

B

Back bar 33, 42
Back pressure, compensated flow
　　　　meter 138, 139f
Baffles 153
　　in plenum 154f
Bag mount 180
Bag valve mask 64
　　face mask 66
　　nonrebreathing unidirectional
　　　　valve 66
　　self-inflating bag 66
　　unidirectional inlet valve 66
Bain's breathing system 178, 187, 189f
Bain's system 186
　　parallel 190f
　　with block assembly 190f
Baralyme 197
Barotrauma 41
Beer's law 275
Bend test 72, 73
Bernoulli's principle 22, 22f, 23f
Bimetallic strip valve 157, 158f
Bivona fome cuff 235

Blades of turbine 131
Bleed valve 180
Bobbin 127, 130
　　annular orifice around 129f
　　flow of gas around 128
　　shaped 130
　　used in flow meters 130f
Bodok seal 33, 36f, 37, 38f, 82-84
Boiling point 6, 145, 146
Bougie used for aiding difficult
　　　　intubation 244f
Bourdon gauge 37, 39
Boyle's
　　anesthesia machine, safety
　　　　features in 59
　　apparatus 28
　　F machine 132f
　　law 17, 17f, 18f
　　machine 29, 30f, 31f, 36
　　　　back bar of 43
　　　　two primitive versions of 29
　　　　type of 46
Brachial plexus block 301
Breathing
　　bag 206
　　circuit type of 46
　　resistance to 206
　　system 44, 48
　　　　configuration to 193
　　　　resistance in 184
　　　　respiratory requirements 183
Broken inner tube, test for identifying 191
Bronchial cuff 237, 238
Bronchospasm, expiratory
　　　　obstruction 287f
Bronchospirometry 236
Broolle's indicator, modified 310
Bubble through device 154
Bullnose
　　type of valve 88
　　valves different varieties of 88f
Bupivacaine 310

C

Calcium hydroxide 196
Calorie 5
Capillary tube 310
Capnography 197, 199, 273, 280, 281f
　　components 280
　　end-tidal CO_2 monitoring 281
　　factors that decrease $EtCO_2$ 284

infrared analyzer 280
interpretation of values 283
mainstream CO_2 analyzer 282
normal capnogram 284
principle of 280
sidestream CO_2 analyzer 282
uses 281
Carbon 70
Carbon dioxide 15
Carbon dioxide absorption 195, 196
Carbon steel alloy
 advantages 71
 features of ideal cylinders 71
 high 70
 low 70
Cardiorespiratory status assessment 278
Cardiorespiratory system, noninvasive monitor for 273
Carinal hook 237f
Carlen's double lumen tube 236, 237f
Carlen's double lumen tube, modified 238
Catheter mount 215f
Catheter mount and connectors 214
Cauda
 equina 308f
 epidural 307
Ceiling
 mounted pendants, types of 106f
 outlets, types of 106
 reel outlets different types of 106
 pipeline supply
  advantages of
   asepsis 93
   economical 94
   efficient 94
   psychological effects 94
   reliable and safe 94
   saves space 94
Central reducing valve 101
Central vacuum
 suction 107
 unit 108f
Cesarean sections 313
Channeling 201
Charles' law 20f, 20
Chloroform 145, 173
Choledochscope 224
Chondrodendron tomentosum 295
Chromium 71
Circle absorber 204f, 205f
 essential components of 202

methods to check the integrity of 207
 with double canister 209f
Circle system 201
 advantages of 202
Circuit breakers 61
Circular facemasks 212f
Circulation monitoring 288
Coaxial systems 187
Cobb's suction union 241, 242f
Cole's tube 238, 239f
Collar index 103
Color coding 77
Combined spinal epidural
 anesthesia 312
 needle 312, 313
 technique of 313
Common gas outlet 47, 174
Compressed medical air 108
Connell meter 133, 137, 138f
Continuous breathing system pressure 61
Continuous epidural 311, 314f
 analgesia 311
 infusion pumps for 313
 technique 311
Continuous positive airway pressure, amount of 193
Control panels, modern 100
Copper kettle
 for ether vaporization 145
 vaporizer 160
Corrugated
 breathing hoses 173, 180, 204, 206f
 tube 178
Cowl 151
 for directing gas surface of liquid 153
Coxeter bobbin 133
 flow meter 136f
Cuff different, types of 229, 230
Cuff
 pressure 230
 volume 272
Cyclopropane 6
Cyclopropane 79
Cylinder 59
 A- and B-type 76
 cautions and rules to be strictly followed with 86
 cracking 87
 decanting or filling of 89
 engraved on the shoulder of 79
 indicates the status of 87
 key 80

label on body of nitrous oxide 78
outlet valves 80
oxygen and nitrous oxide 76
parts of 74
   shoulder of 74
   steel-carbon fibers 75
pressure 56, 113
size 79
spanner 36f, 81
structure 199
transfilling of 97f
with bullnose valve 96f
with protective cover 72f
Cylindrical with a head and tail 130
Cyprane inhaler 148, 149f
Cytotoxic drugs intrathecally 304

D

Dalton's law
   application of 14
   partial pressures of 13
Datex-ohmeda 166
Defibrillation, principle of 291
Defibrillator 290
   paddles on the chest wall 292f
   unit with ECG monitor and recorder 291f
Deflated cuff 260
Depolarising block 296f, 296, 298
Desflurane 44, 145, 165, 167
Desflurane filling system 166, 169, 170
Diaphragm
   elastometal 117
   large 116
   rubber 117
   small 116
Dicrotic notch 273f
Digital nerve block 301
Disc with rod 130
Dogliotti's technique 307
Double burst stimulation 295, 299, 300
Double needle double interspace method 312
Double-canister absorbers 208
Dropper type 156
Dural cuff 308f
Durren's sign 310

E

Easy-fil 168, 169, 170
   filling system 171f

Electrical
   cardioversion 291
   stimulation 296
   stimulations, types of 295
Electrocardiogram monitor 285
Electronic
   device 54
   mechanisms 49
Elwyn tubes 233
Emergency oxygen flush 30f, 33, 43, 46, 47, 47f, 48, 61
Endobronchial tube
   green and Gordon's 237
   reinforced or armoured 233f
Endotracheal
   connectors 239
   tube 66, 224, 227, 258, 282
      double lumen 236
      for laser surgeries 235
      for special purposes 231
      indications for 227
      size of 230
      used to connect 239
End-tidal carbon dioxide monitoring 281
End-tidal CO_2 287
Enflurane 164, 167
Entonox 85, 86
Epidural anesthesia 307
   equipment for 301
   technique of 307
Epidural catheter 308, 309f, 310
   with sterile dressings 311f
Epidural needle 307, 309f, 313f
Epidural set 309f
Epidural space 308f, 313f
   anteroposterior diameter of 313
   methods for identifying 310
Epiglottis 222, 253
Epispinal 301
Ether 6, 9, 142, 145
   inhaler model of 173f
Ethyl
   chloride 145
   violet 197
Ethylene oxide 79
Evaporation, process of 142

F

Facemask 178, 182, 209, 214
   latex-free mask 212

Index 321

pediatric masks 212
Rendell-Baker-Soucek mask, for neonates 213
Fentanyl 313
Fiber-optic intubating
   bronchoscope 224
      parts of 225
      principle and design 224, 225f
   laryngoscope 225f
Fick's law 14
Field block 301
Filling ratio 91
   critical pressure 91
   critical temperature 91
   practical significance 92
Filling systems 169
Filum fermin de interna 302, 308f
Fine-graduated polyvinyl catheter 311
Fish mouth valve 68f
Fixed orifice 127
   dry type 133
   dry type flow meter 134
   variable pressure difference type 126
   wet type 133
   with variable pressure difference 133
Fixed outlet pressure, type of 120
Fixing the breathing system 47
Flattening test 72, 73
Flexi-tip laryngoscope 221f
Flow control valve 56
Flow meter 43, 60, 123, 127
   bank 44f, 131, 132f
   classification of 126
   in anesthesia machine 125
   principles and types 123
   safe arrangement of 140f
Flow-splitting device 150, 151f
Flow test 207
Fluorescent plate 132
Fluotec mark 2 162
   characteristics 162
   limitation 162
Fluotec mark 3 163
   characteristics 163
   vaporizer 45f
Flush valve 35f, 80, 86
Foregger flow meter 134, 135f
Forrester spray 26
Fresh gas flow 192
Funnel filling 169

G

Gamma ray sterilized 311
Gas 4, 6, 7
   bubbles 145
   chemical symbol of 78
   cylinders labels of 79f
   delivery 57
   diffusion of 14f
   flow 123
      inlet 173
      pattern in circle-breathing system 203f
   laws 16
      conversion 20
      diffusion 21
      filling ratio 18
      practical applications 17
      specific volume 16
      vapor and gas 16
   manifold and control panel 94
   mixture 44
   power outlet 56
   specific feeding connectors 60
   supplies 35, 57
   withdrawal line 111
Gay-Lussac's law 21
Genitofemoral nerve, femoral branch of 301
Globular surface, liquid gas interface 144
Goldman
   halothane vaporizer 45f
   vaporizer 161
   molecular weight 3
Granule
   from braking 198
   size 198
Grease 86
Guedel type airway 259
Gum elastic bougie 243
Gwathmey machine 28

H

Halothane 6, 27, 44, 145, 164, 167, 170
Hanging drop 310
Heat 4
   boiling points of 6, 7
   critical
      pressure 6
      temperature of various gases 6

energy in calories 146
specific 5, 146
unit of heat 5
Heidbrink flow meter 137*f*
Heidbrink's expiratory valve 179
Heidbrink's spring-loaded valve 181
Heidbrink's valve 185
Heidbrinks meter 133, 137
Helium 21
Hollow square tubular structures 34
Hospital for oxygen 112
Hot climate 92
Howland lock 220
Howland lock 221*f*
Huber point 309*f*
Hydraulic
 flow meters 133
 force 116
 sight feed meter 135
Hydraulic test 72, 73
Hypotension, onset of 310
Hypovolemia 279
 indicate 280
 state 278
Hypoxic
 drive 26
 guard device 51*f*

I

Iliohypogastric nerve 301
Ilioinguinal nerve 301
Impact test 72, 73
Indicators and alarms 100
Infiltration block 301
Inflatable rim 211
Inflation tube 258
Infraglottic airway 244
Infrared absorption
 spectrometry 280, 282
Infusion pumps 314*f*
Inguinal herniorrhaphy 301
Inhalational anesthetic agents 142, 174
Injector device 154
Inspiratory capacity 200
Inspiratory down stroke 284*f*, 285
Inspired oxygen concentration 61
Intergranular space 197
Interlock system 169
Interspinous ligament 304
Intrathecal block 301
Intrathecal injection 304

Intubating bronchoscope, single use flexible 226
Intubation
 position of head and neck for 219
 technique of
  advantages 226
  disadvantages 226
Iron 70
Isoflurane 27, 44, 145, 164, 167, 170

J

Jackson Rees, modification of Ayre's t-piece 178, 194*f*
Jaw thrus, maneuver of 246*f*
Joule-Kelvin, principle of 8
Joule-Thomson's, effect of 8
Junker bottle for insufflation technique 173

K

Keyed filling 169
 adapters 171*f*
Knob of oxygen flow meter 60
Kuhn bag 193

L

Lack's system 178, 186
Lambert's law 275
Laminar and turbulent flow 124*f*
Laminar flow 124
 pressure difference 185*f*
Laryngeal mask airway 257
 accessories to 268
 adverse effects 262
 classic and the parts 257*f*
 contraindications 261
 different size of 258
 directions for removal 259
 flexible 262, 263*f*
 indication 259, 271
 intubating 264
 method of inserting 260*f*
 method of using 258, 270
 modified versions of 262
 precautions 261
 proseal 266
 proseal anatomical relations of 268*f*
 proseal and parts of 267*f*
 proseal with introducer and deflator 268*f*

short tube 263
sizes and specifications 261, 262
standard 257
supreme 269, 270f, 271
technique of using 265
unique 263, 263f
Laryngeal reflexes 271
Laryngeal spray 26
Laryngectomy tube 239
Laryngoscope 217
Laryngoscope
Bullard fiberoptic 222, 223f
endotracheal tubes and airways 217
Patil-syracuse 222, 223f
polio 222, 222f
traditional screw type 218
types of 219
position of 220
Laryngoscopy, technique of 218, 223
Laryngospasm 253
Laser-flex tube 235, 236f
Latex
allergy 253
rubber armoured tubes 232
rubber tube 232
Law of volumes 20
Leak test 207
Ligamentum flavum 304, 310
Like's spring-loaded syringe 310
Limb
expiratory 191
inspiratory 191
Link 25 safety device 53f
Liquid 4
and gas 2, 2f
anesthetic agents, volatility of 145
drops 9
ether 147
gas interface methods 143, 144f
increasing the surface area of 153
O_2 89
oxygen 109, 112
precautions for 112
withdrawal line 111
Local anesthetic
eutectic mixture of 301
injection of 308f
Lumbar
dural puncture 304
epidural 301, 307
puncture position of 303
region 313
Lung anesthesia 238, 238f

M

Macintosh's
blade, curved blade 220f
indicator 310
laryngoscope 217
needle 310
spray 25f
spring-loaded needle 310
Magill's
breathing system 29f, 173, 178, 179, 183
components of 179f, 181, 182f
components of 180
connector 214, 215f, 240
flow in 85f
endotracheal tube 228, 240f
forceps 267
intubating forceps 244, 245f
red rubber endotracheal tube 228f
suction union 241, 242f
Magnetic field, unit of measurement of 57
Mainstream analyzer adapter 283f
Malignant hyperthermia 286
Mallinckrodt laser 235
Manganese 70
Manifold room 94
bulk gas cylinders 99
control panel 96
gas manifold and control panel 94
oxygen pipeline 95
partial automatic system 97
safety precautions in a manifold room 99
Mapleson's
A configuration 179, 186
B system 186, 187f, 200f
C system 187f
classification 178, 178f
D system 186, 188
E system 191
F system 192
Mask and inflation line 257
Master switch 56, 61
Matter
compound 1
element 1
molecular movement 1
molecule 1
Maximal current 293
McCoy laryngoscope 220
tip of 221

McKesson meter 138, 138f
Medical air, tank for supplying 110
Medical compressed air 109
Medical gas
  cylinders 70
  pipeline system 93
Metal
  ball electrodes 294f
  bellows 157, 158f
  connector 240
  ring 83
  spiral reinforced tubes 232
  tube 137f
Methyl orange 197
Microbacterial filter 311
Miller straight blade
  laryngoscope 218, 220f
  pediatric laryngoscope 217
Minimum contact gauge 97, 98f, 100
Mixed spinal nerve 308f
Moisture content 196
Molecular weight 2
Molecules 2, 124, 142
  number of 3
  solid of 2f
Molybdenum 71
Monitors multiparameter 273
Monoatomic 21
Murphy' safety eye 229f, 230, 234

N

Nasal tube plain 234f
Nasopharyngeal airway 244
  assessing size 253
  different types of 252
Necrosis of nasal mucosa 253
Needle beside needle single interspace
  method 312
Needle valve 125
  flow meter of 126f
Negative intrapleural pressure,
  transmission of 310
Negative pressure sign 310
Neonates and infants, anatomical
  differences of 219
Nerve block 301
Neuromuscular block
  during anesthesia 294
  monitoring 293
  types of 295
Nitrogen in atmospheric air 15f
Nitrous oxide 49, 132

Nitrous oxide 90
  cylinders assessing the contents of 40
  round knob for 133f
Nondepolarising blocks 296, 296f
Noninvasive airway management
  device 257
Noninvasive blood pressure 273
Nonkinkable tubes 232
Noseworthy connector 241, 241f
Nylon
  heads 87f
  reinforced 117

O

Oblique expiratory upstroke 285
Odom's indicator 310
Oil-free air compressors 110f
Opioids 313
Oral airways different 247
Orifice 124
  fixed pressure difference type 126
  type 135
    wet type 135
    dry type 136
Oropharyngeal airway 244
Outlet points from ceiling 104
Outlet pressure type 120
Outlet valve 79
  construction of 88
Oxford tubes 233, 234f
  connectors for 235f
Oxygen 27, 70
  bottling unit 89
  cylinder 32f, 90
  dissolved in blood, amount of 273
  failure alarm 48
    checking the anesthetic
      machine 54
    fail-safe system 49
    features of an ideal device 48
    limitations 50
    link 25 52
    minimum ratio gas system 51
    prevent hypoxic gas mixtures 49
    principle of 50f
    safety devices 49
    three pressure' systems 55
  flow meter 132
    problems related to the position
      of 141
    safety of positioning 140f

flush valve 56
  manifold in manifold room 95f
Oxygen pipeline 95
  pressure failure alarm 56
  reservoir bag 68f
  saturation 275
    continuous monitoring of 278
    in hemoglobin 273
  supply failure alarm 61
Oxy-hemoglobin levels 274

P

Paddles placement of 293
Partial pressure of
  gases in air 13f
  oxygen 15f
Perfusion bar, purpose of 279
Perfusion indicator 277, 279
Peripheral nerve 301
  different types of 297f
  stimulator 294, 294f, 295
Peripheral perfusion 289, 290
Peripheral pulse 289
Pethick test 191
Pharyngeal cavity 258
Phenolphthalein 197
Photoplethysmography 276
Physics 123
Pilot balloon 258
Pin index 86
  safety system 33, 38, 59, 84
Pin valve 60, 125
  and flow of gas 128f
Piped medical gas and vacuum 93
Pipelines and isolation valves 102
Pipes end in wall outlet units 102
Piping up to flow meter 56
Plastic
  armoured tubes 232
  catheter mount 214, 215f
  endotracheal tubes 228
  hammer 87f
Plateau, expiratory 285
Plenum 150, 161
Plethysmograph 276, 278, 279
Plexus block 301
Poikilothermic 4
Polycarbonate 66, 211
  facemasks with flap rim 211f
  mask 210
  transparent mask 211

Polysulfone 258
Poppet valve 117
Position oxygen flow meter 60
Postanesthetic care unit 102
Postdural puncture headache 305
Postspinal headache 305, 310
Post-tetanic count 295, 299f
Potassium hydroxide 196
Power failure indicator 61
Poynting effect 21
Pressure 12, 12f
  atmospheric pressure 15
  critical 6
  difference 127, 129
  gauge 33, 38, 56, 59
    for oxygen and nitrous oxide
      cylinders 39f
    in oxygen cylinder and in nitrous
      oxide cylinder 40f
    practical significance of 40f
    types of 134
  limiting valve 68f
  partial pressure 13
  reducing valve 41, 56, 59, 113, 114, 122f
    mechanism of 117
    simple design of 115f
    two-stage 121f
    types of 120
  regulator 41, 59, 113
    basic principle 114
    benefits of 113
  release valve 42, 43, 119, 120f
  relief device 56, 60
  relief valve 60, 202
  sensors 100
  switches 97
  system
    high 56
    intermediate 56
    low 56
Pressurizing effect 172
Proximal end of the catheter 311
Pulmonary embolus 287f
Pulsatile blood flow in the arterioles 275
Pulse oximeter 273, 273f, 279
  features 275
  finger probe of 275
  fingertip 274
  functional saturation 275
  functioning of 276
  important information 278

measure 289
working principle 274
Pulse plethysmography 289
Pulse rate 273
Pulse waveform 273, 276, 279
Pumping effect 172

Q

Quick-fil 169, 170
Quinke point 305

R

Radial pulse 289
Rebreathing system 194, 199
   advantages 195
   functioning 194
   principle 194
Reducing valves, type of 116
Regulator
   multistage 121
   two stage 121
Reserve bank reducing valve 101
Reserve power 61, 173
Reservoir bag 178, 180
   purpose of 183
Resistance signs, loss of 310
Respiration 273
Respiratory cycle 184f
Resuscitator bag
   child size 67f
   infant size 67f
   self-inflating 64, 65f
   three sizes of 69f
Rigid material, reservoir of 58
Ring Adair tubes 233
Robert Shaw double lumen tube 238f, 238
Rotameter 127, 129, 133
Rotameters 43
Rotor 131f
Rowbotham's connector 240, 240f
   flow in 185f
Running bank reducing valve 101
Ryle's tube, size of 272

S

Sacral epidural 301
Safety devices 57
Saturated vapor pressure 8f, 146
Scavenging system 57
   collecting system 57
   disposal system 58
   receiving system 58
   transfer system 58
Schimmelbusch mask 147, 148f, 173
Schrader
   self-sealing valves 103, 104
   type self-sealing valves 103f
   valve socket 103
Screw threaded
   hose connections 104f
   noninterchangeable 37, 104
Segmental epidural 307
Select-A-tec mounting 168, 168f
Semi-closed breathing system 179
Sevoflurane 27, 44, 145, 167, 170
   cassettes 168
   decomposition 199
Sheila Anderson laryngoscope 217
Shuttle valve 97
Silica 196
   traces of 196
Silicon 70
   masks 210
   rubber flap brim 66
Single needle single interspace
   method 312
Slave control valve for N_2O 51
Slender glass tube fixed 134
Sniffing position 218
Sodalime 196, 197, 208
   canister 203, 204f
   caution about 198
   clinical indicators of exhausted 198
   composition 196
   exhaustion of 202
   granules 197f
   indicators 197
   methods to find out exhaustion of 199
Sodium carbonate 196
Sodium hydroxide 196
Soft silicon round facemasks 213f
Solid drawn cylinders 71
Spill valve 204f
Spinal analgesia 302
   equipment for 301
   ideal sitting position for 303
   positioning for 304
   positioning for right lateral 304
   positioning for sitting position 304
Spinal column, sagittal section 302
Spinal needle 304

different types of tip of 306
disposable with transparent and lock 306f
parts of 305
structures passed through 305f
tip of 305
Splitting ratio 170
Stainless steel shell, inner 111
Steel-carbon fiber cylinder 75f
Sterile disposable sets 311
Stout metal plates 122f
Strict formula of composition 71
Striking point 27
Stylet 242
types of 243f
Subarachnoid block 301, 302
Subarachnoid central neural block 302
Subcutaneous tissue 304
Submaximal 293
Succinylcholine 295
Sufentanil 313
Sulfur 70
Superheater 111
Supramaximal 293
Supraspinous ligament 304
Suxamethonium chloride 295
Switches 100
Swivel mount
for endotracheal connectors 243
with suction port 242
Swivel pendant 106, 107f
Syringe infusion pump 314f, 315

T

Tec 4 164
Tec 4, characteristics 164
Tec 5 164
Tec 6 165
Tec 7 166
Tec 7, vaporizer 167
Temperature
and pressure, standard conditions of 7
compensated vaporizers 161
compensation 156
critical 6
gas flowing of 157
liquid of 157
near the boiling point 156
Tensile test 72, 73
Terminal outlets 102

Tetanic stimulation 295, 298
Thermal capacity 146
Thermal conductivity 146
Thoracic epidural 301, 307
Throat soreness 262
Tracheobronchial stimulation 299
Transient dysarthria 262
Trichloroethylene 148
Trilene 145, 199
vaporizer 157
Tube
fluid pathway 123
from incisors, length of 231
Tuohy needle 311
Turbulent flow 124, 185f

U

Unequal pressures, points of 123
Unidirectional valves 204
Universal F
breathing system 210f
circuit 209
Upstroke, expiratory 284f, 285
Urine output 290
Urine production 289

V

Vacuum-insulated evaporator 110, 111f
Valve
expiratory 173, 178
modern adiabatic compression 118
modern advantages 118
modern dangers 118
modern main features 118
nonrebreathing 150
Vapor 145
Vapor and gases 7
adiabatic compression 12
evaporation of liquid in a closed container 8
explanation of latent heat of vaporization 9
fall of temperature of evaporating liquid 11
latent heat of
condensation 11
crystallization 11
liquefaction 11
melting 11
vaporization 8
sublimation 10

Vapor, formation of 10
Vapor, pressure 145
Vaporization 7, 8f
    factors modifying the rate of 157
    latent heat of 146
    means to enhance 143
    methods to improve the rate of 150
Vaporizer 44, 142, 145, 158
    backpressure compensation 158
    bubble through 155f
    classification of 147
    draw over 147
    dropper type 157f
    EMO 148
    flow compensation 158
    flow-over 150
    fully calibrated 158
    injector type 156f
    inside circuit 30f
    interlock system in 169f
    mounting device 56
    safety features in 172
    stable 159
    temperature compensation 158
Venous blood 16
Ventilation
    adequacy of 274
    controlled 188
    spontaneous 188
Ventimask 24
Venting gas 42
Ventricular fibrillation, treatment of 291
Venturi device
    construction of 24
    ventimask working with 25f
Vernier effect 125
Versatile inventions 273
Video laryngoscopes 223, 224f
Vital organs perfusion of 289
Vital parameters 27
Volatile anesthetic agents 44
    concentration of 174
Volatile anesthetic liquid 142

W

Wall mounting suction unit 109f
Wall outlet
    for vacuum 108
    of pipeline 102
    series of 105
    units, two types of 105f
Wall-Rail mounted designs 57
Water
    depression meter 134
    jacket method 73
    manometer 134
    sight feed meter 133, 135, 136f
    vapor condensation of 9f
Waterproof plasters 311
Waveform
    interpretation of 277
    pulse oximeter of 277f
Wet flow meters 136f
Wick-in-jar 161
Wicks 153
Wood's metal 82
Wooden hammer 87f
Workstations
    fail-safe valve, safety features in 62
    flow meter, safety features in 62
    hypoxia preventing devices, safety features in 62
    oxygen analyzer, safety features in 63
    oxygen failure protection device 62
    pipeline wall outlets, safety features in 62
    pressure sensor shut-off valve 62
    safety features in 61
    scavenging system, safety features in 63
    vaporizers, safety features in 63
    ventilators, safety features in 63

X

Xenon 21
Xomed laser 235
Xylocaine 301, 310
    ampule 304
    fixed proportions of 301
    heavy spinal ampule 304

Y

Yoke 37, 59
    assembly and A-type cylinders 80f
    for oxygen 85f
    hanger assembly 56
    of anesthetic machine 82